# DR. APPLE'S SYMPTOMS ENCYCLOPEDIA

## *The Reassuring Guide to Self-Diagnosis*

## Dr. Michael Apple
## and Dr. Jason Payne-James

Edited by Drs. Robin Fox, Hugo Hammersley,
George Moncrieff, and K. S. Pandher

**Basic Health**
PUBLICATIONS, INC.

The information contained in this book is based upon the research and personal and professional experiences of the authors. It is not intended as a substitute for consulting with your physician or other healthcare provider. Any attempt to diagnose and treat an illness should be done under the direction of a healthcare professional.

The publisher does not advocate the use of any particular healthcare protocol but believes the information in this book should be available to the public. The publisher and authors are not responsible for any adverse effects or consequences resulting from the use of the suggestions, preparations, or procedures discussed in this book. Should the reader have any questions concerning the appropriateness of any procedures or preparation mentioned, the authors and the publisher strongly suggest consulting a professional healthcare advisor.

### Basic Health Publications, Inc.

28812 Top of the World Drive • Laguna Beach, CA 92651
949-715-7327 • www.basichealthpub.com

**Library of Congress Cataloging-in-Publication Data**

Apple, Michael.
  Dr. Apple's symptoms encyclopedia : the reassuring guide to self-diagnosis /
Michael Apple and Jason Payne-James ; editors, Robin Fox . . . [et al.]. —2nd ed.
    p. cm.
  Rev ed. of: Symptoms and early warning signs. 1994.
  Includes bibliographical references and index.
  ISBN 978-1-59120-251-6
  1. Symptoms—Encyclopedias. I. Payne-James, Jason. II. Fox, Robin.
III. Apple, Michael. Symptoms and early warning signs. IV. Title.

  RC69.A66    2009
  616.07'503—dc22

                                                        2008044424

Editor: John Anderson
Typesetting/Book design: Gary A. Rosenberg
Cover design: Mike Stromberg

Printed in the United States of America

10  9  8  7  6  5  4  3  2  1

# Contents

# Preface

*"Every patient carries her or his own doctor inside."*
—ALBERT SCHWEITZER, FRENCH PHILOSOPHER
AND PHYSICIAN (1875–1965)

We all like to feel well, so much so that we take our bodies for granted until something goes wrong. Then we enter the uncertain world of symptoms. Some symptoms matter, some don't—the skill is to tell the difference. And it is at this point that knowledge, such as found in this book, really begins to count, because it helps us understand what is going on; only then can we begin our journey to recovery.

However, *Dr. Apple's Symptoms Encyclopedia* aims to do a little more than just provide the facts. It aims to make sense out of symptoms, an ambitious task since the subject is so huge. We believe that this can, nonetheless, be done by revealing how a doctor thinks when faced by patients telling their stories. How does a doctor think? By ranking the possible diagnoses in terms of probability, which is exactly what has been done in this book.

We hope that this book helps people to engage positively in the process of diagnosis and, with luck, put their illnesses and subsequent management into perspective.

# Introduction

This book has been designed to be extremely easy to use. Please read what follows carefully, as there are two different ways to use the book, depending on whether you want to arrive at a diagnosis based on your symptoms or find out more about an illness you may already have.

For the first time in a popular medical guide, all the symptoms you could reasonably expect to encounter are put into perspective. A diagnosis may be possible in the presence of only some of the listed symptoms. It is not necessary to experience all the symptoms in order to confirm a diagnosis.

We divide the diagnoses into:

• What is **probable**: the common causes of the symptom such as would immediately spring to a doctor's mind. Most of these probable diagnoses occur commonly and doctors see them regularly.

• What is **possible**, once the probable causes have been excluded. Some of these diagnoses are not uncommon, but they may require testing to establish them without doubt.

• **Rare** causes: however, it would be misleading to define how rare. The frequency of these diagnoses is extremely variable. Unless your symptoms happen to match closely the features listed, these diagnoses are unlikely.

Extensive testing may be required to establish these diagnoses and, in some cases, doubt may remain.

## USING THIS BOOK

Mostly, you will find it best to start with your symptom or symptoms. If it is easy to put a name to the symptom, such as headache or painful wrist, look for this in the index, which lists all of the symptoms, and which will refer you straight to the relevant page numbers.

If your symptom is not quite so obvious, or easily defined, you need to decide if it can be isolated to a single part of the body, such as the knee or ab-

1

domen, or whether it is a "general," whole-body symptom, such as fever or weight loss. In the case of symptoms clearly occurring in one part of the body, or in one body system, go straight to the relevant section and look through it. You will find that:

• Each part of the body has its own section. The sections are arranged in a logical order, starting at the top of the body (with the eyes) and moving downward toward the feet. It ends with "general" symptoms that cannot be easily isolated to any one part of the body or any one of the body's systems. (The abdominal symptoms are an exception to this rule and are divided between the digestive system and urinary system.)

• Within each section, the order generally echoes that of the book as a whole: the specific come first and the general come last. Also, symptoms that are obvious to others—revealed by clear visual signs such as a rash or a limp—are placed first. Inwardly experienced symptoms, or those which only you are likely to know about, such as loss of sense of smell, come last within a section. (The psychological and nervous symptoms in the Brain and Nervous System section are an exception to this rule, following an alphabetical sequence.)

• In addition, symptoms are grouped like with like, so that, for instance, in the listing for a common cold, shivers, chills, and sweating all occur within the same few pages. Simply browse through the relevant section looking for the symptom, or combination of symptoms, that fits your condition and, if necessary, follow the cross-referencing, which has been introduced to avoid too much unnecessary repetition.

If your symptom(s) cannot be isolated to a single part of the body, go to the "General" Symptoms section, which comes last in the book. We use quotes around the word *general* because although such symptoms may appear to be general, they may on closer inspection be specifically related to a problem in one part of the body or in one of the body's systems. Within this section, symptoms are again ordered like with like, and as far as possible they proceed from the obvious and noticeable to the "internal" and private.

The second way to use this book is when you already know or suspect that you have a particular illness and want to find more information about its symptoms. Simply look up the illness or disease in the index, which will send you straight to the page(s) where it is covered.

# THE EYES

The eyes are extraordinary structures: delicately built, yet durable, and highly sensitive. Just as remarkable are the mechanisms within the brain that interpret the visual impulses traveling to it from the eyes.

Even now, our understanding of how the eyes work is only sketchy. The study of the eyes is one of the most specialized branches of medicine. There are, however, only a few common symptoms of eye disease—symptoms such as blurred vision or a red eye. Most family doctors have a good working knowledge of eye disease, enough to make a confident diagnosis of everyday problems, but detailed assessment of more serious eye conditions should be referred to an eye specialist for thorough assessment.

Eye problems are common in modern life. Children are especially prone to eye infections; adults to eye injury; and the elderly to deteriorating eyes.

Report all but the most trivial eye problems to your doctor, especially pain or blurred vision. If there is eye disease such as glaucoma in your family, you should have regular eye exams.

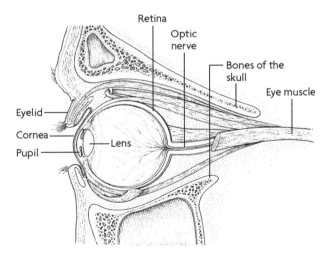

3

## SKIN CHANGES AROUND THE EYE

Brief color changes are probably due to minor infections. Here are other possibilities to explain more long-lasting color changes.

### PROBABLE

#### ■ Injury

Any injury causing bruising of the forehead, or above the eye, will result in a blue/black eye, as the blood in the bruise tracks down the face to settle around the eye. In other words, a black eye need not be caused by injury directly to the eye area.
• At first, redness and pain.
• Black eye appears after a few hours.
• Fades over seven to ten days.

#### ■ Eczema

The skin of the eyelids and below the eyes is especially sensitive.
• Red, itchy skin.
• Dry and flaky.

Those suffering from eczema elsewhere on the body are particularly prone to this problem. Commonly, it is caused by an allergy. The skin around the eye is so delicate that it can react with dermatitis to, for example, makeup, fragrances, or even nail polish. Often, an allergy test is needed to confirm the cause.

#### ■ Xanthelasma

Yellowish, slightly raised nodules usually on the skin on the nasal side of the eye or around the lower eyelid, in adults.
• Painless.
• Grow very slowly.
• Similar nodules may be found on elbows, hands, and knees.

If you notice these, have a cholesterol test, since xanthelasma can be a sign of elevated blood fats.

#### ■ Milia

These are small, pinhead-sized white-yellow spots on the skin near the eye. They are very common and entirely harmless. Essentially, they are just blocked grease glands and can easily be pricked out with a sterile needle.

### RARE

#### ■ Rodent Ulcer

Also known as basal cell carcinoma. A slow-growing skin cancer often found on the face, by the bridge of the nose or the outer margin of the eye's orbit. More common in the elderly.
• Begins as a slightly raised spot, which can ulcerate.
• Sometimes crusts as it grows, but usually has a pearly appearance.
• May bleed.

Cure can virtually be guaranteed if treated early.

## RING AROUND CORNEA

### PROBABLE

■ Corneal Arcus

A white circle around part or all of the cornea, common in those over sixty. Typically, most marked in lower half of the cornea. If seen in a younger person, it may be associated with raised blood cholesterol, which should be checked. Otherwise, it is of no significance.

### POSSIBLE

■ Iron Ring

Grinding or hammering can result in a tiny fragment of metal implanting into the cornea. This is instantly painful and will cause marked watering of the eye. If the fragment is incompletely removed (or left for many hours), a brown ring stain may be left on the cornea.

### VERY RARE

■ Copper Ring

Also called Kayser-Fleischer ring. A green-brown ring associated with the rare condition of Wilson's disease, in which copper builds up in the body. A childhood disease.

• Liver disease (swelling, easy bruising, jaundice).

• Tremor of the limbs.

• Dementia.

Early detection and treatment generally means a good outcome.

■ Calcium

A chalky white deposit can develop as a fine line at the junction between the cornea and the white of the eye in conditions where the calcium level in the blood is abnormally high. This can be quite an irritant and cause some redness of the eye. Important to have a blood test to measure the calcium level.

## RED AND PAINFUL EYE

Never ignore this symptom, which may be a sign of a disease that threatens loss of vision. Seek immediate medical attention.

### PROBABLE

■ Severe Conjunctivitis

The conjunctival membrane covers the white part of the eye. Inflammation causes a mass of red blood vessels running over the eyeball. It is highly contagious, so it tends to spread rapidly among close contacts.

- Initially, itching.
- Both eyes become red.
- The redness is greatest around the outer part of the eyeball.
- Bright light is mildly irritating.
- A yellow discharge.
- Crusted eyelids.

Antibiotic eyedrops or ointment are often recommended and probably render bacterial causes less contagious. Sometimes the symptoms are confined to one eye only, in which case, a doctor will need to exclude other diseases.

### ■ Arc Eye

A variety of acute keratitis *(see right)*. Prolonged use of an arc welder, without adequate strongly tinted eye protection, can result in this miserable condition developing, often several hours after exposure.

- Intense weeping from both eyes.
- Light aversion resulting in the patient keeping their eyes tightly closed.
- Red eyes.

There is little treatment other than pain relief, padding the eye, and using drops to relax the iris. Fortunately, the condition is self-limiting and symptoms usually settle after a few hours. Few people make the mistake a second time! A very

similar condition can occur from exposure to natural ultraviolet (UV) light, for example, skiing without eye UV protection ("snow-blindness").

## POSSIBLE

### ■ Acute Iritis

This is inflammation of the colored part of the eye, the iris, or associated structures. Iritis is not a final diagnosis in itself, since it can be caused by many diseases, in particular arthritic disorders and connective tissue disorders.

- Usually only one eye is affected.
- Moderately painful and red.
- Redness is greatest around the iris.
- The pupil is smaller on the affected side.
- Vision is reduced, blurred.
- The pupil may appear irregular after repeated attacks.
- In severe cases, a milky collection of pus can collect in front of the iris behind the cornea.

### ■ Acute Keratitis

Once again, this is not a final diagnosis, but a complication of several diseases affecting the cornea of the eye. The most common are rosacea *(see Skin, page 98)*, an ulcer on the cornea, or injury.

- Rapid onset of symptoms.
- One eye affected.
- No change in vision.

- Profuse watering; blinking.
- Light irritates the eye.

There are now highly effective antiviral drugs to counter the herpes virus, which is often the cause of this problem, but early treatment is essential. Sometimes steroid eyedrops are recommended, so referral to a specialist is advisable.

## RARE

### ■ Acute Glaucoma

The eyeball contains fluid that circulates via tiny channels. In glaucoma, this fluid builds up pressure, causing changes in the field of vision. However, the changes usually happen so gradually that nothing is noticed until a late stage in the disease. For this reason, screening for glaucoma is strongly advisable in anyone with a family history of the problem, and anyone over the age of sixty. Sudden, rapid rise in pressure can, on rare occasions, occur because of blockage in the channels, or perhaps if a drug dilates the pupils. This is acute glaucoma.

The early symptoms of glaucoma are:
- None at all.
- Possibly vague aching in the eyeball.
- Halos around lights at night.
- Tunnel vision *(see page 34)*.

Acute glaucoma is a medical emergency causing:
- Sudden, excruciating pain in the eye.
- Vomiting as a result of the pain. Indeed, sometimes the patient is just non-specifically unwell with vomiting, and the eye symptoms can be overlooked, resulting in the diagnosis being missed.
- Redness around the iris.
- A hazy cornea.
- Vision severely reduced.

Urgent treatment is needed to reduce pressure within the eye and to save sight.

## SLIGHTLY REDDENED EYE, OR RED EYE WITHOUT PAIN

These are unlikely to signify any serious underlying cause, unless there is also blurred vision or light hurts the eyes.

### PROBABLE

### ■ Conjunctivitis

An infection of the conjunctiva, the thin membrane that covers the white of the eye.
- Eyes may feel itchy or sore.
- Redness appears rapidly, due to many dilated blood vessels.
- The redness is least next to the iris, greatest at the sides of the eyeballs.

- Yellow discharge.
- Eyelids may be crusted.

Conjunctivitis is usually a straightforward diagnosis, but be cautious if redness affects only one eye, when other possibilities need to be considered. Antibiotic eyedrops or ointment are usually effective.

### ■ Allergy

Recurrent, mildly red eyes raise the possibility of allergy. Common causes of allergies (allergens) are pollens or animal dander.

---

Contact lenses are frequently a cause of eye problems. Keeping soft lenses in your eyes for prolonged periods means that you are seventeen times more likely to have an eye infection or conjunctivitis. It is much better to use short-use, hard, gas-permeable lenses. Exposure to the air is crucial for the cornea's oxygen supply. A contact lens acts as a barrier and can result in damage to the surface cells of the cornea, if this barrier remains in place for too long.

A frequent cause of infection is inadequate cleaning of lenses or (equally important) the lens case or out-of-date (and thus no longer sterile) fluid.

---

- Mildly red, itchy eyes.
- May be seasonal, typically associated with sneezing and a runny nose.
- May be related to exposure to allergens.
- Discharge, if any, tends to be clear and not yellow.
- Undersurface of eyelids may appear grainy.

Several effective anti-allergy treatments can help, though for some this becomes a long-term problem.

### ■ Irritant

Smoky atmospheres and air pollution can cause an irritant reaction in the eye, resulting in a sore red conjunctiva.

### POSSIBLE

### ■ Subconjunctival Hemorrhage

An extremely satisfying condition for a doctor to diagnose, since the patient can be totally reassured that no harm will come of it.

- Painless, so the condition is often pointed out by someone else.
- One eye has a bright red patch, which is essentially just a minor bruise. This remains bright red for a few days as the blood is oxygenated from the air.
- The patch may cover half or more of the white of the eye.
- Stops short at the iris.

• Fades away toward the sides of the eye.

It may look alarming, but it is simply due to bleeding from a tiny blood vessel and will fade away over a couple of weeks. In the elderly, it may be prudent to check for high blood pressure.

If, however, it occurs after a blow to the head, expert assessment is needed to check whether there is damage to the eye further back in its socket.

### ■ Feverish Illness

Many febrile illnesses will cause slightly red eyes.

Measles typically causes a viral conjunctivitis affecting both eyes (other features include a troublesome cough and a rash that first starts on the head and neck and spreads down the body over a few days. The lesions are raised reddish bumps, which fade to leave a brownish mark.)

### ■ Kawasaki Disease

A little-understood form of vasculitis that affects many organs, particularly the heart and blood vessels.

• Usually occurs in a young child (two to five years old).
• Very high fever.
• Bumpy red rash.
• Sore throat and dry cracked lips.

• The glands in the neck can become quite large.
• Both eyes become red and sore, but no discharge.
• After a few days, there may be some peeling of the skin on the hands.

Needs urgent hospital admission to prevent long-term complications.

## RARE

### ■ Scleritis/Episcleritis

An inflammatory disease of the white outer part of the eye.

• Part of the white of the eye is red.
• Prominent blood vessels are seen to cause the redness.
• Slight discomfort.
• Often recurrent.

This condition is notable since it tends to be associated with other diseases, especially joint problems. It needs further investigation.

### ■ Meningitis

A few red flecks suddenly appearing on the whites of the eyes may be the earliest signs of meningitis in a baby or child. There may also be:

• A high-pitched cry.
• If old enough, the child will complain of a terrible headache.
• Drowsiness.
• Photophobia (sensitivity to light).

• A bulging, soft spot (fontanelle) on the baby's scalp.
• A red rash elsewhere on the body, which doesn't blanch on pressure (glass test).

Severe meningitis can occur without any of these signs, so the absence of one of these features in an ill child should not be relied on to exclude this life-threatening condition. This is a medical emergency: rush the baby or child to the hospital.

## ABNORMALLY SMALL PUPILS

The pupils are the apertures through which light enters the eyes. Their size is controlled by nerves that make the pupils open and close. Those nerves are affected by changes within the brain and, surprisingly, these nerves course through the chest. It is not always obvious whether one pupil is abnormally small or the other pupil is abnormally large.

It is normal for both pupils to become smaller in bright light. In the elderly, the pupils tend to be smaller than those of young adults. An unconscious young person with pupils like pinpoints should immediately arouse suspicion of a narcotic drug overdose.

### PROBABLE

#### ■ Long-Sightedness

Small pupils are normal in the long-sighted.
• Both pupils are small.
• The pupils react briskly to light and dark.

### POSSIBLE

#### ■ Drugs

Many drugs, and typically pilocarpine and timolol eyedrops used to treat glaucoma *(see page 35)*, constrict the pupils. Small pupils may also be a side effect of the powerful narcotic painkillers such as morphine, dihydrocodeine, and pethidine or drugs of misuse such as heroin.

#### ■ Iritis

*(See page 26)* Suggested by finding:
• Affected eye may have a small, irregular pupil.
• Pain.
• Redness around the iris.
• Reduced vision.

### RARE

#### ■ Horner's Syndrome

A combination of:
• One abnormally small pupil.
• Partially drooping eyelid on that side.

- Decreased sweating on the same side of the face.

The significance of Horner's syndrome is that it demonstrates a problem in one of the nerves controlling the pupil somewhere along its route from the brain, down the chest, and up again to the eye.

Damage to the nerve could be caused, for example, by a brain disease (such as multiple sclerosis), a lung tumor, or enlarged glands within the chest. So, although Horner's syndrome is uncommon, its significance is great and all the more so if there are associated symptoms such as:

- Chest pain.
- Coughing blood.
- Unsteadiness of gait.
- Blurred vision.

### ■ Brain Stem Stroke

An unconscious person (usually middle-aged or older) with bilateral pinpoint pupils may have sustained a stroke in this critical part of the brain.

- Irregular or very reduced breathing.
- Extreme sweating.
- Incontinence.

The patient should be rushed to the hospital by emergency ambulance.

## ENLARGED PUPILS

Young people typically have larger pupils and their size gradually reduces with age.

### PROBABLE

### ■ Emotion

Both pupils will dilate in response to emotional triggers such as fear, excitement, and anxiety.

Accompanying symptoms include:
- Rapid pulse.
- Thumping heartbeat.
- Dry mouth.
- "Stars" in the eyes; but this is controversial.

### ■ Drugs

Commonly prescribed eyedrops, such as atropine and homatropine, are used to treat iritis and are intended to dilate the pupil.

### POSSIBLE

### ■ Third Nerve Palsy

*(See page 19)* The third nerve is one of three nerves controlling eye movements, and it also carries nerve fibers controlling pupil size. If the nerve is damaged:
- The eye turns outwards.
- The eyelid droops.
- The pupil enlarges.

### ■ Injury

A blow to an eye severe enough to damage its internal structure will upset movement of the pupil. This is a particular risk in games using a small ball, such as baseball or squash.

- Probably bruising around the eye.
- Enlarged pupil, unreactive to light.
- Blurred vision is likely (the lens can become dislocated or there can be bleeding within the eye).

Clearly, this needs immediate treatment.

### ■ Coma

A severe head injury or other serious disease affecting the brain, such as a stroke, may cause dilated pupils.

- Deep unconsciousness.
- Breathing is irregular and shallow.
- No response to painful stimulus.

At the worst, dilated pupils in both eyes that do not respond at all to light signal brain death.

### ■ Adie's Pupil

A harmless condition:

- One enlarged pupil, which constricts in reaction to bright light, but more slowly than usual.
- Vision and health otherwise normal.

### ■ Blindness

Depending on the cause of blindness, the pupil in a blind eye may be larger than its companion because the normal reflex response to bright light is absent.

Indeed, any condition that diminishes the perception of light in an eye (e.g., corneal scar, cataract, detached retina, or damage to the optic nerve) will result in the affected eye not responding rapidly to a direct light.

## RARE

### ■ Irritation of Nerves to Eyes

The same process that produces Horner's syndrome *(see page 10)* can, in its early stages, stimulate the nerve, causing a dilated pupil.

Accompanying symptoms which raise suspicion therefore include:

- Chest pain.
- Coughing blood.
- Unsteady gait.
- Blurred vision, numbness of hands.

## IRREGULAR PUPILS

Normal pupils are round or slightly oval, but minor irregularities are common. Their significance depends on the individual's overall state of health.

## PROBABLE

### ■ Normal Variant

Minor degrees of irregularity are almost

certainly of no importance and may well be hereditary.

- No pain or visual disturbance.
- No change with passing of time.
- Otherwise sound health.

## POSSIBLE

### ■ Iritis

*(See page 26)* A small, irregular pupil is a particular feature of this painful condition, especially after repeated attacks.

## RARE

### ■ Multiple Sclerosis

A neurological disease often beginning in early adult life.

- A common initial feature is sudden loss or blurring of vision in one eye.
- Numbness and weakness of different parts of the body.
- Tremor, unsteady gait.

A definite diagnosis of multiple sclerosis can only be made once the individual has had further changes in the brain or spinal cord and this may never happen or only happen after several years have passed.

## VERY RARE

### ■ Syphilis

Years ago, small, irregular pupils would immediately have brought very late-stage, untreated syphilis to mind. Other features would be:

- Brief, severe limb pains.
- Unsteady gait.
- Loss of pain sensation in joints, leading to gross distortion of knees, ankles.
- Drooping eyelids on both sides.

## ENLARGED EYEBALL

### PROBABLE

### ■ Hyperthyroidism

Strictly speaking, this causes not enlargement but protuberance of the eyeballs.

- Both eyeballs affected, though not always symmetrically.
- Sweating, weight loss.
- Fine tremor, hyperactivity.
- Racing heartbeat.

Though treatment controls the general effects, the eyes often remain a little protuberant.

### RARE

### ■ Tumor

- Progressive swelling of one eyeball (in children or adults).
- Squint, loss of vision, pain.

Only after expert assessment can treatment be decided upon.

### ■ Congenital Glaucoma

Raised pressure inside the eye gives rise to a child with:
- "Bull eyes."
- Cornea appears to bulge.

### ■ Thrombosis

A risk in cases of meningitis and severe dehydration. Blood clots in the structures behind the eyes rapidly cause:
- Painful protruding eyes.
- Restricted eye movements.
- Eyes that look swollen.

## COLORED PATCHES ON EYEBALL

Doctors often check the eyes as a matter of routine because the eye may be an indicator of disease elsewhere in the body, for example, jaundice or anemia. The Possible and Rare causes of colored patches are really very infrequent.

### PROBABLE

### ■ Pterygium

A sheath of blood vessels and accompanying tissue grows out along the white of the eye toward the cornea. The term derives from the Latin for "flies' wings," to which the condition does have a superficial resemblance. It is thought to be due to chronic exposure to the elements (especially the wind), so it is most common in cyclists and sailors.
- Appears usually in the middle-aged.
- Small, triangular-shaped white tissue, blood vessels within.
- The broad base points away from the cornea.

A pterygium rarely causes anything other than a cosmetic problem, or possibly slight irritation; but it can be removed if it threatens to grow over the cornea.

### ■ Pinguecula

The name derives from a term meaning "to do with grease." These yellowish discolorations are, again, little more than cosmetic nuisance. Usually only found in the elderly.
- Yellow, opaque raised lumps in the white of the eye.
- Triangular-shaped, with the broad base closest to the cornea.

### POSSIBLE

### ■ Scleritis

In between episodes of inflammation, these groupings of blood vessels simply form a flat, discolored area to one side of the eyeball. *(See page 9)*

## RARE

### ■ Growths

Any of the lumps and bumps—warts, cysts, moles, and cancers—that grow on skin anywhere on the body may appear on the white of the eye. Diagnosis is a specialist matter. Report any recently noticed spot to your doctor. Remember, the appearance of any of these on the eye is very rare.

## DISCHARGE FROM EYES

Eyes may discharge tears or pus, or often a combination of both.

### PROBABLE

#### ■ Conjunctivitis

• Red eyes develop over a day or so.
• Constant discharge of small amounts of yellow pus.
• Eyelids stick together in the mornings with crustiness.

Minor infections are soothed by bathing the eyes with tepid water; severe infections, especially in children, need antibiotic drops. *(See also page 7)*

#### ■ Allergy

Suggested by a combination of:
• A clear discharge from both eyes.
• Itching.
• A blocked nose with clear nasal discharge and sneezing.

May be seasonal (hay fever) or perennial (e.g., due to animal dander, etc.).

### POSSIBLE

#### ■ Blocked Tear Duct

In babies up to one year of age, this is a common cause of a constantly running eye and sometimes of repeated episodes of conjunctivitis. The tear duct is too narrow for tears to drain normally into the nose. (Newborn babies cannot normally produce tears, so this usually becomes manifest after about one month old.)
• Usually only one eye is affected.
• Eye runs tears even when the baby is perfectly well.

Most babies grow out of this by their first birthday. If necessary, it is possible to dilate the tear duct by probing it in an outpatient procedure.

#### ■ Ectropion

A lower eyelid sags and turns outward so that tears spill over; common in the elderly.

## CONSTANT TWITCHING MOVEMENTS OF THE EYES

The technical term for this is nystagmus. It is not always an abnormality, as some people show a few beats of nystagmus if they look to the extreme of their gaze.

### PROBABLE

#### ■ Cataract

This is an opacity of the lens, sometimes visible as the pupil having a white-gray glint.
• Gradually worsens vision.

Usually a disease of later life, but it can be present at birth *(see below)*. Standard treatment is to replace the offending lens with an artificial lens.

#### ■ Injury

Any serious injury to the cornea will leave an opaque patch, which may obscure vision, depending on its position.

### POSSIBLE

#### ■ Congenital

Several unusual inherited conditions can cause a cataract or lead to deterioration of the cornea during childhood.

Diagnosis only established by a specialist examination.

### RARE

#### ■ Trachoma

Though rare in developed countries, this infection is one of the most common causes of blindness.
• Swollen eyelids.
• Undersurface of eyelids is granular.
• Gradual opacity of the cornea.

#### ■ Vitamin A Deficiency

Also known as keratomalacia. Worldwide, this is a serious and avoidable cause of blindness, especially in children. Rare in developed countries.
• Hazy cornea with a thickened, coarse appearance.
• Night blindness.

#### ■ Infection

Yet another hazard to vision now confined mainly to underdeveloped countries. Possible sources of infection are parasites, gonorrhea, and syphilis, complications of each giving rise to a clouded cornea.

#### ■ Acute Glaucoma

Gives a clouded cornea, but in a red, excruciatingly painful eye *(see page 7)*.

#### ■ Tumor

In young children, the earliest sign of a tumor within the eye may be that the pupil appears opaque. (The "red-eye" effect of flash photography is lost and the pupil of the affected eye has a white or black appearance instead.)

- Rarely, both eyes are affected.
- May be hereditary.

- A newly appeared squint is also cause for suspicion.

Needs very urgent hospital treatment.

## CATARACTS

A cataract is an opacity within the lens of the eye. It cuts down the amount of light that can enter the eye and whatever light does enter is made hazy and blurred. An early cataract will not cause any symptoms and will only be spotted on examination of the eye; but a mature cataract is visible as a whitish haze on the lens. Between these two stages, there will be variable symptoms.

Most cataracts are the result of aging. Occasionally, they occur following injury or disease. On rare occasions, a child can be born with a cataract because of a few rare metabolic diseases or certain maternal infections during pregnancy.

### PROBABLE

#### ■ Aging

Most people over sixty will have some opacity of the lens, but if it is not interfering with vision, it is probably best left alone.
- No other general disease.
- Vision deteriorates slowly.
- Eyes are pain free.

Cataract surgery is highly effective.

#### ■ Injury

A penetrating injury to the eye (most commonly a high-velocity fragment, for example, from hammering or drilling) can damage the lens and trigger cataract formation.
- The size of the opacity remains unchanged.
- Disturbance of vision depends on its size.

### POSSIBLE

#### ■ Diabetes

Those suffering from diabetes have an increased risk of developing cataracts in later life.

#### ■ Steroids

Steroids are invaluable drugs used in the treatment of many diseases, including severe asthma, joint diseases, and inflammatory eye diseases such as iritis (see page 26). However, their long-term uses can cause many side effects, including early formation of cataracts. This problem is most likely to result from long-term use of high doses of oral steroids; however, it can also result from steroid eyedrops, which should only be prescribed under specialist supervision.

### RARE

■ **Congenital Rubella**

Rubella ("German measles") caught during the first four months of pregnancy will cause multiple abnormalities in the developing baby. These include:

- Cataracts.
- Mental retardation.
- Heart disease.
- Deafness.

These tragic consequences are avoided by routine vaccination of girls against the disease.

■ **Metabolic or Congenital Disease**

Several unusual conditions may explain cataracts in children, usually in association with failure to thrive and, with some, epilepsy or developmental delay.

## TWITCHING EYELID

For some reason, this symptom generates much anxiety; it is not clear why this should be so. Although Hollywood uses it as cinematic shorthand for an impending nervous breakdown, it is harmless.

- Brief repeated twitching.
- Same lid is affected.
- Worse when tired or stressed.
- Rarely lasts for longer than a few days.

## DROOPING EYELIDS

### PROBABLE

■ **Ectropion**

Sagging of the lower eyelids, very common in the elderly.

- The red undersurface of the lid is exposed.
- Tears spill out easily on the cheek.
- Increased risk of conjunctivitis.

Really bad cases can be corrected by a simple operation.

### POSSIBLE

■ **Bell's Palsy**

A paralysis of the facial nerve.

- The lower eyelid on the affected side droops.
- Sudden onset.
- The eye cannot be completely closed. Normally, when the eye closes, the eyeball looks up into a resting position with the cornea out of harm's way. In this con-

dition, because the eyelid fails to cover the eyeball, a rather disturbing feature is the eye looking toward heaven, whenever the patient blinks.

- The face sags on that side.

Recovery takes time and is often incomplete. Medical assessment is a priority as this is most commonly caused by the herpes simplex virus and early aggressive treatment can significantly improve the recovery. It is also necessary to exclude a stroke, which can result in a very similar weakness, but with a subtle difference.

### ■ Congenital

The probable diagnosis in a child with drooping upper eyelids.

- Normal eye movements.
- Normal muscular power.

## RARE

### ■ Third Nerve Palsy

Refers to the third cranial nerve, which is damaged (for example, by pressure).

- Paralysis involves one eye only.
- Eye turns outward.

- Enlarged pupil.

Specialist investigation is needed to determine the underlying cause, which may be a brain tumor, diabetes, or an enlarged artery in the brain pressing on the nerve.

### ■ Myasthenia Gravis

A treatable condition causing rapid tiring of the muscles.

- Drooping eyelids are an early feature.
- Both upper eyelids are affected.
- Muscles elsewhere grow fatigued abnormally fast, sometimes resulting in slurred speech, swallowing difficulties, or double vision.

### ■ Syphilis

The late stage of untreated syphilis (which may be up to twenty years or more after the first infection) causes widespread nerve disorders.

- Tingling feet.
- Brief shooting pains in the limbs.
- Unsteady movements.
- Pain sensation is diminished.
- Drooping eyelids on both sides.

## EYELIDS INFLAMED OR ITCHY

Localized inflammation is probably due to infection. More generalized itching is usually allergic.

## PROBABLE

### ■ Blepharitis

An irritating condition in which the margins of the eyelids just by the roots of the eyelashes become chronically inflamed.

- Constant raw appearance.
- Crusting near the roots of the eyelashes.
- Flaking skin on eyelids.
- Irritation.

The problem is often associated with eczema elsewhere on the body. All doctors have their favorite treatments, a sure sign that none guarantees a cure, but hot saline soaks are probably as good as anything.

This common condition may be thought of as a type of dandruff *(see Skin section)* affecting the eyelids. Some people find it helps to wash their eyelids nightly with a diluted solution of shampoo on a cotton swab.

### ■ Allergy

Both eyelids are involved, causing a persistent mild irritation and desire to rub.

- Skin is slightly reddened.
- Dry, flaking skin.
- Often causes eczema elsewhere.

This is another minor but annoying condition, often due to an allergic contact reaction. Possible triggers include hair spray, eye makeup, or even nail polish, but the reason often remains obscure even after allergy testing. The skin around the eye is so delicate that it reacts to minimal exposure, when other areas of the skin tolerate an agent without and problem (e.g., nail polish).

## POSSIBLE

### ■ Insect Bites

A common reason in the summer and autumn.

- Localized, raised red bumps.
- Itchy for a few hours.

### ■ Pubic Lice

Lice will happily make a home in any hairy area with the right density of hair, which happens to include the eyelids. A diagnosis to be delivered with tact.

- Tiny round insects seen adhering to the root of the eyelashes.
- May also inhabit the eyebrows.

Treatment is to suffocate the lice with a copious application of Vaseline (petroleum jelly).

## RARE

### ■ Trachoma

An infection common in the Third World causing:

- Swollen eyelids.
- Grainy red undersurfaces of the eyelids.

One of the most common preventable causes of blindness. *(See also page 16)*

## LUMPS ON EYELIDS

### PROBABLE

■ **Stye**

• Infection at the root of a single eyelash.

• Often preceded by a day of mild discomfort.

• Pus may appear.

The most important treatment is regular, hot saline soaks. Antibiotic drops may help.

■ **Infected Meibomian Cyst**

The meibomian glands are helpful little structures that produce a greasy lubricant for the eyelashes. Infection reaches them via hair roots.

The important difference between this condition and a stye is that the lump is behind the root of the eyelash, on the flat part of the eyelid. It can be felt and seen as a small, pea-like lump below the skin.

• Pain, redness inside an eyelid.

• Small, tender lump appears.

Treatment is same as for a stye, although an oral antibiotic is often required. Often, an unsightly lump remains, which may need to be removed later.

### POSSIBLE

■ **Molluscum Contagiosum**

A long name for a benign, wart-like condition that appears in mini-epidemics among children.

• Small, rounded, slightly raised lumps that usually dimple in the center.

• Likely elsewhere on body.

Harmless, though cosmetically a nuisance; best left to clear spontaneously as messing with them can cause the virus to spread.

### RARE

■ **Dacrocystitis**

Infection in the tear duct, which drains tears from the inner corner of the eyelid into the nose.

• Pain, swelling near bridge of nose.

• Skin becomes red and tender.

• Pus discharges from eye.

A fairly serious condition that needs early treatment. *(See also page 23)*

■ **Rodent Ulcer**

A slow-growing form of skin cancer, commonest in the elderly who have led an outdoor life.

• Begins as a small, pearly lump.

• Grows slowly.

• Center may ulcerate and bleed.

Considered curable, but needs attention as early as possible. *(See also page 22)*

## SWOLLEN EYELIDS

The loose skin of the eyelids easily swells to an alarming degree, but rarely for any serious reason.

### PROBABLE

#### ■ Allergy

An allergic reaction of the skin of the eyelids to various agents, including fragrances, makeup, hair spray, and nail polish. Often, the cause remains unknown. Usually both eyes are affected.

• Painless.
• Mild itching, flaking skin.
• Looks worse after sleep, because swelling worsens when lying flat.

#### ■ Stye

Although a stye is a boil at the root of an eyelash, large ones may cause generalized swelling of the rest of the eyelid. *(See also page 25)*

• Only one eye affected.

#### ■ Blepharitis (Chronic)

Prolonged inflammation of this kind *(see page 19)* eventually makes the eyelids permanently slightly swollen.

### RARE

#### ■ Orbital Cellulitis

A spreading infection involving the skin of the eyelids and the surrounding parts of the face.

• Confined to one eye.
• So much swelling that the eyelids cannot be opened.
• Red, tender eyelids.
• Malaise, fever.

Needs vigorous and immediate treatment with antibiotics to prevent it from spreading deeper behind the eye.

#### ■ Nephrotic Syndrome

A very rare condition nowadays, most commonly due to an immune reaction in the kidneys following a streptococcal infection.

• Swelling around the eyes with initially markedly reduced amount of urine being passed, which is dark.
• Loin pain.

Needs urgent assessment, usually in a hospital.

## PAIN OR ACHING IN THE EYE AREA

### PROBABLE

#### ■ Eye Strain

This familiar symptom arises after hours of close work, especially under poor or glaring light, especially if appropriate corrective eyeglasses are not used.
- Vision is undisturbed.
- Aching in and around eyes.
- Relieved by a few hours of rest.

Recurrent eye strain means that you should have an eye test, or consider adjustment to the lighting where you work.

#### ■ Nasal Congestion

Along with common cold there is often:
- Aching behind and around the eyeball.
- Blocked, runny nose.
- Mild headache.

The symptoms settle after a few days.

#### ■ Conjunctivitis

Conjunctivitis gives a prickling sensation, together with:
- Red eyes, worse around the margins.
- Mildly irritated by light.
- No loss of vision.
- Often a crusty deposit on the eyelashes.

### POSSIBLE

#### ■ Glaucoma

(See page 35) This serious, but treatable condition frequently causes no other symptoms than a vague ache in and around the orbit.

It is easily detected with a simple eye exam by an optician.

#### ■ Dacrocystitis

An infection in the tear duct at the inner corner of the eye.
- Pain and swelling.
- A red lump appears.
- Eye runs with tears and pus.

Early treatment with antibiotics is advisable.

#### ■ Flu-Like Illness

Aching in the eyes is a frequent accompaniment to a feverish illness, including the common cold or flu.
- Vision unaffected.
- Slight redness of eyes.
- Fever, aching muscles.

Within a few days, the underlying cause is clear.

#### ■ Sinusitis

A very common cause of aching in and around the eyes.

- Usually develops after a common cold.
- Pain or pressure felt across the forehead and in the morning.

Sinusitis responds to steam inhalations. Occasionally, a steroid nasal spray or oral antibiotics may be necessary.

## RARE

### ■ Tumor

Needs to be considered in case of persistent pain, especially with children.
- Bulging eye.
- Disturbed vision.
- Newly appeared squint.

## DRY EYES

A constant feeling of irritation in the eyes.
- Frequent, mild conjunctivitis.

## PROBABLE

### ■ Aging

The eye's natural ability to lubricate itself with tears decreases with age. "Artificial tears" in the form of eyedrops are effective, but have to be used regularly.

> Regular use of a computer monitor can cause uncomfortable or dry eyes. There is static electricity between the eyes and the screen. Dust is attracted to the eyes and can cause irritation. Tip: have your own antistatic wipes and use them to keep the area around your workstation as free from dust as possible.

## POSSIBLE

### ■ Dry Atmosphere

Many people complain of dry eyes during the winter, when central heating systems are on, or after prolonged periods of time in an air-conditioned atmosphere.

## RARE

### ■ Sjögren's Syndrome

Production by the tear gland is dramatically reduced as well as reduced saliva production in the mouth, leading to a dry mouth. It may be associated with rheumatic disorders or with autoimmune disorders, giving rise to:
- Joint pains.
- Swollen joints.
- Rashes.

Blood tests are usually necessary to establish the diagnosis.

## FEELING SOMETHING IN THE EYE

Considering how much dust flies around the average street, it is remarkable how rarely anything gets into the eyes.

- A sudden, prickling feeling in one eye.
- Rapid blinking.
- Tears, aversion to light.
- Mild discomfort.
- The feeling that you must get something out of your eye.

### PROBABLE

#### ■ Foreign Body

Typically dust. Often a helper can see and remove the foreign body. But beware of a foreign body involving high-speed fragments, for example, while hammering concrete or drilling.

Continuing symptoms, or signs of infection, deserve specialized examination in case a foreign body has lodged deeper into the eye.

#### ■ Conjunctivitis

It is common during the early stages of conjunctivitis before the redness is noticeable to feel that something is lodged in the eye. Some cases of conjunctivitis may actually begin with a small foreign body, which then creates infection.

### POSSIBLE

#### ■ Ingrowing Eyelash

A constant feeling of irritation in one part of the eye suggests that you should scrutinize the eyelids for this frequently overlooked cause.

#### ■ Allergy

A recurrent feeling of irritation may be caused by allergy. *(See also page 15)*

- Mild redness.
- Itching, rather than pain.

#### ■ Stye

An infection at the root of one of the eyelashes.

- Visible as a yellow swelling.
- The eye becomes red.
- Swelling of the eyelid is common.

Hot saline soaks allow drainage of infection, otherwise antibiotic ointment treatment may be necessary.

## MODERATE TO SEVERE PAIN IN EYE

With the exception of an obvious foreign body, any such degree of eye pain needs expert assessment since neglect may damage sight.

### PROBABLE

#### ■ Foreign Body

Dust, grit, or ingrowing eyelashes cause irritation out of all proportion to the size of the foreign body.
- One eye affected.
- Sudden onset of feeling something in the eye.
- Intense irritation and watering.
- Light irritates the eye.
- Vision unaffected, though may be blurred by tears.

The eye's own protective mechanisms sweep out the foreign body in most cases.

#### ■ Ulcer or Abrasion of Cornea

An ulcer can quite easily occur on the delicate cornea, due to damage from a foreign body or from infection.
- Intense discomfort in one eye.
- Builds up over a few hours.
- Light causes much discomfort.
- Redness around the iris.

### POSSIBLE

#### ■ Iritis

An inflammation of the iris. It may be as-sociated with a variety of rheumatic dis-orders, which need to be considered in recurrent cases.
- One eye affected.
- Redness, greatest around the colored area.
- Marked aversion to light.
- Blurred vision.
- Small pupil on affected side.

Treatment with eyedrops, though quite straightforward, is necessary to prevent permanent damage to the iris.

#### ■ Episcleritis

Irritation in the white part of the eye (sclera).
- Redness in one obvious area of the white of the eye.
- Prominent blood vessels.
- Pain is moderate.
- Moderate aversions to light.
- Vision is unaffected, apart from blur-ring due to tears.

#### ■ Shingles

Every doctor has a tale to tell of being fooled by early stages of this condition, which is caused by the chicken pox virus.
- At first, discomfort around one side of the face with no skin changes.
- After a few days, the rash appears.
- Crusting sores develop over the eye-lids, side of the nose, and forehead.

- Accompanied by severe pain.
- If spots appear on the side of the nose or inside the nose, there is an increased chance of the eyeball being infected.

The worry about this otherwise harmless condition is ulceration of the cornea. Fortunately, there are now powerful antiviral drugs that reduce this possibility, but they need to be given early in the illness.

## RARE

### ■ Acute Glaucoma

*(See page 7)*

### ■ Retrobular Neuritis

Inflammation of the optic nerve, especially associated with multiple sclerosis.
- Rapid loss of vision in one eye.
- Moderate pain when the eye is moved.

### ■ Thrombosis

A blood clot in the skull behind the eyes, causing:
- Sudden pain behind both eyes.
- Eyes to protrude.

### ■ Corneal Ulcer

A possibility if only one eye is inflamed. These uncommon infections begin with:
- Itching in one eye.
- Intense photophobia.
- Redness, mainly around the iris.

Contact lens wearers should be especially aware of this problem, which can be due to overuse of the contact lens.

A doctor will check for an ulcer using a fluorescent stain. The usual cause is the herpes virus. Specialist assessment and early vigorous treatment with antiviral eyedrops is essential.

## EYES ABNORMALLY SENSITIVE TO LIGHT

Any existing irritation of the eyes will cause some discomfort in bright light. Persistent or severe sensitivity to light is called photophobia.

## PROBABLE

### ■ Conjunctivitis

Mild redness around the outer parts of the whites of the eyes, plus:
- Sticky discharge.

- A mild gritty feeling in eyes.

Antibiotic eyedrops or ointment is usually advisable to reduce the spread of the condition as much as anything. *(See page 7)*

### ■ Allergy

Recurrent photophobia suggests an allergy, especially in someone with other signs of an allergic constitution, such as:

- Eczema.
- Runny nose, sneezing on exposure to pollens, animal hair.
- Itching eyes on exposure to dust or in specific environments.
- Vision is not affected, other than by the watering produced by the allergy.

Treatment is typically a combination of antihistamine tablets and anti-allergic eyedrops.

## POSSIBLE

### ■ Iritis

*(See page 26)*

### ■ Damaged Cornea

A clinical picture similar to iritis, but with:

- Less severe pain.
- Redness around the cornea.
- History of abrasion or ulcer in the eye.

Needs appropriate treatment.

### ■ Measles

An increasing rarity in developed countries, where vaccination programs are leading to its eradication, measles is still found in the Third World, where it can kill up to 20 percent of children.

- Aversion to light is prominent feature in the days before the rash appears.

- High fever for four days.
- Bloodshot eyes.
- Runny nose, cough.
- Blotchy red rash appears behind the ears and spreads over the whole body.
- Temperature remains high for another three to four days.

## RARE

### ■ Meningitis

Aversion to light is a significant symptom of meningitis, but there will usually be associated symptoms, including:

- Headache.
- Resistance and pain on attempting to bend the neck.
- Nausea.
- Drowsiness, or confusion.
- In babies, a bulging, soft spot on top of the skull.

If you suspect meningitis, don't delay seeking medical advice.

### ■ Albinism

Due to lack of pigment, albinos have a special sensitivity to bright lights. Nystagmus (abnormal eye movements, *see Constant Twitching Movements of the Eyes, page 16*) and squint are also common features.

## BLURRED VISION

The everyday experience of the world being somewhat out of focus can nearly always be put down to just that—in other words, you need glasses.

Temporary blurring will result from any eye irritation causing tears to flow, for instance, conjunctivitis. Persistent or recurrent blurring may result from the following.

### PROBABLE

#### ■ Uncorrected Vision

With time, the power of the lens of the eye changes, as does that of the muscles that change its shape in order to focus on objects at different distances from the eye.

- A very gradual change.
- Can be corrected with glasses.

Adults are aware of the process. This may not be the case in children, who may not realize that they have a problem; hence, the importance of eye exams during childhood.

### POSSIBLE

#### ■ Macular Degeneration

A deterioration of part of the retina in the elderly, causing loss of fine vision to a variable degree, not correctable with glasses. *(See page 35)*

#### ■ Cataract

The interference with light caused by the cataract may be misinterpreted as blurred vision. *(See page 17)*

#### ■ Effects of Drugs

Many drugs affect the muscles in the eye, causing blurred vision. It is a question of relating the symptoms to taking the drug. Common culprits include those drugs given to control bladder function and antidepressants.

### RARE

#### ■ Diabetes

Swings in the bloodstream's sugar level can cause blurred vision.

- A temporary symptom, fading within minutes.
- Undiagnosed diabetes causes thirst, excess urine production, and tiredness.

## DISTORTION OF VISION

Objects look too small or too large, and straight lines appear curved. Not a common symptom and, if persistent, needs expert assessment.

### PROBABLE

■ **Unknown Cause**

The sensation of distortion of size or shape sometime happens for just a brief moment. An object may suddenly seem to be distant.

- Vision otherwise unaffected.
- Recovers within moments.

### POSSIBLE

■ **Detached Retina**

Light fading on the crinkled, detaching retina is seen as distorted.

- Preceded by many floaters. *(See page 33)*

- The classic symptom is often described as a "curtain coming down to obscure the sight."
- Many flashing lights.

Seek medical help immediately, since early intervention can prevent loss of vision. *(See page 37 for further details)*

### RARE

■ **Distortion of the Retina**

Just as the distortion of the screen alters the film projected on it, so distortion of the retina has the same effect. This may be caused by tumors, bleeding, or inflammation.

- Other symptoms of retinal detachment *(see above)*.
- A bulging eye.
- Loss of vision.
- In children, a white appearance to the lens.

## DOUBLE VISION

Movements of the eyes are delicately coordinated by an automatic process of the brain. The process has to be learned, accounting for the alarming gyrations of the eyes that occur in newborn babies until they have developed the necessary coordination. Once achieved, we experience stereoscopic vision. When things go wrong, we start seeing two of everything, since the brain is no longer able to merge the output from the two eyes into one image.

Don't confuse this symptom with blurred vision, which raises quite different possibilities.

## PROBABLE

### ■ Using Extremities of Gaze

It is normal to experience double vision if the eyes are swivelled to the extreme left or right, up or down.

### ■ Paralysis of Eye Muscles

The eye is moved by six muscles, each of which turns the eye in a particular direction. Paralysis of any of those muscles results in double vision because the affected muscle is unable to move one eye as well as the other eye can move.

The pattern of weakness gives a clue as to which muscles are affected, being some combination of:

• The affected eye turning inward or outward.

• Eyelid may droop.

• Pupil on that side may be wider than the unaffected side.

Many cases are unexplained. A head injury is a common cause and will be obvious. Other possibilities are meningitis, infections, and botulism, but these give rise to further dramatic symptoms that overshadow the double vision, for instance:

• Severe headache.

• Confusion, drowsiness.

• The eye hurt by light.

## POSSIBLE

### ■ Multiple Sclerosis

A disease of the nervous system often beginning in early adult life. Double vision results from partial weakness of the eye muscles.

• Vision may also be blurred.

• Slight discomfort in the eye.

• Unsteadiness in walking.

• Tremor or weakness in the arms or legs.

• Numbness of the limbs.

The double vision usually recedes over a few weeks.

## RARE

### ■ Displacement of Eyeball

Caused by something pushing the eye forward and interfering with its movements. Bleeding behind the eye, or thrombosis, would be suggested by:

• Sudden onset.

• Pain in the eye(s).

• Eye(s) suddenly protruding.

Graves' disease, associated with an overactive thyroid gland, or a tumor behind the eye, would produce:

• Slower onset of symptoms.

• Gradual protrusion of one or both eyes.

• Sweating, rapid pulse, and weight loss.

### ■ Myasthenia Gravis

An unusual disease in which the muscles anywhere in the body tire rapidly. Eye symptoms are an early feature.

- Eyelids droop.
- Double vision may occur in any direction of gaze.
- Both eyes are affected.

The diagnosis is established by the individual's reaction to certain injected drugs.

### ■ Disease of One Lens

The apparently impossible symptom of double vision affecting one eye may, in fact, be due to disease in one lens, which splits the image as a prism does.

## FLASHING LIGHTS

Caused by individual light receptors firing off in the retina.

### PROBABLE

### ■ Normal

Flashing lights are frequently experienced after a blow to the head or after suddenly getting up from a squatting position, when blood flow is briefly disturbed.

- Both eyes affected.
- You feel light-headed briefly.
- Return to normal within seconds.

### POSSIBLE

### ■ Migraine

Flashing lights shimmering in one section of the field of vision are a typical warning of the onset of migraine. *(See also page 38)*

- Usually both eyes are affected.
- Nausea.
- Headache.

### RARE

### ■ Detached Retina

*(See page 37)*

- One eye affected.
- A shower of flashes.
- Numerous floaters.

These symptoms need urgent specialist attention.

## FLOATER (FLOATING SPOTS BEFORE THE EYES)

The interior of the eye is a liquid, in which it is normal for clumps of cells to float around, hence the term "floater." An alternative medical term is muscae volitantes, meaning "flying flies."

### PROBABLE

#### ■ Normal

A floater is probably harmless if:
- There are only one or two.
- Vision is otherwise normal.
- The eye is painless.

### POSSIBLE

#### ■ Severe Short-Sightedness

This can cause the release of more than usual numbers of floaters.

### RARE

#### ■ Detached Retina

*(See page 37)* Before complete detachment, warning signs include:
- Large numbers of floaters.
- Shower of lights.

If you have these symptoms, you need urgent specialist attention.

#### ■ Damage to Retina

Inflammation or bleeding within the eye causes:
- Many floaters in one eye.
- Blurring of vision.
- Pain.
- Redness.

Treatment depends on the causes.

## SEEING HALOES AROUND LIGHTS

This happens if the cornea becomes waterlogged, as in glaucoma, or if something within the lens is scattering the light.

### PROBABLE

#### ■ Glaucoma

*(See page 35)*
- Haloes, seen especially at night.
- Tunnel vision.

Untreated, glaucoma progressively destroys sight, producing little by way of symptoms until the disease is well advanced. So, it is important to have your eyes examined if a close relative suffers from glaucoma, while those over sixty should be checked regularly anyway.

### POSSIBLE

#### ■ Cataract

*(See page 17)* The haziness in the lens acts like a prism, scattering light so that objects appear to be surrounded by haloes and rainbows.

## TUNNEL VISION

Loss of the outer field of vision: you seem to look at the world through a tube. The brain is so adaptable that the condition can progress remarkably far before you notice a problem.

### PROBABLE

■ Glaucoma

*(See page 35)* Suggested by the combination of:
• Tunnel vision.
• At night, bright lights appear to be surrounded by haloes.
• Sometimes, aching in eyes.

### POSSIBLE

■ Retinitis Pigmentosa

*(See page 36)*

■ Migraine

• Symptoms develop over a few minutes.
• Visual field appears to shrink.
• Followed by severe headache, nausea.
• Vision recovers.

### RARE

■ Brain Tumor

Can cause tunnel vision by increasing the pressure inside the brain or by a direct destruction of the parts of the brain required to interpret vision. There are likely to be other symptoms such as:
• Severe headache, typically on waking at night.
• Persistent nausea.
• Change of personality.
• Altered awareness.

■ Syphilis

Years after infection, the widespread damage wrought by this disease also causes a multitude of symptoms including:
• Severe shooting pains in limbs.
• Unsteady gait.
• Drooping eyelids.
• Loss of pain sensation in limbs, leading to grossly deformed joints.
• Some degree of mental disturbance.

## BLINDNESS

There can be no glossing over the fact that many causes of blindness remain untreatable. It is, therefore, of little consolation (but nonetheless important) to know which causes of blindness are treatable or at any rate controllable. People with high blood pressure, diabetes, or a family history of glaucoma should take special care of their eyes and heed any warning signs, including flashing lights, pain in the eyes, and pain in the temples.

## PROBABLE

### ▪ Cataract

A white patch seen in the lens of the eye and nearly always due to the aging process.

• Very gradual loss of clear vision.

• The awareness of light is not lost, only clarity.

Cataract surgery is surely one modern medicine's unqualified successes. *(See page 17)*

### ▪ Macular Degeneration

The retina of the eye is made up of a sandwich of light-sensitive elements. The macula is a small area of the retina where these elements are most concentrated and where the sharpest vision is achieved. "Degeneration" means decrease in function—part of the natural process of aging. This is the most common cause of deterioration of eyesight in the elderly.

Disease in the macula has a serious effect on vision, but does not cause total loss of sight. The usual reason for its deterioration involves the blood supply or the nerves to or in that area. Unfortunately, little can be done to halt established degeneration, but recent advances can help some people with macular degeneration.

• Gradual, painless loss of vision.

• Central vision deteriorates, making reading, for example, impossible.

• Vision, especially close vision, is blurred and not improved with corrective lenses.

• Outer vision is unaffected.

• Objects may look distorted or small.

There is never complete loss of vision, because the outer parts of the retina are spared.

### ▪ Diabetic Eye Disease

One long-term effect of diabetes is degeneration of blood vessels within the retina. This causes loss of vision that can be gradual or sudden, depending on the pattern of degeneration. Diabetics, therefore, need regular checks on their retinas. It is possible to treat blood vessels that appear diseased with a laser beam. There are no symptoms of this condition, so it has to be assessed by an expert.

### ▪ Glaucoma

Raised pressure inside the eye, a common condition that should be screened for in the elderly and earlier in those with a family history of glaucoma. The features on blindness caused by this insidious disease are:

• Painless.

• Peripheral vision is lost, giving rise to tunnel vision.

• Occasionally, aching in the eyes.

• At night, bright lights appear to be surrounded by a halo.

## POSSIBLE

### ■ High Blood Pressure

This may increase the likelihood of macular degeneration *(see page 35)* and should be treated. Mild to moderate high blood pressure has no symptoms. Very high blood pressure over a long period may cause:

• Severe headaches.

• Symptoms due to strain on the heart such as breathlessness, ankle swelling, palpitations, or chest pain.

### ■ Choroiditis

The choroid is one of the layers that makes up the retina. Inflammation in the choroid results in a gradual, but permanent, loss of vision corresponding to the site of damage. The reason for most cases of choroiditis is unknown, although there is proven association with toxoplasmosis, an infection that causes illness similar to glandular fever. Syphilis used to be a more common cause.

• You may recall an episode of disturbed vision in one eye.

• You then become aware of an area of blindness in that eye.

• Only one eye affected.

• The area is fixed, and neither grows nor shrinks.

### ■ Retinitis Pigmentosa

A degenerative condition affecting the retina and so called because of the dark pigment that is visible over the retina through an ophthalmoscope. This tends to be an inherited condition and nothing can be done to stop it.

• Symptoms begin in adolescence.

• Gradual loss of the peripheral field of vision, leading eventually to tunnel vision.

• Night blindness.

## RARE

### ■ Trachoma

Worldwide, trachoma is a common cause of blindness, but it is rare in the developed world. The infection causes:

• Extremely sore, puffy eyes.

• Runny eyes.

• Scarring of the cornea, resulting in partial or total blindness.

## SUDDEN BLINDNESS

Unusual, but when it does occur, this usually has a serious underlying cause.

### PROBABLE

■ **Blockage of Central Retinal Artery**

This artery supplies blood to the back of the eye, and blockage may occur because of a tiny blood clot or because the artery constricts to the point where it cuts off blood flow:

- Sudden, total blindness.
- No pain.
- One eye affected.

If the blockage is a result of a spasm of the artery, there is a chance of vision returning after an hour or so. Otherwise, there is no treatment. It is important to search for the causes that may threaten the sight of the other eye, for example, a source of blood clot in the heart or temporal arteritis *(see page 38)*.

■ **Blockage of the Central Retinal Vein**

This vessel carries blood away from the eye. Blockage is usually caused by pressure from a diseased retinal artery, which runs very close to the vein. The elderly and those with diabetes or high blood pressure are at increased risk.

- Loss of vision is rapid, but not instant, as in arterial blockage.
- Usually, light can still be seen.

Sometimes partial vision returns, though this can take a few weeks.

■ **Detached Retina**

It may come as a surprise to know that the retina is not firmly attached to the back of the eye but is held in place by the pressure of fluid within the eye. The retina can tear, allowing fluid to leak behind it and to peel it off the back of the eye. A blow to the head or (rarely) a tumor growing at the back of the eye may also dislodge the retina.

- Most common in the very short-sighted.
- Multiple flashing lights may be a warning of detachment.
- A shadow appears to fall over the field of vision, sometimes described as like a curtain falling.

With early treatment, the retina can often be anchored back into place.

■ **Amaurosis Fugax**

Mini-stroke causing a blockage of the central retinal artery; however, the blood clot rapidly dislodges.

- Sudden, painless loss of vision in one eye.

- Vision returns after a few minutes.

Your doctor must search for the site where the blood clots originate. It is usually in the carotid artery, which runs up the neck.

### ■ Stroke

A stroke is caused by blockage of blood flow within the brain. If the blockage happens to involve the part of the brain that processes information from the eyes, the result is blindness.
- Sudden, painless onset.
- Vision is usually lost in both eyes at once.
- Sudden paralysis of one side of the body.
- In severe strokes, unconsciousness follows.

The exact nature of the loss of vision can give a clue as to where in the brain the damage has occurred. *(See also Blind Spots, page 40)*

### Possible

### ■ Temporal Arteritis

This cause of blindness should be better known because it is treatable.
- It is almost always confined to people over the age of fifty-five or sixty years.
- The artery on the side of the scalp becomes exquisitely tender, making brushing the hair or wearing a hat intolerable.

- The blood supply to the muscles used for chewing can be compromised, so the individual has to stop eating every few minutes.
- General malaise.

The condition responds dramatically to steroid drugs, which can save sight if the condition is recognized in time.

It is associated with a condition known as polymyalgia rheumatica *(see page 278)*, which also only occurs in the elderly.
- Gradual appearance of a vague weakness and malaise.
- Muscular tenderness, especially around the shoulders and neck.

### ■ Migraine

Visual disturbances, including temporary blindness, are common in migraine. Commonest in, but not confined to, the young and middle-aged.
- Shimmering lights in the eyes.
- Nausea.
- One-sided temporary blindness.
- Possibly slurred speech, loss of use of one hand.
- As symptoms fade, a severe headache begins.

The first time this happens, it may seem like a stroke. Many doctors recommend further tests, since occasionally there is a cause for the migraine within the brain.

## ■ Optic Neuritis

Inflammation of the optic nerve, usually in a young adult.

- Sudden loss of vision in one eye.
- Usually, the loss is confined to the central field of vision, so the individual can still see "at the edges of vision."
- The eye may ache.

Recovery after a few days. Optic neuritis can be a warning sign of multiple sclerosis. Other underlying causes may be syphilis, diabetes, and lack of B vitamins.

## ■ Vitreous Hemorrhage

Bleeding into the fluid within the eyeball. Associated with diabetes and with general arterial disease.

- Mild cases give rise to multiple floaters *(see page 33)*.
- Otherwise painless partial loss of vision in one eye.

The condition is confirmed by looking at the interior of the eye with an ophthalmoscope. There is rarely any treatment. The outcome depends on the size of the bleed and any underlying disease.

## ■ Acute Glaucoma

*(See page 7)*
   Suggested by the sudden onset of:
- Excruciating pain in one eye.

- Vomiting.
- Red eye.
- Glazed appearance of the eye.

Requires emergency treatment.

## RARE

## ■ Methyl Alcohol

Drinkers of methylated spirits are at risk of sudden blindness in one or both eyes. It may be total.

## ■ Injury

A head injury can cause sudden blindness by damaging the part of the brain involved in vision, or by causing retinal detachment *(see page 37)*.

## ■ Hysteria

Blindness of psychological origin is suspected if the back of the eye appears normal and if tests show that visual stimuli are reaching the brain. The individual has usually exhibited other odd physical symptoms, such as:

- Unexplained paralysis.
- Loss of speech.
- Abnormal gait.
- Does not show expected emotional reaction to blindness, when for most people it is a devastating event.

There is often a previous psychotic history.

## BLIND SPOTS

You may become aware of an area of your field of vision where the vision is dim or absent altogether. Wherever you look, that patch remains fixed in relation to the rest of your visual field. This is known as a scotoma. A scotoma that suddenly appears draws attention to itself, whereas a slowly enlarging scotoma can be entirely overlooked—you are aware only of unspecific blurring of vision—until it is of considerable size.

Scotomas in both eyes are usually due to damage to the optic nerves somewhere in the brain. A scotoma in one eye is nearly always due to a cause within that eye.

A scotoma should not be confused with the blind spot which everyone has: an area of absent vision that might possibly be noticed if one eye is covered and an object slowly moved to the side. There is a point at which the object briefly disappears from vision. This corresponds with the part of the retina where the optic nerve leaves the eye and where, therefore, there are no visual receptors.

### PROBABLE

#### ■ Macular Degeneration

Age-related deterioration of the eye causing a fixed area of dim or absent vision. *(See page 35)*

• One eye is affected more than the other.

• A loss of vision in the center of the field.

• The area of loss may increase very slowly.

#### ■ Stroke

A stroke affecting the back of the brain causes:

• Loss of part of the field of vision.

• Both eyes are affected.

• Other features of a stroke, such as paralysis, confusion.

*(See also page 415)*

#### ■ Injury

A blow to the head severe enough to damage the eye or brain may cause loss of vision.

• Usually both eyes are affected.

### POSSIBLE

#### ■ Pituitary Tumor

The pituitary gland is a structure in the brain that lies close to the nerves coming from the eyes. Any tumor in the gland presses on those nerves, producing a characteristic blind spot.

• Painless.

• Loss of the outer field of vision.

• Mild headache.

There may be other symptoms as a result of abnormal hormone production: for example, excessive height, absent menstrual periods, breasts constantly leaking milk.

## RARE

### ■ Poisoning

Tobacco, ethyl alcohol, and lead are some of the many poisons that may affect the optic nerve.
• Gradual loss of the central field of vision.
• Vision is generally dimmed.

• Loss of vision may be abrupt after a binge.

Recovery depends on how long-standing the damage is.

### ■ Carotid Aneurysm

Caused by the effect of pressure from a swollen carotid artery within the brain, which presses on the optic nerve.
• A blind area in the outer field of vision.
• Affects one eye at first.
• Gradually involves both eyes.

## NIGHT BLINDNESS

### PROBABLE

### ■ Retinitis Pigmentosa

*(See page 36)* Suspected in a young adult with:
• Night blindness.
• Tunnel vision.

### POSSIBLE

### ■ Severe Short-Sightedness

• Difficulty seeing when the light is poor.
• Blurred vision helped by glasses.

### ■ Congenital

Occasionally, poor night vision is present from birth.

### RARE

### ■ Vitamin A Deficiency

Vitamin A is required for vision, this being the basis for the parental wisdom that eating carrots, a rich source of vitamin A, will help night vision. It is a fair bet that this explanation will leave children unimpressed and carrots uneaten, but children should at least be aware that lack of this vitamin is a major cause of blindness in the Third World.
• Night blindness is an early symptom.
• The eyes appear leathery and the lenses clouded.

Given soon enough, high doses of vitamin A save sight.

## COLOR BLINDNESS

A condition affecting about one in twelve males and about one in 200 females. In the commonest form, red-green vision is partly or completely absent; less commonly, blue-green vision is affected. Total absence of any color vision is very rare. So adaptable is the brain that it is possible to reach adult life without any suspicion of a problem. The individual appears to distinguish colors by noting subtle differences in brightness and grayness. Context also helps; for example, the lowest traffic light is green, because that is what everyone else calls it. The writer has even known a successful color-blind interior designer. Normal color vision is needed in certain occupations, such as pilots and train drivers, where it is essential to see color absolutely correctly.

Occasionally, someone with previously normal color vision finds it deteriorating for one of the following reasons.

### PROBABLE

#### ■ Cataract

This common problem, typically experienced as haziness in the lens, does not really destroy color vision but makes colors less easy to distinguish. *(See page 17)*

#### ■ Damage to the Retina

Many retinal diseases can affect color vision by damaging the receptors respon-

sible for seeing color. Other symptoms, considered fully elsewhere in this section, may include:

- Gradual loss of vision.
- Sudden loss of vision.
- Blind spots.

It is not possible to be more specific without medical assessment of the eye, optic nerve, and the parts of the brain responsible for vision.

### POSSIBLE

#### ■ Malnutrition

Lack of vitamins and protein needed for the visual receptors can cause color vision to deteriorate. It is a possibility among the severely malnourished, alcoholics, those with wasting diseases, or the mentally disturbed.

There is likely to be also:
- Night blindness.
- In children, failure to grow.
- Hair loss, loss of skin color.
- Swollen ankles.

### RARE

#### ■ Toxic drugs

This includes a massive overuse of tobacco and alcoholism.

Overdosage of digoxin, as used for heart disease, can make the world look yellow or green.

## SQUINT

A squint is the result of the eyes being out of alignment: they appear to point in different directions. Often a squint is suspected as an impression rather than definitely seen: you may have a feeling on looking at someone that their eyes are not quite in line. If that someone is a child, please do not ignore that feeling, for squint is an important symptom and should never be ignored.

Forget the old wives' tale of children growing out of a squint; it does not happen. What does happen is that the child experiences double vision and gradually the brain learns to ignore the vision from one eye in an effort to overcome the defect. If unrecognized, this leads to permanently damaged vision in one eye. Symptoms that suggest a squint are:

• Obvious deviation of one or both eyes.

• Head held in an unusual posture to compensate.

• Squint noticed if child is tired.

The assessment and treatment of squint is a complex area. In most cases, the cause is either muscle imbalance or different strengths of lens in each eye. Both causes are treated by surgery or glasses.

### PROBABLE

■ **Muscle Imbalance or Inequalities of Vision**

If the head is held at an unusual angle, it suggests the likelihood of muscle imbalance underlying the squint. You may also notice that one eye cannot turn beyond a certain point. Otherwise, it is likely that one eye is long-sighted or (less commonly) short-sighted compared to the other. Usually, however, it is a matter of specialist assessment to differentiate these problems.

### POSSIBLE

■ **Prominent Skin Folds**

In children, the folds of skin by the bridge of the nose may be unusually wide, giving the impression that the eyes turn in. Even if this happens to be the case, the child should still be checked.

### RARE

■ **Nerve Palsies**

It has been mentioned *(see Paralysis of Eye Muscles, page 31)* that six muscles control the movements of the eyes. Each muscle is subject to paralysis for a variety of reasons. Nerve palsy is probably the cause if there is:

• A drooping eyelid.

- Changes in size of the pupil *(see pages 10–11)*.

Nerve palsies have a variety of causes, which themselves need further investigation.

### ■ Tumors of the Eye or Socket

These can occur at all ages, producing a squint by pressure on one eyeball. So, don't ignore a newly acquired squint, especially in children.

- The eye protrudes more and more.
- There is a pain behind the eye.
- The pupil may appear white if the tumor is inside the eye.

# THE NOSE

## NOSE IS AN ODD SHAPE

There is, of course, no such thing as a "normal" shape for a nose. The "one-off" factors that can deform it are considered here.

### PROBABLE

#### ■ Injury

Typically, the nose is flattened or made crooked (you may hear doctors describe the latter as "deviation"). This is likely to be accompanied by swelling and bleeding and indicates a fracture of the nose bone.

It is normal to wait for a week to allow swelling to go down before deciding whether the nose needs straightening by surgery.

• Nasal bone fracture.
• Flattening of the nose.
• Deviation of the nose.
• Swelling.
• Bleeding.

### POSSIBLE

#### ■ Rhinophyma

Also known as "potato nose" or "bottle-nose." Caused by overactivity of the sebaceous gland of the nose. It takes some years to develop. It is relatively common, affecting men more often than women, and is usually seen in older age groups and in patients with a high alcohol intake.

• Large, bulbous nose.
• Purplish red in color.
• Irregular "pitted" surface: the pits mark the entrances to the glands.

Can be treated easily by surgery and long-term antibiotics can be given to reduce occurrence.

### RARE

#### ■ Nasal Septal Necrosis

A blow to the nose may not break the nasal bones but instead damage the

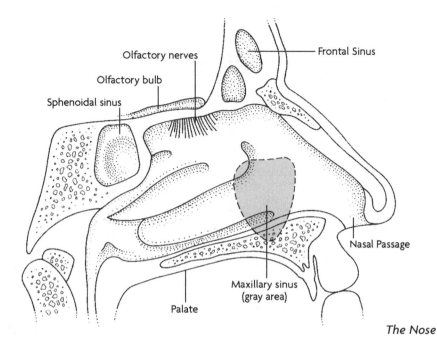

*The Nose*

nasal septum (a thin layer of cartilage separating the two sides of the nose). Pressure from a blood clot under its mucous membrane covering causes:
• Headache.
• Local pain at the tip of the nose.
• Apparent widening of the tip of the nose.
• Loss of sensation over the skin of the nose.
• Destruction of septal cartilage over a matter of weeks, causing the nose to dip at the bridge.

### ■ Leprosy
Causes collapse of the nose due to septal ulceration. This is one of several obvious symptoms which will be apparent.

### ■ Cancer of the Nose
Any irregular sore on the nose that enlarges over months or years, that bleeds, ulcerates, or is painful could be malignant. Enlargement of local lymph nodes suggests malignancy.

## REDDENED NOSE

### PROBABLE

■ **Staphylococcal Infection**

An infection of the skin in a part of the nose.

- Local swelling.
- Local redness.
- Local pain.
- Local heat.

May require antibiotics.

### POSSIBLE

■ **Acne Rosacea**

A rash caused by overactivity of the sebaceous glands.

- Associated with facial flushing.
- Redness from small blood vessels.
- Rash covers nose, brow, face, and chin.
- Small pustules may be evident.
- May persist for years.

Treatment is available, usually with antibiotics for the long term, but can be difficult.

■ **Erysipelas**

A bacterial skin infection.

- Associated with a break in the skin, often near eye, nose, or mouth.
- Fever.
- Malaise.
- Hot, reddened swelling all over affected area.
- Painful.
- Blisters may appear.

Need to see a doctor immediately. Antibiotics will treat this effectively if given at an early stage.

■ **Rhinophyma**

*(See page 45)*

## STREAMING NOSE

### PROBABLE

■ **Common Cold**

There are many different types of common cold virus. As you throw off each new one, you develop a natural immunity to it. Children often have a "perpetual runny nose" because they are being exposed to new viruses every day at school. The elderly rarely get colds for

they have built up immunity to so many of the viruses.

■ **Vasomotor Rhinitis**

Some individuals suffer from overreaction of the nasal lining. This leads to an excess of the usually small amounts of "normal" nasal discharge. Some drug treatments taken as nasal sprays, which can be obtained over the counter, may help this condition. Its features are similar to those of allergic rhinitis.

### ■ Allergic Rhinitis

In the same way that hay fever is caused by pollen, many allergens can cause a runny nose. Locally applied steroid nasal sprays can be effective in preventing the reaction.

## POSSIBLE

### ■ Sinusitis

Nasal discharge will often be yellow or green, sometimes thick. There may be an associated headache.

### ■ Foreign Body

Discharge is foul-smelling and on one side only.

The foreign body needs to be removed by a doctor.

### ■ Nasal Polyp

Polyps, which are benign fleshy growths, can appear inside the nose. As well as obstructing the nasal passages and blocking the nose, they can cause an increase in the volume of secretions, which will appear as a runny nose.

Treatment is medical management (use of topical nasal steroids) or surgical removal of the polyps.

### ■ Drug Withdrawal

A clear, runny discharge is a common symptom when withdrawing from a "hard" drug such as heroin, or its substitute, methadone. Other signs include:

- Running eyes.
- Sweating.
- "Goose flesh."
- Yawning.
- Stomach cramps.
- Diarrhea.

## RARE

### ■ Cancer of the Nose

Any tumor of the nose or in the spaces around the nose may cause a nasal discharge.

Recurrent nosebleeds or bloody streaks in the discharge may be a feature. Discuss with your doctor.

## NOSEBLEEDS

Also known as epistaxis. A particularly common problem in children, although most adults have episodes of bleeding from the nose at some time. There are many causes, some due to local disease and some indicative of systemic, or "whole body," disease. Most nosebleeds can be treated by continuous, firm pressure across the fleshy part of the nose just below the bridge. Pressure should be maintained for as long as ten minutes in severe cases. Sit forward with the head supported and breathe through your mouth. Local application of ice at the bridge of the nose may also help. Only in rare cases is medical or surgical intervention required. But see your doctor or local hospital emergency department about any profuse or prolonged bleeding.

## PROBABLE

### ■ Minor Infection

The most common cause of persistent and recurrent nosebleeds is a minor nasal infection. This brings blood vessels very close to the surface on the inside of the nose. The slightest disturbance will then set off a nosebleed. Antibiotic ointment used inside the nose over a few days can have dramatic results.

### ■ Nose Picking

Probably the most common cause in children. The finger, or the fingernail, damage an area of skin, known as Little's area, situated at the entrance to the nose.
- Occasionally, profuse bleeding.
- Often occurs at night.
- Almost always cures itself after applying pressure.

- May be recurrent.

### ■ Injury

If the nose is clearly deformed or misaligned as a result of a blow, see a doctor. There could be an underlying fracture.

### ■ Common Cold

Nosebleeds are a surprisingly frequent symptom of common colds. The inflammation compromises the fine blood vessels.

Repeated nose blowing to clear mucus may also bring on bleeding.

## POSSIBLE

### ■ Foreign Body

A toddler or young child can push a bead or some other small object into a nostril, which may remain unrecognized for days, weeks, or months. Inflammation develops, causing:
- Discharge from one nostril.
- It may be purulent, yellow-green.
- Possibly bloodstained and smelly.

Removal may require a general anesthetic.

### ■ Chronic Sinusitis

The linings of the bony sinuses become chronically infected.
- Profuse discharge back into throat, rather than out through the nostrils.
- Obstruction of the nose.

- Head pain, particularly in the forehead or under the eyes.
- Loss of sense of smell.
- Nosebleeds, often with excessive nose blowing.

### ■ Drug-Induced

A number of drugs—typically warfarin, which thins the blood, and some drugs used to treat arthritis—may cause nosebleeds.

If nosebleeds occur while you are taking warfarin, it may indicate that you are taking too much, so consult a doctor.

### ■ Benign Tumors, including Nasal Polyps

These can bleed from time to time, particularly after nose picking or blowing.
- Obstruction of the nose.
- Associated sinusitis.
- Discharge of mucus.
- Loss of sense of smell.

## RARE

### ■ Hereditary Hemorrhagic Telangiectasia

*(See page 80)*

### ■ Disorders of Blood Clotting

The most common are factor VIII deficiency (true hemophilia), Christmas disease, and von Willebrand disease. Common features include:
- Persistent bleeding after minor cuts and abrasions.
- Marked bruising.
- Bleeding after extraction of teeth.
- Bleeding into joints, causing eventual degeneration.
- Spontaneous bleeding, including nosebleeds.

Simple blood tests will determine whether there is any abnormality of clotting. It is particularly important to know if you have a disorder before dental treatment—if in doubt, check.

### ■ High Blood Pressure

More common in the middle-aged and elderly. An otherwise fit individual who suddenly gets recurrent nosebleeds must have blood pressure measurements and tests to check clotting ability.

### ■ Cancer of the Nose

There are several potential symptoms:
- Obstruction of the nose.
- Discharge from the nose.
- Associated sinusitis.
- Nosebleeds.

It is *very* rare for anyone to present nosebleeds to their doctor as a symptom of cancer of the nose.

## NASAL-SOUNDING SPEECH

Any disease or injury that blocks the nose or distorts the nasopharynx will alter the quality of the sound produced. The most frequent causes are the common cold, septal deviation *(page 53)*, "adenoids" *(page 52)*, and injury. Less common, but worth considering, are cleft palate *(page 81)*, a foreign body *(page 49)*, chronic sinusitis *(page 49)*, and benign tumors, including polyps *(page 50)*.

## SNORING AND SLEEP APNEA

An all-too-common problem, rarely reported to doctors by snorers. It happens when the tongue obstructs air flow, setting up vibrations of structures in the mouth, particularly the uvula (the fleshy, wriggly bit that hangs down between your tonsils), soft palate, and tongue. Most common in drinkers, the obese, those over forty and male, and those with nasal obstruction or misshapen noses. Sleeping on the side rather than the back will probably help. If you find your partner's snoring is making you seriously dissatisfied with him (or her), you will not want a doctor to tell you to be understanding because snorers cannot help it. However, you should be interested in the fact that some snoring, some of the time, is inevitable.

Exceptionally severe, persistent snoring justifies surgery. A modern operation known as a uvuloplasty, which reshapes the soft palate at the back of the mouth, can transform the lives of severe snorers.

For less severe cases, one trick that is said to work is to sew a hairbrush inside the back of your pajama top. This wakes you when you roll on to your back (the snoring position). Also try adjusting pillows and bedding, changing the ventilation in your bedroom, and eating bedtime snacks—all of which are said to have made a difference to some people's snoring.

Sleep apnea is defined as an episode of cessation of breathing during sleep. This can occur many times per night and the resulting sleep deprivation causes daytime lethargy, poor concentration, poor memory, and falling asleep during the day.

• The person is usually overweight and has a short, thick neck.

• In children, the tonsils may be so large that they meet or "kiss" in the middle.

This requires specialist referral.

## BREATHING THROUGH THE MOUTH: A BLOCKED NOSE

The effects of an obstructed nose depend somewhat on the cause, but may include:
- Pain in the nose.
- Discharge from the nose.
- No sense of smell.
- Breathing through the mouth.
- Snoring.
- Dry mouth.
- Bad breath.

For details, see the sections concerning those symptoms.

Causes of obstruction include the following.

### PROBABLE

■ **Adenoids**

Perhaps the most common reason for "mouth breathing." The adenoids are lymph tissue lying at the back of the nose and pharynx near the soft palate. They are prone to acute or chronic infection.

Acute infection gives:
- Pain behind nose.
- Catarrh.
- Nasal obstruction (due to enlargement).
- Enlarged neck lymph nodes.

Chronic infection gives:
- Enlarged adenoids.
- Chronic catarrh.

- Persistent cough.
- Breathing through the mouth.
- Ear infection, possibly leading to impaired hearing.

Both types of "adenoiditis" cause alteration in the quality of speech. As the adenoids perform no essential function, removing them is a common and usually very helpful operation (common, of course, in childhood).

This operation used to be carried out frequently. Current understanding of how both the adenoids and the tonsils develop is that there is a natural shrinkage of these tissues as a child reaches his or her tenth birthday. An operation can be avoided if symptoms are not too troublesome.

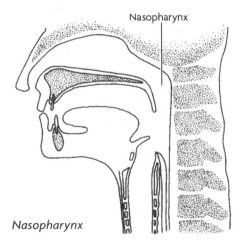

Nasopharynx

*Nasopharynx*

■ **Septal Deviation**

The septum is the thin layer of cartilage separating the two sides of the nose. "Deviation" may occur during birth (1 to 2 percent of babies have permanently deviated septa). It may also occur as the result of injury at a later age. The result is obstruction of one of the nostrils, either partially or completely. *(See Nose Is an Odd Shape, page 45)*

■ **Injury and Common Cold**

*(See page 45 and page 47)*

■ **Vasomotor Rhinitis and Allergic Rhinitis**

*(See page 47 and page 48)*

**POSSIBLE**

■ **Foreign Body, Chronic Sinusitis, and Benign Tumors including Nasal Polyps**

*(See page 48, page 49, and page 50)*

## PAINFUL NOSE

This is such a general symptom that analyzing it in its own right is not helpful. There will always be some other accompanying factor(s) to pin it down. Is there nasal discharge or bleeding? Is the speech affected? Is the nose misshapen? Does the nose itch? Has the sense of smell gone? These are all covered in detail in neighboring pages and will give proper insight into "pain in the nose."

## TINGLING NOSE AND SNEEZING

Look for an outside cause first: is it the smell of a houseplant or an animal? Or a chemical? Or chili powder or pepper? Some people sneeze in bright sunlight. There are many different causes, a large number unique to individuals. Failing these, consider vasomotor rhinitis *(see page 47)* or allergic rhinitis *(see page 48)*.

## LOSS OF SENSE OF SMELL

**PROBABLE**

May be due to smoking, common cold, vasomotor rhinitis, or allergic rhinitis. These diagnoses are either self-evident or covered in detail elsewhere. With a common cold, the loss is transient *(see page 47);* vasomotor rhinitis *(see page 47)* and allergic rhinitis *(see page 48)* cause intermittent loss, which may become long term.

## POSSIBLE

### ■ Obstructive Lesions of the Nose

*(See Breathing Through the Mouth: A Blocked Nose, page 52)*

### ■ Breathing Through the Mouth

*(See page 52)*

### ■ Sinusitis

*(See page 49)* Acute sinusitis may lead to transient loss and chronic sinusitis to long-term loss of smell.

## RARE

### ■ Head Injury

A blow to the head may sever the fila-ments of the cranial nerve in the roof of the nose. As the nose is pushed in, or the forehead struck, there is a bony displacement that can cut the nerve responsible for sensing smell, causing permanent loss of smell.

### ■ Meningioma

A tumor of the sheath covering the brain. It can press on the olfactory nerve (responsible for smell), causing progressive loss of smell and other symptoms, such as headache.

### ■ Frontal Lobe Tumor

This can cause pressure on brain tissue involved in sensing smell, and it can damage the pathways conducting sense of smell. Loss is progressive and other symptoms will be apparent.

# THE EARS

The ear has something in common with an iceberg: there is so much more to it than you see. There are three parts to the ear: the outer, the middle, and the inner ear.

The visible ear is cartilage, covered with skin, and it is subject to any of the problems that affect skin elsewhere: bruising, infections, and eczema. Hidden from view is the eardrum, which guards the inner ear, a beautifully intricate structure that turns sound waves into the electrical impulses for transmission to the brain. The inner ear also contains

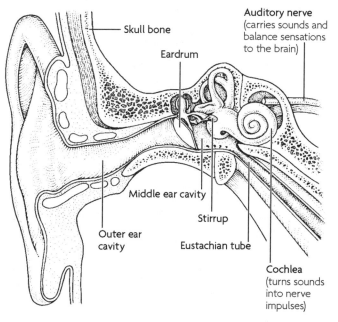

*The Ear*

the fluid-filled semicircular canals, which give you your sense of balance and orientation. Then there are the passages connecting the inner ear to the back of the throat: they allow equalization of air pressure on both sides of the eardrum, without which you experience pressure or "popping" in the ears. Skin, nerves, bones, fluid—it's little wonder that there are many minor diseases that can afflict the ear, and a few serious ones.

## BLEEDING EAR

Blood from the ear, usually mixed with pus, is a common symptom, not often due to a serious cause.

### PROBABLE

#### ■ Middle Ear Infection

This problem is inescapable in childhood, occasional in adults, and usually accompanies a common cold. The eardrum becomes red and bulges. If the drum bursts, pus and blood ooze from the ear for a few days.

• Pain in the ear for a day or two.
• Then, suddenly, a smelly, bloodstained discharge.
• The pain goes.
• The discharge lessens over a few days.

There is evidence that most ear infections are viral in nature. Most will resolve with analgesic and doctors do not like prescribing antibiotics for the first three days.

The eardrum nearly always heals, but your doctor will want to watch progress in order to be certain.

### POSSIBLE

#### ■ Boil

Just like a pimple elsewhere, a boil in the canal of the ear may burst, discharging a few specks of blood.

• An extremely tender spot, just inside the ear canal.
• Bursts after a day or two.
• Symptoms then rapidly vanish.

#### ■ Polyp

These fleshy lumps can form deep inside the ear if there is recurrent infection. They are painless, but may ooze or bleed and can be seen through an otoscope (an instrument used for seeing inside the ear).

#### ■ Injury

A severe blow to the head may rupture the eardrum and cause bleeding.

### RARE

#### ■ Cancer

Growths within the ear canal or within the inner ear are unusual.

- Intense, persistent pain in the ear.
- Constant discharge of pus mixed with blood.

- Partial paralysis of one side of the face.

## BOIL IN THE EAR

Boils form at the root of the tiny hairs lining the ear canal. They cause pain out of all proportion to their tiny size because the skin of the ear canal is unable to stretch much without intense pain.

- Localized, throbbing pain.
- You may be able to feel a tender lump.
- Reaches a peak after a day or two.
- Discharges small amounts of blood and pus for a couple of days.

Will usually clear by itself, but antibiotic drops help. Sometimes oral antibiotics are necessary.

### POSSIBLE

■ **Herpes Simplex**

A cold sore in the ear canal will give symptoms similar to a boil, but:

- The pain is more prolonged and recurrent.
- The sore is filled with clear fluid, rather than pus.

■ **Ramsay Hunt Syndrome**

*(See page 61)*

## LUMPS AND BUMPS ON THE EAR

### PROBABLE

■ **Resolved Boil**

The aftermath of a boil.

- Initially, pain and redness from the boil.
- May discharge pus.
- Becomes smaller over a few days.
- Firm lump left at the site. Usually the lump disappears, but this can take months.

■ **Cauliflower Ear**

This is the permanently enlarged, fleshy, misshapen ear left after injury. It results from permanent scarring of the cartilage that makes up the external ear and is an occupational hazard of boxers and rugby players.

### POSSIBLE

■ **Auricular Appendage**

A small, painless outgrowth between the

ear canal and the cheek. It is present from birth, harmless, and removable.

## ■ Wart

Can occur on the ear as on other parts of the skin.

• Appears rapidly, then stops growing at about 5 mm in length.
• The end is rough, with black spots.

Removable but complete cure can be difficult.

## ■ Gout

A disorder of body chemistry leading to the appearance of crystals of uric acid (tophi) in many parts of the body, especially the joints.

• Firm, irregular lumps called tophi in the outer ear.
• These become extremely painful.
• Pain in other joints, classically the big toe.

## ■ Tumor

A slow-growing skin cancer can involve the ear.

• Begins as a small, crusted spot.
• Develops a rolled edge.
• May bleed.
• Does not heal.
• Gradually enlarges.

This is a form of cancer, but can be treated. See a doctor.

## DISCHARGING EAR

### PROBABLE

## ■ Ear Infection

*(See page 62)* Gives pain, pus, and blood for a few days.

## ■ Otitis Externa

Eczema of the skin lining the ear canal. The skin of the ear canal is as prone to eczema as is skin elsewhere in the body.

Aggravating factors include swimming pool chemicals, poking about in the ear with pencils or earbuds, and even medicated eardrops. Frequently, bacteria or fungi invade the eczema, giving a mixed picture of infection and irritation, which is difficult to cure.

• Intensely itching ear canals.
• Persistent thin, watery discharge.
• Discharge thicker if infection occurs.
• Pain on pulling the ear signifies an infection.

Treatment is with antifungal, anti-inflammatory eardrops and oral antibiotics.

## ■ Chronic Otitis Media

Chronic infection of the inner ear, with pus discharging for weeks on end through a hole in the eardrum. There is usually a previous history of repeated ear infection.

- Yellowish discharge.
- Quantity varies from day to day. Treatment involves eradicating infection, getting air into the ear, and, eventually, repairing the hole in the eardrum.

## RARE

### ■ Cholesteatoma

This is a mass of abnormal cells that forms usually as a result of recurrent ear infections. The cells destroy surrounding tissues, causing symptoms of:

- Deafness.
- Discharge.
- Vertigo.

Treatment consists of surgically removing the cholesteatoma and refashioning the inner ear. This is a complex operation.

### ■ Polyp

A fleshy, non-cancerous growth arising from a cholesteatoma and causing discharge, sometimes bloodstained.

### ■ Rupture of Eardrum

Caused by injury and resulting in:

- Deafness, which may be partial or total.
- Ringing in ears.
- Bloody discharge.

An injury serious enough to fracture the skull near the ear means that the fluid which surrounds the brain may leak out of the ear. This significant condition causes the above symptoms plus:

- Painless, persistent leakage of clear fluid.

## EARACHE

Pain in the ear is usually caused by a relatively minor problem within the ear. It nonetheless keeps doctors on their toes because it can be a symptom of disease elsewhere.

## PROBABLE

### ■ Ear Infection

*(See page 62)* Pain, pus, and discharge arising over a few hours or days. A routine symptom in children with common colds.

### ■ Eustachian Catarrh

This condition may be described by your doctor as "eustachian tube dysfunction." If fluid builds up inside the inner ear, it muffles hearing. This condition is common for a few days or weeks after a common cold. Chronic catarrh is also familiar to those who suffer from hay fever or sinusitis. It is particularly important to pick up in childhood since it can cause deafness severe enough to interfere with speech and to hinder progress in school.

- Hearing is muffled.
- A feeling of pressure inside the ear.
- Yawning relieves pressure temporarily.
- In children, delay in learning to speak.

Adults rarely need any treatment other than decongestants; children suffering deafness may need surgery to drain the fluid.

> The eustachian tube is a ventilation pipe that goes from the back of the throat to the inner ear. Air passes through the tube to equalize the pressure on either side of the eardrum. This is why swallowing relieves popping ears. The tube is narrowest in childhood and it is then that most problems occur.

### ■ Wax

A block of hard wax may eventually become painful and give rise to muffled hearing. People vary enormously in how much earwax they produce and often recognize for themselves when so much has built up that they need their ears cleared by syringing with warm water. If possible, however, leave your ears alone.

The ear is a self-cleaning organ. It is rarely necessary to have ears syringed. Small hairs move the wax to the outer ear where it can be wiped away.

Avoid cleaning your ears with cotton swabs—it causes more problems than it cures. Always try simple earwax softening drops first, and try to allow the ear to clear naturally. Ear syringing is rarely required.

### ■ Boil

(See page 57) A pimple in the ear canal, causing a remarkable amount of pain for such a small object.

## POSSIBLE

### ■ Throat Infection

A throat infection (including tonsillitis) may seem obvious and recognizable, but often the throat symptoms are overshadowed by earache. Common in young children.

- Sore throat.
- Pain on swallowing.
- If there are white patches on tonsils, it may signify tonsillitis.

### ■ Teeth Problems

The large molar teeth, if decayed, may cause aching that appears to radiate into the ear. In children, eruption of the back teeth can cause a combination of symptoms easily taken for an ear infection:

- Feverish, unhappy child.
- Rubbing ear.
- Dribbling.

## ■ Mastoiditis

The mastoid bone is the prominent swelling behind the ears and it was once common for ear infection to spread into that area. With the use of antibiotics, this is now unlikely.

- Pain behind the ear.
- Tender, red swelling of the mastoid bone.
- Fever and malaise.
- Heavy yellow discharge from the ear.

The condition urgently needs surgical drainage of the mastoid bone.

## ■ Perichondritis

Occasionally, the outer ear, which is made up of cartilage, becomes inflamed, typically after a knock or in cold weather.

- Throbbing pain over part of the outer ear.
- Skin is reddened.

Symptoms resolve of their own accord over a few days, just occasionally needing antibiotic treatment.

## RARE

## ■ Rodent Ulcer (Basal Cell Carcinoma)

A form of skin cancer that can occur anywhere on the ear or in the ear canal.

- Starts by looking like a small sore that does not heal.
- Grows very slowly.
- May bleed and cause pain.

Cured by treatment given at an early stage.

## ■ Tic Douloureux

The medical term for this is trigeminal neuralgia. An unpleasant condition arising from irritation of the nerve that supplies feeling to much of the face and the ear. The cause is unknown. Commonest in the late middle-aged and elderly.

- Sudden, severe shooting pains across ear, face, nose.
- Pains set off by eating, the cold, or other triggers.

There are several drug treatments for this miserable, though harmless illness.

## ■ Ramsay Hunt Syndrome

This is a form of shingles that can be a puzzling cause of pain.

- Pain in one side of throat and the ear on that side.
- Hearing may seem hypersensitive.

- Loss of taste on that side of the tongue.
- Small, crusting spots appear in the throat and ear after a week or two.

### ■ Cancer of the Ear

Cancer of the ear canal or inner ear is unusual.

- Intense, prolonged pain.
- Bloody discharge.

### ■ Cancer of the Tongue

It is important to check the back of the tongue in cases of persistent earache in which there appears to be no cause within the ear itself.

- A persistent, shallow ulcer on the back of the tongue.
- Most common in smokers.
- Gradually enlarges, with pain and bleeding.

### ■ Cancer of the Tonsil

Another unusual cancer, most common in old age.

- One tonsil is enlarged.
- Earache.
- Pain on swallowing.

## EAR FEELS "FULL"

A familiar sensation, variously described as fullness, cotton wool between the ears, pressure in the ears, or muzziness in the head. The basic features are slight deafness and muffled hearing due to some physical obstruction to hearing. The causes are often obvious and readily treatable.

### PROBABLE

### ■ Eustachian Catarrh

*(See Earache, page 59)* Caused by buildup of fluid within the inner ear as after a common cold. Treatment, if needed, consists of decongestants and aromatic inhalations.

### ■ Wax

Probably the most common cause of a slight feeling of fullness, often accompanied by dizziness, discomfort, and mild earache *(see page 60)*.

Simple earwax softening drops often allow the ear to clear naturally.

### ■ Infection

Rather than causing the painful picture described elsewhere *(see, for example, Earache, page 59)*, infections sometimes run a less obvious course with:

- Vague mild discomfort.
- Fluctuating, mild deafness.
- Feeling of pressure in ear.

The diagnosis has to be made by a doctor or nurse who can see the eardrum.

## POSSIBLE

### ■ Hay Fever

Causes fullness as a result of swelling of the lining of the nose and ears.
- Seasonal sneezing, sore eyes.
- Persistent runny nose during the pollen season.

- Often associated with eczema and asthma.

## RARE

### ■ Chronic Otitis Externa

Severe cases give rise to chronic swelling of the ear canal, which also becomes blocked up with debris. Cleansing is needed for an extended period. *(See page 67)*

## DEAFNESS OR HEARING DIFFICULTIES IN ADULTS

Adult deafness or loss of hearing is, to a large extent, a normal part of the aging process. The hearing loss can gradually worsen, unnoticed, until it interferes with work or social relationships, at which point it is suddenly seen as a "new" problem. Special attention should always be given to sudden deafness, deafness affecting one ear only, or when it is associated with pain, giddiness (vertigo), or ringing in the ears (tinnitus).

## PROBABLE

### ■ Wax

An extremely common cause for a mild degree of hearing loss.
- Often causes sudden, partial hearing loss.
- "Blocked" feeling in ears.

### ■ Chronic Otitis Media

Long-term infection within the ear leads to:
- Deafness.
- Persistent discharge of pus-like material.
- Sometimes pain and vertigo.

Treatment is meticulous cleansing of the ear in a specialist clinic. The sudden appearance of pain and vertigo calls for urgent specialist assessment: this could indicate a deterioration of the condition. Normally, continuous cleansing of the ear will allow healing.

### ■ Otosclerosis

A condition causing increasing stiffness of one of the bones that transmits sound waves from the eardrum.
- Often runs in families.

- Most common in women, and gets worse during pregnancy.
- Progressive deafness, starting in early adulthood.
- Ringing in the ears is common.

Surgery can help, but usually a hearing aid is the simplest treatment.

### ■ Presbyacusis

This is the familiar hearing loss that comes with age, caused by degeneration of the pathway that turns sound waves into electrical impulses for transmission to the brain.
- Typically noticed in late sixties.
- Both ears affected.
- Pain free.

## POSSIBLE

### ■ Ménière's Disease

Suggested by repeated attacks of deafness along with vertigo and ringing in the ears.

### ■ Acoustic Trauma

Repeated loud noise damages hearing. It is said, however, that five years of exposure is needed for any significant damage to occur, by which time the most dedicated nightclubber may well have moved on to embroidery.

Actually, deafness from loud music at clubs is usually temporary, but prolonged and repeated exposure to loud noise can result in some loss of hearing. Ringing in the ears is common after hearing loud noises. Workers exposed to loud noise should wear ear protection and have regular hearing checks.

Prolonged use of personal stereos at high volume damages ears. The direct application of earphones, delivering high-volume sound, has been shown to significantly affect young people's hearing. If others around you can hear it, it is too loud.

### ■ Arteriosclerosis

Poor blood flow to the arteries supplying the ear can cause a range of symptoms; usually confined to the elderly.
- Fluctuating deafness, giddiness, ringing in the ears.
- Symptoms may vary, depending on the position of the neck. There is no specific treatment.

## RARE

### ■ Infection

Deafness is a rare and unpredictable complication of certain infectious illnesses, notably measles and mumps. It is also a possible consequence of meningitis and syphilis.

Children who have recurrent ear infections may have decreased hearing. *(See also Deafness or Hearing Difficulties in Children, page 65)*

### ■ Acoustic Neuroma

A slow-growing tumor on the nerve of hearing. Though rare, it is suspected frequently on the basis of the following suggestive symptoms:

- One-sided progressive deafness.
- One-sided tinnitus.
- Vertigo.
- Later numbness of face, unsteadiness.

A brain scan allows for quite precise localization, improving the chances of successful removal by surgery.

### ■ Skull Fracture

A fracture could damage the nerve of hearing and disrupt the delicate bones that transmit sounds, causing sudden loss of hearing.

### ■ Drugs

The nerve of hearing is sensitive to several drugs, the most common of which is aspirin taken in overdose.

- Tinnitus is an early warning sign.
- Giddiness.

### ■ Paget's Disease

A not uncommon condition of later life in which:

- Bones become tender.
- Bowing of the legs.
- Enlargement of the head.
- The deafness is caused by a squeezing of the nerve of hearing by enlarged bone.

This disease is frequently unrecognized until characteristic signs are noticed on an x-ray.

## DEAFNESS OR HEARING DIFFICULTIES IN CHILDREN

Hearing difficulties in childhood are difficult to detect, but every effort must be made to do so. Specialized testing of the newborn is becoming increasingly routine. Suspect a hearing problem if there is no startled reaction to sudden, loud noises, or if, as he or she develops, the baby does not turn to a sound. Later, delay in starting to speak should arouse suspicion. Later again, a schoolchild's performance may deteriorate for no obvious cause; once more, consider the possibility of loss of hearing. You cannot be too careful.

### ■ Wax

Simple to detect, and simple to remedy with drops to soften the earwax.

Most specialists advise against syringing in young children.

### ■ Serous Otitis Media

This is a common reason for hearing loss in children who have recurrent ear infections leading to a buildup of fluid within the inner ear. The condition is also known as glue ear because the fluid can be thick and sticky. The condition often cures itself over a few months. The symptoms are:

- Deafness, which may be partial or total.
- Occasional pain in ear.

Certain typical changes in the appearance of the eardrum will alert a doctor to the condition. As a remedy, grommets may be inserted.

## POSSIBLE

### ■ Congenital

Always to be considered in children born deaf, in whom there may have been a failure of development of the organs of hearing. Sometimes deafness runs in the family; sometimes the mother has been exposed to drugs that damage the ear *(see right)* or has had German measles (rubella, see below).

There are also many syndromes in which deafness is one of several abnormalities, but this is a matter for specialist assessment. In most cases of congenital deafness, however, no cause can be found.

## RARE

### ■ Congenital Rubella (German Measles)

A rarity since vaccination has become generally available. Rubella contracted in the first four months of pregnancy wreaks havoc on the developing child. As well as deafness, it can cause:

- Poor development of the brain and mental retardation.
- Cataracts.
- Heart defects.

This tragic outcome is rare thanks to national immunization programs against rubella. Check on your rubella immunity before you get pregnant.

### ■ Infection

Deafness is an unusual and unpredictable complication of certain infectious illnesses, notably measles and mumps, both of which are increasingly rare, thanks to immunization. It may also be a consequence of meningitis.

### ■ Neonatal Jaundice

Severe jaundice in the days after birth can cause brain damage, including deafness. Hence, the vigorous treatment given to babies who develop the condition.

### ■ Drugs

The nerve of hearing is sensitive to several drugs, the most common of which is aspirin taken in overdose. Another is the antibiotic gentamicin, now reserved for life-threatening disease such as meningitis, where the risk of damage to hearing is outweighed by the risk to life.

- Tinnitus is an early warning sign.
- Giddiness.

If a potentially harmful drug has to be used, blood levels should be monitored to avoid damage.

### ■ Congenital Hypothyroidism

An underactive thyroid gland can lead to a child with:

- Coarse features.
- A gruff cry.
- Enlarged tongue.

In many countries, there are screening programs to detect this curable illness as early as possible in newborn babies.

## ITCHING EAR

### PROBABLE

### ■ Otitis Externa

A form of eczema affecting the skin of the ear canal. Common in adult life, typically in those with eczema elsewhere.

- Intense itching.
- Skin of ear canal and ear itself is flaking, crusting, swollen.
- Ear feels wet, with a thin, clear discharge.

Like any other area of skin, the ear can become sensitized to chemicals. Common among these are chlorine in swimming pools, hair spray, and the antibiotics in the very drops used to treat otitis externa.

### POSSIBLE

### ■ Fungal Infection

Organisms known as fungi can invade skin that is already broken down by otitis externa.

- Symptoms of otitis externa.
- Black spores may be visible in the discharge.

Treatment is with antifungal drops.

## NOISES IN THE EAR

Noises other than ringing in the ear are very common and very rarely due to serious underlying causes. They nearly always pass within two weeks. Many cases remain unexplained, the symptoms going as mysteriously as they came. If noises occur in a particular location, check for a cause as simple as the hum from central heating, power lines, or similar noise source. *(See also Ringing in the Ear, page 69)*

## PROBABLE

### ■ Eustachian Catarrh

Blockage caused by fluid building up inside the ear, often experienced with a common cold.
- Muffled hearing.
- Popping or crackling inside the ears.
- Slight discomfort from a feeling of pressure in the ears.
- Swallowing gives temporary relief.

### ■ Acute Inner Ear Infection

Causes noises for similar reasons as does eustachian catarrh *(see above)*.
- Rapid onset of pain.
- Deafness.
- Crackling inside ears.

Antibiotics are usually given for this condition.

## RARE

### ■ Heart Murmur

The sound arising from a diseased valve in the heart may be heard inside the head when there is no competing noise.
- A whooshing noise.
- In time with heartbeat.

Needs to be assessed by a doctor.

### ■ Anemia

If extreme, anemia is said to cause noises in the ear. This symptom is likely to be overshadowed by other features of anemia, such as:
- Pallor.
- Tiredness.
- Sore tongue.
- Dizziness on standing.

A blood test will quickly confirm the diagnosis.

## TENDERNESS BEHIND THE EAR

Immediately behind the ear is a bone known as the mastoid, felt as a prominent swelling. Pain and swelling in this area is always to be taken seriously.

## PROBABLE

### ■ Acute Ear Infection

Although the infection is confined to the middle ear, occasionally there is a mild degree of tenderness over the mastoid bone. Middle ear infections are usually treated with an antibiotic, which should prevent further spread.

## POSSIBLE

### ■ Mastoiditis

Though now uncommon, this was once a feared consequence of ear infections, since infection can spread from the mastoid region into the brain.

- Begins with an ear infection.
- Redness, swelling over mastoid bone.

- Yellow/green discharge from ear.
- Fever, pain, malaise.

Urgent surgical treatment is needed.

## RINGING IN THE EAR (TINNITUS)

Of all ear diseases, this causes the most misery because of its persistence. It is usually described as a ringing noise, but sometimes it is lower-pitched than that —more of a hum. As an occasional symptom, it is quite common, no more than a nuisance.

Chronic tinnitus is another matter. Treatments vary from drugs to devices that mask the sound, but there is no real cure. Brief episodes of tinnitus may be caused by a blow to the head, wax in the ears, a foreign body, infection, or sudden changes in air pressure. Prolonged cases may be due to the following.

### PROBABLE

#### ■ Otosclerosis

This is a common cause of deafness *(see page 63)*. Tinnitus tends to be the earliest symptom of the condition, which is due to increasing stiffness of one of the bones that transmit sound.

#### ■ Ménière's Disease

The classic symptoms of this disease are varying combinations of:

- Tinnitus.
- Vertigo.
- Deafness.

#### ■ Presbyacusis

Hearing loss as part of the aging process is frequently accompanied by tinnitus. *(See page 64)*

### POSSIBLE

#### ■ Arteriosclerosis

The blood supply to the brain and ear arrives via major arteries in the neck, which, with age, can get furred up. This is thought to underlie cases of tinnitus in the elderly associated with:

- Giddiness on standing up.
- Giddiness set off by head movements, especially looking up.
- Deafness.

It helps to take your time when getting up and to avoid sudden, extreme movements of the neck.

#### ■ Drugs

Common drugs that can cause tinnitus include aspirin, quinine, and streptomycin.

## ■ Psychological

Occasionally, tinnitus or other noises in the ears are actually hallucinations in someone suffering from serious mental disease. Suspicion should be aroused by reports of:

- Bizarre noises.
- Voices commenting on the individual's activities.

The individual may also appear:

- Unusually suspicious.
- Moody to an exaggerated degree.

This situation needs sensitive, expert assessment.

## RARE

## ■ Paget's Disease

A disease of bone that can squeeze the nerve of hearing, resulting in:

- Deafness.
- Tinnitus.

*(See also page 65)*

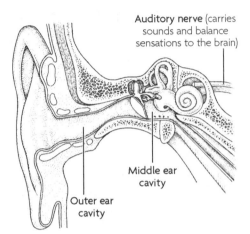

Auditory nerve (carries sounds and balance sensations to the brain)

Middle ear cavity

Outer ear cavity

---

## VERTIGO

Vertigo means a sense of rotation. Giddiness is a mild form of the same symptom. They are frequently caused by disorders of the ear, although the connection may not be obvious since there may be no other features of ear trouble such as pain, discharge, or tinnitus. For that reason, vertigo/giddiness is covered in detail elsewhere in this book *(see The Brain and Nervous System)*. The following conditions are, however, relevant to the ear.

## PROBABLE

## ■ Catarrh

The congestion that accompanies a cold often also causes mild giddiness for a few days.

- Nasal congestion.
- Slight pressure in ears.

- Mild deafness and ringing in the ears.

## Labyrinthitis

A common, alarming, but harmless condition, occurring in mini-epidemics. It may be due to a viral infection of the balance organ, which is located in the ear. It is increasingly thought to be due to shifts in crystals that line sensitive structures within the ear. The nerve endings that normally transmit messages telling us how we are balanced become inflamed and send off inaccurate and confusing messages. This causes acute loss of balance and intense true vertigo, with the room spinning round.

- Abrupt, disabling vertigo: you may even find it impossible to stand up.
- Usually noticed on attempting to get up in the morning.
- Nausea or vomiting are common.
- Vertigo returns each time you move your head.

This is a panic-inducing illness, but rest assured that the symptoms will fade over two or three weeks. Minor recurrences are possible for several months afterwards.

## Ménière's Disease

Vertigo can be an early symptom of this condition. Later, there is:

- Ringing in the ears (tinnitus).
- Deafness.

## POSSIBLE

## Chronic Otitis Media

*(See page 63)* Persistent yellow or green discharge from one ear, together with:
- Discomfort.
- Deafness.

Needs specialized treatment to clean the ear and to eradicate infection.

## Otosclerosis

A cause of deafness in middle life, but as early features there can be:
- Tinnitus.
- Vertigo.

## Wax

Wax is a convenient scapegoat for many ear problems, perhaps too convenient. However, if there is just mild giddiness, with no other symptoms except that the ears are full of hard wax, it is reasonable for a doctor to suggest clearing the wax with drops to soften it or, if necessary, syringing the ears to exclude wax as a cause of vertigo.

## RARE

## Acoustic Neuroma

*(See page 65)* This growth on the nerve of hearing is suspected if, as well as vertigo, there is progressive:
- One-sided deafness.
- One-sided vertigo.
- One-sided tinnitus.

# THE MOUTH

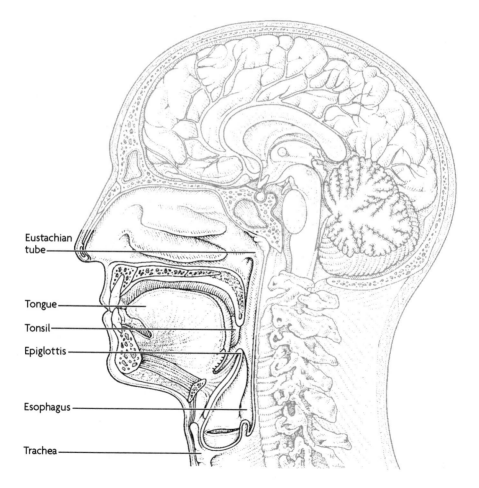

Eustachian tube

Tongue

Tonsil

Epiglottis

Esophagus

Trachea

## BLUISH-PURPLE LIPS

A feature of cyanosis *(see page 438)*, it can be caused by low body temperature. But long-term cyanosis suggests that blood oxygen levels are low. Similar discoloration may be noticed in the ear lobes, all the mucous membranes, the tongue, and anywhere that blood flows close to the surface of the skin, such as the beds of the fingernails. In general, cyanosis suggests either heart or lung disease.

### PROBABLE

#### ■ Low Temperature

Commonly seen in shivering children on the beach or other places outdoors. It may, however, also be present in the elderly. Consider hypothermia if there are other symptoms, such as:

• Confusion.
• Slowness of thought.
• Decreased movement.

The individual should be warmed gradually: layers of blankets are best. Hot drinks, such as tea, may be given. Avoid alcohol, which increases heat loss. In all cases, seek medical help urgently—hypothermia must be dealt with in a hospital.

#### ■ Chronic Bronchitis

*(See page 216)*

#### ■ Emphysema

*(See page 213)*
• Shortness of breath, which gets progressively worse over period of months and years.
• The chest becomes expanded, as though permanently inhaling.
• May accompany chronic bronchitis.
• Respiratory infections.
• Cyanosis.
• Respiratory failure.

#### ■ Pulmonary Edema

Retention of fluid in the lungs as a result of failure of the heart to pump effectively. Heart failure may have occurred because of either poor blood supply to the heart or a structural abnormality such as disease of the heart's valves. Symptoms include:
• Shortness of breath on exertion and in severe cases at rest.
• Shortness of breath when lying down flat.
• Nighttime shortness of breath.
• Frothy sputum, sometimes pink with blood.
• Cyanosis.
• Fast or irregular heart rate.
• Swelling of ankles.

## POSSIBLE

### ■ Shock

*(See page 420)* Cyanosis is just one of several noticeable features. May be an emergency.

### ■ Pneumonia

Actually, "pneumonias" would be a better term, since there are several types. Cyanosis is a typical feature of all of them. *(See page 438)*

Some types of pneumonia may still be fatal, particularly in the very young or the elderly. See a doctor without delay.

## RARE

### ■ Pulmonary Embolus

*(See page 210)* Bluish lips are just one of several more dramatic features, such as sudden shortness of breath, sudden onset of sharp chest pain, bloody sputum, and collapse.

### ■ Congenital Heart Disease

Cyanosis is a typical and obvious feature of newborn babies with heart abnormalities. The tetralogy of Fallot and transposition of the great arteries are probably the most well known. Heart defects may also accompany abnormalities, such as Down's syndrome or those caused by the mother having rubella during pregnancy. In addition to cyanosis, there may be:

• Shortness of breath.

• Finger clubbing.

• Toe clubbing.

• Polycythemia (excess hemoglobin to compensate for poor oxygenation).

• Malaise.

• Poor growth.

### ■ Airways Obstructed by a Foreign Body

Any object that obstructs the free passage of air in and out of the lungs may result in cyanosis. The sudden onset of blueness, choking in someone eating, or in a child, must be considered as being possibly due to inhalation of a foreign body, perhaps a peanut or a piece of a toy. This is a life-threatening emergency. *(See Heimlich Maneuver, page 206)*

### ■ Laryngeal Edema

An infection (typically diphtheria, epiglottitis) or a severe allergic reaction may cause swelling of the soft tissues of the larynx, preventing air from getting into the lungs.

• Blue lips.

• Stridor (a harsh and frightening noise heard as air is forced past a blockage in the airways).

• Distress.

If caused by an infection of the upper airway, all the usual features will also be noticed. Laryngeal edema is an emergency; get help quickly.

■ **Fibrosing Alveolitis**

Inflammation of the alveoli (tiny air sacs) in the lungs. Tends to develop in middle age and progresses gradually.
- Increasing shortness of breath.
- Dry cough.
- Clubbing.
- Cyanosis.

■ **Pneumoconiosis**

A term used for a number of occupationally related chest diseases, typically associated with work in dusty environments.
- Slow onset.
- Increasing shortness of breath on exertion, and then at rest.
- Intermittent cough.
- Onset of bronchitis.
- Cyanosis.

- Respiratory failure.
- Heart failure.

■ **Extrinsic Allergic Alveolitis**

A disease that develops because of recurrent allergic reactions to dust from animals or plants. Quite common in farmworkers.
- Recurrent brief attacks, up to a couple of days, of shortness of breath, malaise, fever, and cough, when exposed to the dust.

After repeated exposure over the years, a chronic condition develops with:
- Shortness of breath.
- Finger and toe clubbing.
- Cyanosis.
- Respiratory failure.
- Heart failure.

## CRACKING AT CORNERS OF MOUTH

The medical terms for this are angular stomatitis or cheilosis. In isolation, this is normally of no great significance.

**PROBABLE**

■ **Childhood Cracking**

If the corners of your child's mouth are constantly wet, they will be at increased risk of cracking. Children taking bottles or who suck their thumbs may develop inflammation at the corner(s) of the mouth. This may also occur in older children, with no very obvious cause.
- Redness.
- Cracking.
- Pain.
- May develop on one side only.

Clears up of its own accord.

■ **Age**

As individuals age, they can develop a crease running downwards from the angle of the mouth, along which saliva flows, causing skin irritation along with:

- Redness.
- Cracking.
- Pain.
- May be on one or both sides.

Clears up of its own accord.

## POSSIBLE

■ **Brain Injury**

Anyone who has suffered brain injury (stroke, accident) or who has chronic neurological disease may have facial weakness or swallowing problems that allow saliva to pool in the mouth and dribble out.

- Redness.
- Cracking.
- Pain.
- May be on one side only (after stroke) or on both sides if there is a swallowing problem.

Clears up of its own accord.

## RARE

■ **Scurvy and Zinc Deficiency**

*(See page 441 and page 79)* Riboflavin is a water-soluble vitamin present in many foods; deficiency is likely to be a feature only of severe, general malnutrition. Inflammation of the tongue (glossitis) may be present.

## HARE LIP

Colloquial term for cleft lip. *(See Cleft Lip and Palate, page 81)*

## LIPS—CRACKED, SORES, OR PATCHES

Sore, inflamed lips are common in adults and children: the lips look red and are often cracked. The usual cause is intermittent exposure to heat and cold. The skin of the lips loses its natural oil, becoming dry and uncomfortable or "chapped."

Other common causes are lip-licking and lip-chewing. The first is typical of children with colds who develop runny noses and continually lick or wipe their upper lips, causing inflammation. The second is a comfort habit adopted at times of stress.

The lips and the surrounding skin are possible sites of sores or lesions for many diseases. Some are local and some are general; some are permanent and some temporary; and some need treatment and some don't. The following list cannot be exhaustive, but it does highlight examples of all these types.

## PROBABLE

### ■ Aphthous Ulcer

May develop after injury, when the individual is run-down (physically or mentally) or more commonly for no clear reason.

- Exquisitely painful.
- After twenty-four hours, mucous membrane breaks down to form an ulcer.
- Often a grayish/white appearance.
- Ulcer is normally about 3–4 mm in diameter and oval shaped.
- Pain can make, eating, talking, or brushing teeth difficult.
- May be multiple.
- Tend to be on inner aspect of lips.

Healing occurs between five days and two weeks.

### ■ Herpes Simplex

Also known as a cold sore. A virus that infects the skin.

- Often precipitated by upper respiratory tract infection when the individual is run down.
- Also precipitated by weather extremes (heat or cold).

- Initially a slightly irritating patch on the lip or local skin.
- Little fluid-filled vesicles develop.
- These become crusted and a scab develops.

The disease runs its course in ten to fourteen days.

If severe, and recognized at an early stage, it can be helped by antiviral medication.

### ■ Mucocele or Retention Cyst

Blockage of one of the small glands on the inner aspect of the lips, which causes:

- Sudden appearance of a lump, a few millimeters in diameter.
- Painless.
- Translucent/bluish color.
- Suddenly empties.
- Rarely lasts for more than a couple of days.

### ■ Burn

Local areas of pain and ulceration on one lip (particularly in the middle of the lower lip) are often caused by smokers under the influence of alcohol placing the cigarette the wrong way round in their mouth. Often, the individual cannot recall the incident. The patch will heal in about five days.

## Impetigo

A nasty and highly infectious skin infection that can occur anywhere but commonly on the face and lips and other exposed parts. Most common in children.
- Starts with redness.
- Vesicles and bullae (fluid-filled sacs) develop on the skin surface.
- These burst and crusting occurs.
- May spread over a large area of the face.
- Asymmetrical—does not spread evenly over both sides of face.

Needs antibiotic treatment.

## POSSIBLE

### Candidiasis

A "thrush" infection of the lips, typical of the elderly, those with dentures, those who are "run-down," or with diets deficient in vitamins or iron. Treatment is antifungal creams or lozenges.
- Redness.
- Soreness.
- Slight swelling.
- Occasional cracking and bleeding.
- White plaques or patches may be seen.

### Leukoplakia

- White patches on the tongue or lining of the mouth.
- Cannot be scraped off.

- Occasionally disappear leaving a red base.
- Localized hardening under the patch may occur.

It is associated with smoking, spirits, spices, sepsis, sharp teeth, and syphilis.

Leukoplakia may also be an early warning sign of cancer, so long-standing firm white patches on the tongue or in the mouth must not be ignored.

## RARE

### Zinc Deficiency

Any elderly person on a poor diet or with malabsorption or malnutrition problems, who develops intermittent sores on or around the mouth, may be zinc deficient. A blood test may be needed to confirm this, and zinc supplements can be given.

### AIDS

Can give rise to multiple mouth ulcers, as well as:
- General malaise.
- Weight loss.
- Skin rashes.

Blood tests confirm the diagnosis.

### Cancer

Any long-standing ulcer or growth on the lip, particularly in elderly smokers with poor oral hygiene, may be cancerous.

- Persistent ulcer or irregular lump.
- Persistent painless, but enlarged lymph nodes.
- Bleeding from lesion.
- Loss of weight.
- Malaise.

## Hereditary Hemorrhagic Telangiectasia

Also known as Osler-Weber-Rendu syndrome. A hereditary condition.
- Small red vascular lesions on lips and in mouth.
- Similar lesions throughout gastrointestinal tract.
- The gastrointestinal lesions may cause internal bleeding.
- Rarely seen before the age of forty.

## Chancre

The first sign of infection with syphilis. May occur on the lips or in the mouth after oral sex.
- Appears three to four weeks after contact.
- Initially, a hardened, elevated solitary lesion.
- Becomes a shallow ulcer.
- Painless.
- Does not bleed.
- Raised, red edges.
- Local, painless lymph node enlargement.

If suspected, must be seen and treated by a doctor.

## Dermatitis

Any area of skin may develop sensitivity to some irritant. Habitual sucking or chewing of pens or application of some lipsticks or lip balms are examples of agents to which some may react.
- Redness.
- Itchiness.
- Soreness.
- Sometime crusting and weeping.
- Normal lips when the irritant is not being used.

## Behçet's Syndrome

Most common in men from the teens to the early thirties.
- Painful ulceration of the mouth.
- Genital ulceration a few weeks after the oral lesions.
- Eye inflammation (uveitis) with the genital ulceration.

The condition repeats and relapses. Treatment is aimed at relieving the symptoms. This condition is most common in the Middle East.

## Erythema Multiforme

Associated with reaction to drugs or infection. Most common in young males.
- Extensive painful ulcers inside the mouth.

- Lesions can also be found on the skin.
- Gum inflammation.
- Crusting, bloodstained lesions on lips.

Treatment consists of identifying and removing or treating the cause.

### ■ Lichen Planus

Found in those over thirty.
- Multiple, fine white lines on lips, tongue, and the cheek
- Tiny white spots in the same region.
- Sometimes ulcers between the spots and lines.

- Occasionally, fluid-filled sacs form, which then burst, causing painful ulcers.

### ■ Poisons

A number of drugs and other products that contain substances, such as arsenic, bismuth, lead, and mercury, will cause pigmentation of the mouth and lips, in addition to their other symptoms and signs. In the absence of other definite causes for mouth pigmentation, accidental or deliberate taking of such substances should be considered.

## CHAPPED LIPS

Essentially the same as Sore Lips *(see page 77)*.

## CLEFT LIP AND PALATE

These terms cover a fairly wide range of abnormalities that occur during development in the womb. They are quite common—one in 750 births. For some reason, generally unknown, areas of tissue fail to "join" and the resulting gap is seen at birth, sometimes on one side, or in severe cases as a cleft lip and palate on both sides beneath the nose.
- Distortion of the nostril on the affected side.

- In more than half the cases, there is also a defect in the hard palate.
- Speech problems, typically nasal speech, will develop if left untreated.

The trend at present is to repair these deformities by plastic surgery as soon as reasonable after birth so that breast-feeding and speech development are affected as little as possible.

## SKIN AROUND MOUTH LOOKS PALE

This is a very specific symptom, otherwise known as circumoral pallor, associated with scarlet fever. It should not be confused with more general pallor of skin, mucous membranes, and nails associated with anemia or blood loss *(see page 430)*. The symptoms of scarlet fever are:

- Tonsillitis and pharyngitis.
- Red rash, predominantly on trunk.
- Sore and coated tongue.
- Circumoral pallor.
- Otitis media may develop *(see page 58)*.

## BLEEDING GUMS

This is almost always due to overvigorous brushing of the teeth and can be a normal daily occurrence for some people. If bleeding is persistent, or the gums are painful, some degree of gum disease (also known as gingivitis or periodontal disease) may be present *(see page 83)*.

This may resolve without treatment but if there is infection as well, antibiotics may be necessary. The care of a dental hygienist may be beneficial. A very rare cause of bleeding gums is scurvy, caused by vitamin C deficiency.

## FOUL-SMELLING BREATH

Halitosis. Most dentists and doctors would attribute bad breath to poor oral hygiene. This is by far the most common cause of bad breath. There are, however, other causes, related to a variety of abnormalities of the mouth, the sinuses, and the lungs, as well as disease elsewhere in the body.

### PROBABLE

■ Poor Oral Hygiene

The surest way to develop bad breath is to fail to clean your teeth. Even regular tooth brushing may not be enough to prevent the accumulation of food debris, which collects in the cracks between teeth and generates odors as it decays. Dental flossing clears these crevices and helps prevent bad breath.

- Staining between teeth.
- Irregular color to teeth.
- Breath worse in the morning on waking.

In addition to brushing and flossing your

teeth, regular cleaning by a dentist or an oral hygienist can help prevent bad breath.

### ■ Food and Drink

• Individual has recently eaten spiced foods or drunk alcohol.

• No other evidence of disease in the mouth or elsewhere.

• Not present if diet is confined to non-spicy food or if alcoholic drink is stopped.

### ■ Smoking

• Halitosis.

• Stained teeth.

### ■ Dental Caries

Caries means tooth decay. The enamel covering of the tooth is damaged by bacteria. Regular brushing and avoidance of sugary foods may help, as may fluoride—ask your dentist's advice.

• "Sensitive" teeth.

• Painful tooth or teeth.

• Halitosis.

• Worse on drinking and eating very hot or cold foods and drinks.

### ■ Mouth Breathing

Any condition that makes you breathe through your mouth rather than your nose may result in halitosis because of drying up of the salivary secretions, which act as a rinsing agent. Thus, nasal polyps, a broken nose, hay fever, or even snoring may cause halitosis, because they make it difficult to breathe through the nose.

### ■ Mouth or Throat Infection

Any mouth or throat infection may cause bad breath; all may be associated with:

• Pain.

• Fever.

• Malaise.

• Halitosis.

• Unpleasant taste in the mouth.

### ■ Gum Disease

Disease of the gums and tooth sockets, with inflammation of the gums (also known as gingivitis). Caused mainly by poor oral hygiene.

• Bleeding gums, particularly after brushing teeth.

• Sensitive gums.

• Halitosis.

• Often associated with dental caries.

### ■ Dentures

If not cleaned regularly and adequately, food debris or saliva may accumulate on dentures, giving off an offensive smell, even when in the mouth.

### ■ Postnasal Drip

• May be present for some weeks after flu/colds.

• Mucus drips back into throat causing reflex coughing.

- Worse at night.
- General health otherwise good.
- Halitosis may be present.

## POSSIBLE

### ■ Sinusitis

Infection of any of the sinuses may cause:
- Persistent nasal discharge (out through the nose or back into the throat).
- May be green or yellow.
- Possibly headache.
- Occasionally pyrexia (fever).
- Malaise.
- Halitosis.

### ■ Catarrh

A term with many different meanings: some use it to describe a blocked nose (because of nasal inflammation); some use it for large amounts of infected mucus. It often results in bad breath, either because of accompanying infection in the mouth or nose, or because a blocked nose is making you breathe through your mouth.

### ■ Chronic Lung Conditions

*(See also Foul-Smelling Breath and Cough, page 86)* Any lung condition that causes persistent production of mucus, or where the lung has a long-standing focus of infection, may cause halitosis. Patients with chronic bronchitis, tuberculosis, cystic fibrosis, bronchiectasis, emphysema, and other diseases may well complain of halitosis. The main symptoms of the underlying disease usually include:
- Purulent (green/yellow) mucus.
- Cough.
- Fever.
- Malaise.

### ■ Pyorrhea Alveolaris

A disease of gums and tooth sockets, actually a severe, advanced form of gum disease *(see page 83)*.
- Gum margins recede.
- Teeth loosen.
- Pus caused by infection of the tooth socket leaks out between gums and teeth.
- Pain.
- Halitosis.

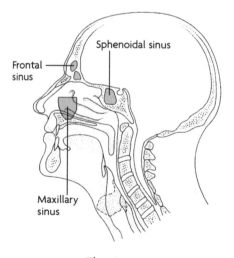

*The sinuses*

(labels: Sphenoidal sinus, Frontal sinus, Maxillary sinus)

### ■ Diabetic Ketoacidosis

Diabetics whose blood sugar is not properly controlled can develop abnormal blood biochemistry called ketoacidosis. This is characterized by a sweetish smell on the breath (some describe it as "sickly").

## RARE

### ■ Vincent's Angina

Also known as "trench mouth," this is a bacterial disease of the tonsils that spreads to the gums. Associated with poor hygiene.

- Fever.
- Sore throat.
- Infected gums.
- Enlarged lymph nodes in the neck.
- Often only one tonsil is affected, with ulceration, and a membrane that may spread to soft and hard palate.

Highly infectious. Responds rapidly to antibiotics.

### ■ Cancer of the Mouth, Upper Respiratory Tract, or Larynx

Halitosis may be an accompaniment to any site of cancer in the mouth, upper respiratory tract, or larynx, particularly if the tumor has become infected and ulcerated. Thus, persistent halitosis, in addition to some or any of the following, particularly in elderly smokers, needs close investigation:

- Persistent, painless enlarged lymph nodes.
- Other lumps developing in mouth/ tongue or palate.
- Change in voice.
- Loss of weight.
- Feeling unwell.
- Persistent pain in mouth or neck.
- Dentures not fitting.
- Anemia.

### ■ Renal Failure

Uremia is present. Urea is a waste product produced by the kidneys and normally excreted in the urine.

- Brown/yellow appearance of skin.
- Bruising.
- Fast rate of breathing.
- Swollen ankles.
- Heart failure.
- Breath smells of urine/ammonia.
- Altered sensation in limbs.

### ■ Liver Failure

This may occur as a result of a number of diseases that damage liver tissue, such as hepatitis or cirrhosis. It may result in a large number of symptoms, including:

- Jaundice.
- Fatigue.
- Mental deterioration.
- Reddened palms ("liver" palms: the fatty parts of the palms are flushed red).

- The appearance of tiny blood vessels in the skin ("vascular spiders").
- Fever.
- Halitosis: sweet and feculent (fetor hepaticus).

■ **Drugs and Poisoning**

Some drugs have characteristic smells, excreted in air exhaled from the lungs. Examples are paraldehyde (now rarely used) and disulfiram (a drug prescribed for alcoholics).

## FOUL-SMELLING BREATH AND COUGH

### PROBABLE

■ **Chronic Bronchitis**

*(See page 216)* The typical picture is:
- Smoker's cough, especially in the early morning.
- Cough in winter.
- Wheezing.
- Sputum varying from white to yellow/green.
- Increasing breathlessness over the years.
- Cyanosis.
- Halitosis.

### POSSIBLE

■ **Lung Cancer**

*(See page 226)* Associated symptoms that may be noticeable include:
- Dry cough.
- Bloody sputum.
- Hoarse voice.
- Shortness of breath.
- Chest pain.
- Infection in the lung.
- Malaise.

- Weight loss.
- Halitosis.

■ **Bronchiectasis**

The air passages are widened, preventing oxygen entering the circulation efficiently. Features include:
- History of recurrent chest infections.
- Lots of yellow/green sputum with or without blood.
- Fever.
- Looking unwell.
- Weight loss.
- Malaise.
- Severe halitosis.

■ **Cystic Fibrosis**

*(See page 144)* Later in infancy, symptoms may include slow growth, offensive diarrhea, and/or respiratory infections, which may be associated with halitosis.

### RARE

■ **Lung Abscess**

A collection of pus lying within the lung

tissue. It may be caused by inhaling infected material, as a complication of pneumonia, or by rare causes such as spread of a liver abscess into the chest. In general, features include:

- A preexisting infection.
- Fever.
- Shivering.
- Sweats.
- Malaise.
- Pleurisy (pain in the chest on breathing in and out).
- Foul sputum.

- Halitosis.

### ■ Pulmonary (Lung) Tuberculosis

Most often found in malnourished or immunosuppressed patients. Features may include:

- Malaise.
- Fatigue.
- Weight loss.
- Cough with sputum, sometimes bloody.
- Chest pain.
- Shortness of breath.
- Halitosis.

## BREATH SMELLS OF URINE

*(See Renal Failure, covered under Foul-Smelling Breath, page 85)*

## BREATH SMELLS SWEET

*(See Diabetic Ketoacidosis and Liver Failure, covered under Foul-Smelling Breath, page 85)*

## ABNORMAL TEETH

Including discoloration and deformity. The following diseases and predisposing factors are worth considering.

### ■ Age

As is well known, teeth tend to become discolored with age. Periodontal disease such as gingivitis causes gum loss, making the teeth appear longer than normal (hence the expression "long in the tooth").

### ■ Smoking

Yellow-brown staining, even with regular brushing. It also hastens the age-related color changes of teeth.

### ■ Betel Nut Chewing

Brownish-red discoloration of all teeth, commonly seen in Asian men and women who are habitual betel nut chewers.

### ■ Transverse Ridges

Transverse ridges on teeth may be seen in people who had scurvy or rickets while the surface enamel of their teeth was forming.

### ■ Chondroectodermal Dysplasia

A congenital disorder. Features include:
• Short stature.
• Short fingers.
• Small teeth.
• Dry skin.
• Scanty hair.

### ■ Hutchinson's Teeth

Rarely seen nowadays; caused by congenital syphilis. The incisor teeth have a

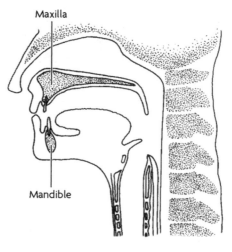

*Maxillary and mandibular teeth*

notch at the lower edge, are small, and taper toward the notched edge. Other signs of congenital syphilis may also be present.

## GRINDING THE TEETH

This is a symptom of more concern to the partner or parent of the affected person. It is observed commonly at night and may be associated with snoring. Some individuals do it habitually. The noise is caused by the opposing movement of the upper (maxillary) and lower (mandibular) teeth against each other. The symptom often disappears spontaneously. Only rarely does it cause permanent tooth damage. If the symptom persists, the advice of a dentist should be sought.

Made-to-measure molds, which fit over the teeth, can be worn at night to protect the teeth and to prevent grinding.

There is an association between tooth grinding and migraine—many people find that they have both conditions.

## DAMAGED TOOTH

If possible, the broken fragment(s) of a damaged tooth should be kept and taken with you to a dentist. If the entire tooth and root has been displaced, it may be possible to reimplant it. If there is a possibility that the jaw is fractured, get professional help quickly. The cosmetic problems of a broken or chipped tooth are less important than underlying bone damage. The bones may need to be realigned *(see Upper and Lower Teeth Not Closing Properly, page 94)*. Cosmetic repair can be undertaken at a later date, once the bone damage has been treated.

## TEETHING PAIN

The first baby teeth, normally the lower central incisors, appear at the age of six to ten months. Teeth continue to appear until about thirty months. Most infants and toddlers will have episodes of crying, fever, and salivation that may be attributed (not always convincingly) to teeth erupting or growing.

Fever is not a prominent symptom in a teething child: if your child has a fever, do not attribute it to teething. Pain and discomfort are the major symptoms, leading to irritability and crying. Just as you would take a painkiller for toothache, it is reasonable to use infant acetaminophen to soothe a teething child.

It is always important to exclude other causes, such as ear or throat problems.

## DRY MOUTH

The Probable causes are, of course, dehydration, mouth breathing, and fear or anxiety *(see page 490, page 83, and page 384)*. Remove the cause, and a normal "wet" mouth returns. If a dry mouth persists, then it might indicate underlying disease.

Anesthetics and antidepressants can also cause a dry mouth.

### POSSIBLE

■ **Salivary Gland Calculus**

Stones (calculi) can form in the ducts of the major salivary glands, blocking saliva. They are most common in the submandibular salivary glands but occasionally occur in the parotids.

• Swelling over the gland on one side.

• Swelling worse at mealtimes or in the presence of food.

• Swelling is uncomfortable.

• Sensation of dryness on the same side of the mouth.

• Swelling suddenly goes down—you may note saliva trickling into mouth.

Sometimes the stones are passed, sometimes they need surgical removal.

## RARE

### ■ Sjögren's Syndrome

Probably an autoimmune disease, most common in middle-aged women.

• Dry eyes, causing a painful, gritty feeling.

• Dry mouth, with halitosis.

• Salivary gland swelling.

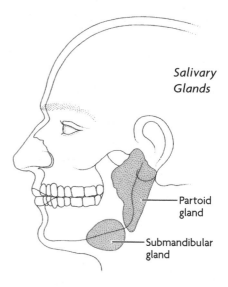

*Salivary Glands*

Partoid gland

Submandibular gland

Other connective tissue disorders may be associated, for example, rheumatoid arthritis.

## GENERALLY INFECTED MOUTH

Severe generalized infection of the oral cavity, including tongue, palate, and gums, is a medical emergency. It is rare and happens if oral hygiene is extremely poor or, indeed, absent.

## RARE

### ■ Vincent's Angina and Vincent's Acute Ulcerative Gingivitis

Named after the infecting organisms; also known as "trench mouth." These are bacterial diseases of the mouth that may originate in the gums between the teeth or the tonsils (Vincent's angina). May spread rapidly to adjacent tissues.

Vincent's angina:

• Pyrexia.

• Local pain.

• Sore throat.

• Enlarged lymph nodes in the neck.

• Often only one tonsil is affected, which is ulcerated with a membrane present.

• The membrane may spread to soft and hard palate.

- Excessive salivation may occur.
- Highly infectious.

Responds rapidly to appropriate antibiotics.

Vincent's acute ulcerative gingivitis—in addition to the preceding symptoms:
- Deep gum ulcers.

■ **Cancrum Oris**

A severe form of the conditions described above, which occurs in poorly nourished children. Even with treatment, gross scarring of the cheek can result, as well as limitation of jaw movement.

## DIFFICULT TO OPEN MOUTH

This is usually the result of a disease affecting structures involved in opening the mouth, causing a combination of either pain or swelling. Pain gives the impression that it is difficult to open the jaw. It is, however, rarely a primary symptom. The diseases listed here are in order of overall frequency, not in order of how often they give rise to difficulty in opening the mouth.

### PROBABLE

■ **Aphthous Ulcer**
*(See page 78)*

■ **Dental Caries**
*(See page 83)*

■ **Dental Infection**
*(See page 136)*

■ **Upper Respiratory Tract Infection**
*(See page 135)*

■ **Tonsillitis**
*(See page 135)*

■ **Mumps**

Inflammation of the parotid glands, often mistaken for lymph glands.
- Both glands affected and markedly swollen.
- Swelling makes opening the jaw uncomfortable.
- Occasionally, pancreas and testes are affected (after puberty).

### POSSIBLE

■ **Infectious Mononucleosis**
*(See page 136)*

■ **Peritonsillar Abscess**
Also known as quinsy. *(See page 137)*

■ **Impacted Wisdom Tooth**
Emerging wisdom teeth, especially if obstructed by existing teeth, may cause

such pain, discomfort, and infection at the back of the mouth that it is difficult to open your mouth. Dental opinion should be sought if suspected.

### ■ Arthritis in Temporomandibular Joint

This joint is where the mandible hinges with the skull. Arthritis can develop with age or after injury.

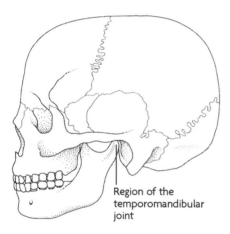

Region of the temporomandibular joint

- Pain localized just in front of the ear.
- Pain may extend across side of face.
- Pain worse on chewing or moving jaw.
- A grinding sensation over the joint may be noted.

- At first, only on one side.
- May eventually affect both sides.

## RARE

### ■ Tetanus

A disease caught by soil penetrating a trivial skin wound and contaminating it with the organism *Clostridium tetani.* It can be fatal.

- Local muscular weakness near the wound.
- Muscular spasms develop.
- Inability to open the mouth, called trismus or "lockjaw."
- The spasms and trismus give rise to a grinning appearance ("risus sardonicus").
- Fever.

Gradually, spasms are caused by the slightest stimulus. In severe cases, the number and frequency of spasms increases until death occurs. Keeping your tetanus immunization up to date is essential.

### ■ Strychnine Poisoning

The symptoms of strychnine poisoning are similar to those of tetanus *(see above)* but without a history of wound contamination.

## TOO MUCH SALIVA

In the absence of any other problems, this is rare. Any condition that causes painful swallowing or a sore throat may lead to an apparent excess of saliva, as the pain prevents the usual frequency of clearing of the saliva from mouth to stomach.

However, there are some conditions in which excessive saliva is a notable feature.

### PROBABLE

■ Smoking

Many smokers, especially pipe and cigar smokers, notice that they salivate excessively when smoking, which is an effect of nicotine. It is unclear why this is not noticed by all smokers.

■ Nausea and Vomiting

Prior to vomiting, the mouth often appears to fill with salty saliva.

■ Tonsillitis

*(See page 135)* Excessive saliva is a typical feature.

■ Pharyngitis

There may be an apparent excess of saliva due to pain on swallowing.

### POSSIBLE

■ Infectious Mononucleosis

*(See page 136)*

■ Brain Injury

*(See page 77)*

■ Peritonsillar Abscess

*(See Swollen Lymph Nodes in Neck, page 137)*

### RARE

■ Cancer of the Esophagus

## IMPACTED TOOTH

A tooth that cannot erupt because it is blocked or otherwise prevented from emerging by other teeth. This applies most frequently in adult life to the wisdom teeth. The unerupted tooth may be covered by a flap of gum that can become infected and painful. Extraction of the unerupted tooth is the usual, and effective, treatment. It may have to be done under general anesthesia.

## LOOSE TEETH

*(See Dental Caries, page 83; Gum Disease, page 83; Pyorrhea Alveolaris, page 84)* These are associated with, or lead to, loose teeth, decaying teeth, and toothache.

## UPPER AND LOWER TEETH NOT CLOSING PROPERLY

The medical term for this is malocclusion. Teeth should snap shut directly opposite each other. Most people have some degree of malocclusion, typically protruding front teeth (overbite), and this needs no further treatment. Some have irregular teeth because as babies their teeth developed too slowly, because of infection or an extra tooth. Dentists can correct deformities to improve function and cosmetic appearance.

Damage to the jaw bones, into which the teeth are bedded, can also cause malocclusion. If bone damage is suspected, specialized treatment is essential. Deformity will give rise to pain around the face and ear *(see Difficult to Open Mouth, page 91)*. Arthritis may develop.

## SENSITIVE TEETH

Most people suffer from sensitive teeth at some time, frequently caused by overvigorous brushing of the teeth, leading to receding gums. This exposes the nerve fibers around the tooth, sometimes producing extreme sensitivity to heat and cold. When a tooth is damaged or infected, again the nerves will be exposed and unusually sensitive. *(See Dental Caries, page 83; Gum Disease, page 83; Pyorrhea Alveolaris, page 84)*

Special toothpastes for sensitive teeth coat the nerves and reduce sensitivity. They will not work in cases where there is gum disease, dental caries, or infection.

## DECAYING TEETH

*(See Dental Caries, page 83; Gum Disease, page 83; Pyorrhea Alveolaris, page 84)*

## TOOTHACHE

*(See Dental Caries, page 83; Gum Disease, page 83; Pyorrhea Alveolaris, page 84)*

# THE FACE

Many symptoms of the face can also appear elsewhere on the body. This section concentrates on conditions most likely to be localized to the face.

## SWOLLEN OR PUFFY FACE

Generalized swelling or puffiness of the face, as distinct from, say, swelling in the neck, is uncommon. Considered here is true, overall facial swelling or puffiness.

For causes of local swelling, see the sections on skin and on the neck.

Because the tissues around the eye are so soft, relatively minor inflammation can cause considerable swelling of the eyelids, which can swell and close the eye.

### PROBABLE

■ **Insect Bite**

• Sudden onset of swelling localized to site of bite and surrounding tissues.
• Often quite itchy.
• Subsides after a day or so.
• Occasionally becomes infected, with swelling becoming red and hot, and fever developing with malaise.

■ **Dental Abscess**

• Painful swelling above or below the lower or upper jaw.
• Whole cheek may be swollen.
• Obvious dental pain or decay (caries).
• Swelling worsens over two to three days.

A visit to your dentist plus a course of antibiotics should provide rapid relief. Dental treatment may subsequently be required.

■ **Trauma**

• Clear history of injury.
• Bruising on the face can cause marked swelling, particularly when the bruise is only a day or two old and begins to change color.

## POSSIBLE

### ■ Angioneurotic Edema

Often associated with urticaria (hives) *(see Skin section)*. Normally caused by an allergy, typically to a food or a drug, but often the cause is not identifiable.

Symptoms may include:

• Swelling of lips and eyes.

• Can involve the tongue and cause some obstruction to breathing, in which case it is a medical emergency.

### ■ Erysipelas

An infection of the skin and underlying tissues. Often, bacteria get in through a minor cut or graze. The word literally means "like lightening" and it can come on remarkably quickly.

• Red, shiny, hot skin.

• Painful.

• Fever.

• Malaise.

Needs antibiotic treatment (sometimes in the hospital via an IV drip).

### ■ Cushing's Syndrome

*(See page 273)*

### ■ Hypothyroidism

Weight gain and other changes associated with this condition may give the appearance of a puffy face, although there is no true swelling. *(See page 351)*

## RARE

### ■ Acromegaly

In this condition, excess growth hormone is produced in adult life. Enlargement of the jaw and forehead is part of the clinical picture of acromegaly and might be mistaken for facial puffiness *(see page 273)*.

### ■ Glomerulonephritis

One of the conditions described under Nephritis *(see page 318)*.

### ■ Nephrotic Syndrome

*(See page 22)*

## FACIAL NODULES OR BUMPS

A possible cause is gout *(see page 284)*. A very rare cause is leprosy *(see page 46)*.

### PROBABLE

### ■ Cold Sore

Common, and caused by a herpes virus. They often develop with or after a febrile illness, or if generally run-down. However, they can also be provoked by anything that causes a rise in skin temperature, such as direct sunlight or even the slight temperature rise that women experience premenstrually.

- Initially, irritation noted on skin usually around mouth.
- Becomes progressively more painful.
- Skin reddens and little vesicles (fluid-filled blisters) appear.
- Vesicles burst and sometimes crusts form.
- Clears up in about two weeks.

A similar type of infection may occur in the genital region.

### ■ Impetigo

A bacterial infection of the skin. Very contagious. May occur in children and adults.

- Blisters may develop in the form that usually occurs in newborn babies.
- Honey-colored scabs develop rapidly.
- Large areas can be infected if untreated.

At some stages, impetigo can be difficult to distinguish from a cold sore (and impetigo can develop on cold sores).

Antibiotics are required: if the condition is mild, treatment is by ointment; but if it is severe, by tablets.

## POSSIBLE

### ■ Eczema

Sometimes called dermatitis. On the face, cosmetics are a common cause, but other causes include hair dyes, nail polish, and some plants.

Features include:
- Redness (where the cosmetics were applied).
- Red, raised spots.
- Small blisters that weep.
- Crusting and scaling.

It is not uncommon for patches of eczema to appear eventually all over the body.

### ■ Shingles

An infection caused by the same virus that causes chicken pox.
- Red, blistering rash.
- Can be very painful (pain preceding the rash).
- May be extensive (typically covering one side of the face).
- Localized to one side of the body's center line.
- Crusting of the blisters.
- Heals in about two weeks, but pain may persist for months or years.

Can occur at any age, including young people; the older the individual, the more severe it usually is.

If the side of the nose (or inside the nostril) is affected, there is a risk that the eyeball can be involved and this demands urgent medical attention.

## RARE

### ■ Rodent Ulcer

A small cancerous sore that virtually never spreads to distant parts of the body. Often appears in the elderly around the nose, eyes, ears, or mouth.

- Starts as a small pink lump.
- After some weeks or months, it may become ulcerated.
- Gradually, if undiagnosed and untreated, it invades underlying tissues, for example, the bones of the nose.

Once diagnosed, treatment is usually straightforward.

### ■ Pemphigus Vulgaris

*(See page 244)*

### ■ Dermatitis Herpetiformis

*(See page 244)*

### ■ Pemphigoid

*(See page 244)*

### ■ Erythema Multiforme and Stevens-Johnson Syndrome

The second is a severe form of the first, where there is involvement of the inside of the mouth. Both are reactions to provocations such as infection or medications. Features include:

- Red rash of different shapes, which may be present all over the body.
- Raised red lesions and blisters may occur.
- Each episode may last two to three weeks.

Stevens-Johnson syndrome may also include:

- Fever.
- Malaise.
- Lung inflammation.
- Kidney damage.

## REDDENED FACE

The probable causes are, of course, embarrassment, heat, and alcohol, all of which can make the blood vessels in the skin widen so that they carry more blood than usual. In each case, the redness may well extend across not only the face and head but also the neck and upper trunk. That the blood vessels can respond to a state of mind is proof, if any were needed, that mind and body are indeed not separate but complementary.

### POSSIBLE

### ■ Acne Rosacea

Most common in the middle-aged and elderly.

- Facial reddening.
- Some inflamed pustules.
- Skin is shiny.
- May become permanent.

Hot or spicy food, alcohol, embarrassment, or temperature changes can exacerbate the reddening.

## ▪ Epilepsy

Epileptics may be aware of facial flushing just before a fit, and observers will often notice it afterwards.

## ▪ Drugs

Several drugs can cause flushing, especially calcium antagonists commonly used to treat blood pressure.

A possibility if the flushing follows a change of medication.

## ▪ Menopause

Flushing is one of the most common symptoms women experience as they approach the "change of life." Symptoms can persist for years.

## RARE

## ▪ Mitral Valve Disease

- Shortness of breath.
- Lung congestion.
- Coughing blood.
- Bronchitis.
- Heart failure.

- Facial flush, very marked below the eyes.

## ▪ Carcinoid Syndrome

A tumor that may occur in many parts of the body. Most of its symptoms are caused by chemicals it secretes, and may include:

- Facial flushing, extending over body.
- Diarrhea, abdominal pain.
- Enlarged liver.
- Wheezy chest.
- Heart problems.

## ▪ Pheochromocytoma

Another tumor that causes symptoms by the chemicals it secretes. It is very rare.

- High blood pressure.
- Diarrhea.
- Nausea.
- Abdominal pain.
- Facial flushing.

## ▪ Systemic Lupus Erythematosus

*(See page 460)*

## ADENOIDAL FACE

A term used for individuals who tend to mouth-breathe rather than breathe through the nose. They tend to walk, move about, and even sit with their mouths permanently open. This is because their enlarged adenoids prevent them from breathing through their nose.

Their voice may also be affected and is often described as "adenoidal." Symptoms may include:

- Breathing through the mouth.
- Snoring.
- Open mouth—the jaw hangs down.
- Nasal speech.

## GRINNING

One of the several symptoms of tetanus *(see page 92)* is spasms, which contort the face in to the so-called "sardonic grin." There is nothing funny about this or the other potentially fatal symptoms, which is why immunization—and keeping your protection up to date—is essential. Gardeners are particularly at risk from skin wounds being contaminated by soil containing the tetanus organism.

## EXPRESSIONLESS FACE

Parkinson's disease is the classic reason for an expressionless, immobile face. However, a number of conditions can give rise to a similar appearance as a result of damage to the part of the brain that controls facial, and other, movement.

### PROBABLE

■ **Parkinson's Disease**

A slowly progressive disease of the middle-aged and elderly.
- Tremor.
- Rigidity and some muscle pain.
- Slow movement.
- Immobile, mask-like face.
- Difficulty in writing.
- Occasional swallowing disorders.

Can be controlled with medication.

■ **Depression**

A depressed person may progressively lose the expression from his or her face. A dull, saddened, flat face is characteristic of depression. *(See also page 399)*

### POSSIBLE

■ **Drugs**

Drugs that may cause some (but not necessarily all) of the symptoms of Parkinson's disease include phenothiazines and butyrophenones. Both these groups of drugs are sometimes used as tranquilizers.

■ **Scleroderma**

A multisystem disease, affecting women more than men, that is likely to have been diagnosed already. *(See page 263)*
- Stiffness of hands leading to rigidity.
- Smooth, hard, shiny skin.
- Difficulty in opening mouth.
- Immobile face with loss of expression.
- Alimentary tract, heart, and kidneys may become involved.

### RARE

■ **Hepatolenticular Degeneration**

Also called Wilson's disease. An inherited disorder, usually showing itself during the teens.

- Parkinson's disease symptoms, plus:
- Liver damage leading to jaundice in some cases.

- Yellow-brown rings on the eyes.

## PART OF THE FACE PARALYZED

Excluded here is immobility of the entire face, covered under Expressionless Face *(see page 100)*.

### PROBABLE

#### ■ Bell's Palsy

The cause is unknown, but the facial nerve is damaged on one side. The affected individual may note the symptoms on waking up one morning, or after having been out in cold weather, or in a draught:

- May be a dull ache on the affected side.
- Cannot close eye.
- Mouth drawn to the side, away from the damaged nerve.
- Saliva may dribble from the affected side.
- Cannot smile properly or bare the teeth.
- Occasionally, taste sensation to one side of the tongue is affected.

With luck, recovery commences within seven to ten days, but may take several weeks.

If you suspect Bell's palsy, see a doctor as soon as possible.

Recent evidence has confirmed that many cases are due to the herpes simplex virus and early antiviral treatment together with steroids can improve the outcome significantly. (Rare causes include a late stage of Lyme disease and Guillain-Barré syndrome.) Some doctors believe that high doses of steroids, given early enough, may improve the chances of recovery.

#### ■ Stroke

Any stroke may damage part of the brain that controls the nerve that makes the facial muscles work. Different types of stroke may affect the face in slightly different ways so that a number of symptoms can be present to a greater or lesser degree. These include:

- Difficulty or inability to wrinkle the forehead.
- Difficulty or inability to blink or close the eye.
- Difficulty or inability to smile symmetrically.

- Difficulty or inability to bare the teeth.
- Difficulty or inability to whistle.
- Saliva may leak out of the affected side of the mouth.
- The body is usually affected on the same side as the face: for example, weakened left hand and face paralyzed on the left-hand side. When the dominant side of the body (right side in right-handed people) is affected, speech is often affected.

Paralysis of the face is unlikely to occur in the absence of other symptoms, which may help to determine the diagnosis.

## POSSIBLE

### ■ Injury

All or part of the facial nerve, which controls movement of the facial muscles, may be damaged, sometimes permanently. The symptoms are the same as for Bell's palsy *(see page 101)*. Knife wounds to the face may be a cause (including surgery, especially on the parotid gland). The facial nerve travels through the ear, just behind the eardrum, and is easily injured at this site too.

### ■ Poliomyelitis

"Polio" can also affect the facial nerve, with similar results to Bell's palsy *(see page 101)*.

## RARE

### ■ Tumors

Primary or secondary cancerous tumors developing in the part of the brain that controls facial movement or that involve or press on the facial nerve, may cause a mixture of symptoms similar to those of stroke *(see page 101)* or Bell's palsy *(see page 101)*.

### ■ Herpes *(Varicella Zoster)*

A herpes infection of the mouth, palate, or ear can damage the nerve supply to the face causing symptoms similar to Bell's palsy *(see page 101)*. This is known as Ramsay Hunt syndrome.

### ■ Guillain-Barré Syndrome

A disease of the neurological system with many different symptoms, ranging from mild to severe. Most cases recover, but this may take many months.
- Altered sensation in the arms and legs.
- Shoulder and back pain.
- Facial palsies.
- Muscles of respiration may be so weakened that artificial ventilation is required.
- Swallowing may be affected and tube-feeding may be needed while recovery progresses.

### ■ Motor Neuron Disease

*(See page 276)*

## FACIAL PAIN

Covered here are causes of pain that have no *visible* symptoms, so, for example, shingles is excluded.

### PROBABLE

■ **Dental Disease**

Check teeth and gums first if local face pain develops with no obvious cause. Is it an abscess? If in doubt, always check with your dentist.

■ **Sinusitis**

*(See page 467)*

■ **Referred Pain**

Because the body's "wiring"—its nervous system—is interconnected, pain arising in one place can travel onward or "be referred" to another. If the teeth and gums appear normal, then pain in the face may arise from elsewhere in the head, for instance, the facial sinuses.

■ **Temporomandibular Joint Dysfunction**

A common cause of pain, particularly if there is any problem with the bite. The patient's partner often complains that the individual grinds their teeth at night.

### POSSIBLE

■ **Migraine**

*(See page 109)* Facial pain can be felt as part of a migraine attack.
• The pain will usually be severe and piercing.
• Only one side of the face will be affected in classic migraine, but can be bilateral in common migraine (the word *migraine* come from the French meaning "half face").

■ **Cluster Headache**

• Intensely severe pain in or behind one eye.
• The eye often looks bloodshot during an episode and there may be some stuffiness in the nostril on the affected side.
• Typically, episodes of pain occur at precisely the same time each day (often in the middle of the night) and clusters continue for a few weeks, before remitting.

■ **Post-Herpetic Neuralgia**

Persistent burning pain at the site of a previous attack of shingles *(see page 26)*.
• Normally occurs in elderly patients.
• Pain is so severe that suicide may be considered.

- Even touching the site may start an attack of pain.

## ■ Trigeminal Neuralgia

Also called tic douloureux. Pain in the face in an area supplied by the trigeminal nerve.

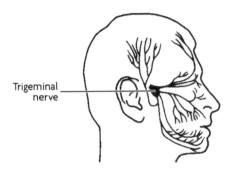

Trigeminal nerve

- Stabbing, intermittent facial pain.
- Can be triggered by touch or for no reason.
- Attacks come in bouts.

Many different treatments have been tried, some with more success than others. A specialist opinion is usually recommended, as the symptoms can be incapacitating.

## RARE

### ■ Malignant Disease

A doctor will consider the possibility of a cancerous tumor of the nose, mouth, sinuses, or pharynx, particularly if the individual is an elderly smoker.

### ■ Eagle's Syndrome

Sharp localized pain to side of jaw, below the ear. Pain can be felt inside the mouth.

Due to an overgrowth of a bony spike (called the styloid process, as it looks like the tip of a pen) from the underside of the skull.

### ■ Paget's Disease

This disease *(see also page 450)* can cause local pain in the bones affected, including those of the face.

### ■ Psychological or Atypical

In a few individuals, no cause of pain is ever found, despite full investigation and assessment. This pain is described as "atypical." Recent research by dental experts and pain specialists has found that tricyclics, a group of drugs generally used to treat depression, can be helpful to patients with "atypical facial pain."

It is certainly worth trying these drugs before accepting that "only psychotherapy will help."

# THE HEAD

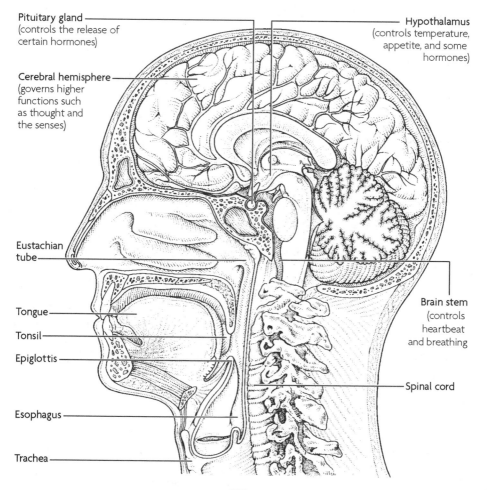

Pituitary gland
(controls the release of
certain hormones)

Hypothalamus
(controls temperature,
appetite, and some
hormones)

Cerebral hemisphere
(governs higher
functions such
as thought and
the senses)

Eustachian
tube

Tongue

Tonsil

Epiglottis

Esophagus

Trachea

Brain stem
(controls
heartbeat
and breathing

Spinal cord

## OVERSIZED HEAD

There are two possibilities: hydroceph-alus and Paget's disease *(see page 450)*.

Hydrocephalus, literally "water in the head," is a problem of newborn and very young babies. Within the brain, large quantities of clear fluid are constantly being produced. This fluid normally cir-culates through cavities within the brain and down the spinal cord, out through tiny holes onto the outer surface of the brain, where it is reabsorbed. Occasion-ally, damage to this circulation results in a backlog of fluid into the cavities of the brain, causing increased pressure and swelling.

- Progressive enlargement of the head.
- Bulging fontanelles (soft spots on the top of a baby's head).

The increased pressure damages the brain and can cause:

- Intellectual impairment.
- Epilepsy.
- Physical impairment.
- Vulnerability to infection.

Hydrocephalus needs specialist treat-ment: the fluid can be drained away, bypassing the blockage, to the stomach (abdomen) by a tube set permanently below the skin on the scalp.

## BULGING OR SUNKEN PLACES ON HEAD

Several causes of bulges in the head are worth considering in their own right, sep-arately from lumps, bumps, and swellings that can occur anywhere on the body, and which are covered in detail in other major sections of this book.

One somewhat specialized area should also be mentioned in this context: the fontanelles. These are the soft "gaps" that can be felt in babies' heads at the points where the skull bones have not yet fused into a consistent bony cover-ing. The smaller, posterior fontanelle

closes soon after birth, while the larger one, the anterior fontanelle, usually closes by one-and-a-half years of age. The size of the fontanelles varies enor-mously from child to child. Your doctor will often feel the fontanelle if your child is unwell. A bulging fontanelle can indicate raised pressure in the head, as in meningitis. It can also mean only that your baby is screaming the house down. It is best to check any changes or con-cerns regarding the fontanelle with your doctor.

## PROBABLE

■ **Dehydration**

A baby who is short of fluid, typically after a bout of diarrhea, will show:

- Sunken eyes.
- Sunken fontanelle.
- Loss of skin elasticity.
- Listless, apathetic behavior.
- Dry lips and mouth.

Dehydration is a serious condition in any baby or child; if you suspect it, see a doctor urgently. It can be effectively treated, but time is of the essence.

## POSSIBLE

■ **Paget's Disease**

*(See page 450)*

## RARE

■ **Hydrocephalus**

*(See Oversized Head, page 106)*

■ **Raised Intracranial Pressure**

A tumor or infection raises the pressure inside the skull. It is normal for the fontanelles to bulge outwards when a baby cries or strains, say when coughing. But if intracranial pressure is increased, the fontanelle bulges permanently. There may well be other symptoms such as vomiting and headache. See a doctor.

When the fontanelle is closed, after around eighteen months, it cannot bulge. After this time, the main features of raised intracranial pressure will be vomiting and headache.

## BLOOD VESSELS STAND OUT IN HEAD

An obvious feature of temporal arteritis *(see page 109)*.

## HEAD TWISTING TO ONE SIDE

*(See Stiffness or Pain in Neck, page 132)*
A common cause is torticollis *(see page 133)*.

## HEADACHE AND FITS OR CONVULSIONS

*(See Convulsions, page 392)*

## HEADACHE

It is so rare for headache to be the symptom of grave underlying disease, such as a brain tumor, that worrying about it, though understandable, is usually a waste of time. Better to worry about other aspects of your health that really might be significant, such as smoking or excess alcohol or cholesterol intake. As a rough rule of thumb, even the most vicious, throbbing headache is in all likelihood "innocent": the headache that signifies a brain tumor is something else entirely and will almost always be accompanied by other symptoms. Ninety-eight percent of all headaches that doctors treat are caused by tension or sinus trouble.

### PROBABLE

#### ■ Tension Headache

Often develops in people with work or family problems. May also arise if an individual finds himself or herself under pressure, whatever the circumstances. The source of tension is not always obvious.
• May be intermittent for weeks and months in a previously fit individual.
• Normal periods in between.
• Band-like, crushing pain around head.
• No other physical abnormalities present.

• Disappears after a variable length of time.

#### ■ Sinusitis

*(See page 467)* Any inflammation of the sinuses (air spaces in the facial bones) can cause headache. This can be due to infection, catarrh, and even hay fever.
• Tends to be a remorseless, low-grade, throbbing pain.

#### ■ Menstruation or Menopause Related

Alterations of body hormone production—naturally, during, before, or after a period—can cause variable headaches. Your doctor may be able to advise you on treatments or checkups from which you might benefit.

#### ■ Infection

Viral infections of any kind are notorious for producing multiple symptoms, of which headache, often dull and persistent, is but one. Other features are:
• Fever.
• Muscle and joint pain.
• Malaise.

These are in addition to other, more specific, symptoms—typically, sore throat.

## POSSIBLE

### ■ Migraine

Recurrent, severe headaches, often but not always accompanied by visual disturbance. Migraines often start in adolescence. Many different symptoms are described, including:

• Vision affected before the headache starts.

• Occasionally, numbness or weakness of one limb before the headache starts.

• Pain starts on one side of the head, but may spread.

• The pain throbs.

• A wish to avoid light.

• Vomiting may occur.

• May last for a couple of days, but normally four to twelve hours.

The cause is not fully understood but is probably related to abnormal blood flow in the fine vessels of the scalp. Some relief is available from modern medications—see your doctor.

### ■ Cluster Headache

• Most common in men.

• Tends to be one-sided.

• Often severe.

• May occur at night.

• Occurs several times within a period of a few weeks, then disappears, returning some months later.

• Is harmless.

### ■ Temporal Arteritis

Inflammation of the temporal artery, which runs along the side of the face. Most common in the elderly.

• Severe pain on the side of the face.

• Skin over the artery is inflamed.

• Artery is thickened and painful to touch.

• There may be fever and malaise.

If suspected, urgent medical treatment is needed, as the eye may become involved.

### ■ Eye, Ear, Nose, Throat, or Dental Disease

*(See those sections for full detail)* All these organs can produce pain that is referred to the head. The pain may be dull and persistent. These possibilities should therefore be excluded if

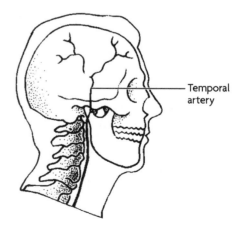

Temporal artery

a headache persists for longer than expected.

### ■ Drugs

Including cigarettes and alcohol. The system is poisoned by the body's inability to eliminate the broken-down byproducts.

Some prescription drugs can cause headache, too. You must reasonably suspect this if the headache is noted after taking the drug. One such drug is the anti-angina medication, glyceryl trinitrate, which gives some people a throbbing headache. Overuse of painkillers containing codeine, found in many over-the-counter remedies, is now a well-recognized cause of chronic headache.

If headaches coincide with taking a prescribed drug, always report it to your doctor—there may well be an alternative to try instead.

### ■ Toxic Fumes

Dry-cleaning agents, tar, and diesel fumes are among regular culprits. Some people suddenly develop a sensitivity to fumes, even having worked with them for years.

Low-grade poisoning with carbon monoxide—for example, from a faulty central heating system—can cause headaches. Other features include drowsiness and an abnormally pink complexion. A very low index of suspicion for the lethal situation is wise.

### RARE

### ■ Meningitis

An infection of the membranes that enclose the brain and spinal cord. If you suspect it, see a doctor immediately.
• Severe headache.
• Stiff neck; bending the neck worsens the pain.
• Reduced level of consciousness.
• Photophobia (fear of light).
• Vomiting.
• Fever.
• Very ill.
• A rash may appear.

### ■ Subarachnoid Hemorrhage

A leakage of blood from a vessel into the liquid that bathes the spinal cord and brain. The following may occur:
• Sudden onset of severe headache, sometimes after a period of exertion— often described as being like a blow on the back of the head. However:
• The headache may have a slower, more insidious, onset.
• Vomiting.
• Stiff neck.
• Mental confusion.
• Speech difficulties.
• Limb weakness.
• Visual disturbances.
• Convulsions.

If suspected, see a doctor urgently.

## ■ Brain Tumor

Because the adult skull is rigid, a growth within it can increase the internal pressure, giving rise to headache. However, not every brain tumor has this effect. Brain tumors can be primary—a pituitary tumor is an example—or secondary, that is, having spread from elsewhere in the body, for example, from a primary breast cancer. There will almost always be a range of symptoms:

- Gradually increasing, dull headache.
- Vomiting.
- Impaired consciousness.
- Pulse becomes slower.
- Respiration rate becomes slower.
- Convulsions may occur.
- Vision may be affected.
- Headache often present when you wake in the morning.

If the first three symptoms develop in an individual, along with other signs of neurological damage—say, weakness or numbness of a limb—urgent medical assessment is needed. The symptoms can be relieved, even if the tumor itself cannot be removed.

## ■ Subdural Hemorrhage

Blood collects between the layers of tissue covering the brain. When this blood breaks down into a bruise, it draws more fluid to it, causing raised pressure. May happen in the elderly after an (apparently) insignificant bump on the head. Symptoms may develop some weeks later and include:

- Headache, often minor.
- Periods of sleepiness and unconsciousness.
- Increased confusion and incontinence.
- Possibly speech difficulties.
- Possibly convulsions.

May often be mistaken for "getting old" —so, should not be discounted if someone has recently received a blow to the head.

## ■ Brain Abscess

Infection enters the brain in one of several ways: a broken skull bone with overlying skin damage; from ear, throat, sinus, and lung infection; or occasionally from facial infection.

- Symptoms of the initial infection, for example, earache.
- Progressive headache.
- Progressive drowsiness.
- Fever.
- Vomiting.
- Malaise.
- Anorexia.
- Convulsions.

## HEADACHE WITH HIGH FEVER

The most common illnesses that give fever combined with headache are common viral infections, such as influenza and glandular fever. There are, however, several rare but dangerous infections that may also be responsible for similar symptoms. Be sure to read the sections on fever *(see pages 453–461)*.

## HEADACHE PLUS CHILLS AND FEVER

*(See Fever, pages 453–461)*

## HEADACHE: BABIES AND CHILDREN

Babies and children can get headaches for the same reasons as adults. But in seeking the cause, you should consider two other factors.

First, babies and young children (up to the age of five or even six years) are notoriously inexact about where pain is coming from. "Head pain" often turns out to be earache or sore throat. So, explore every possibility before settling for headache.

Second, complaining of recurrent headaches can be characteristic of a child who is unhappy or under stress: typically, he or she is going through a bad patch at school. If you can detect no other symptoms, and if illness or disease can really be ruled out, then you should find out what is causing the problems. Removing the cause can make the headaches vanish overnight.

## RECURRING HEADACHE

*(See Headache with High Fever, page 111)*

# The Throat

SLURRED OR UNCLEAR SPEECH

Hoarseness is covered separately (*see page 114*).

Listed here are the main causes of impaired speech; but bear in mind that impaired speech is not always a feature of these conditions, and that their other symptoms usually predominate.

Look up specific entries elsewhere in the book for further details.

## PROBABLE

### ■ Alcohol and Drugs

- Temporary slowness and slurring.
- Deafness.

If an individual is unable to hear their own voice, he or she is unable to create the precise intended sound.

### ■ Septal deviation

- Muffled or nasal quality to speech.

*(See page 53)*

### ■ Nasal Injury

- Muffled or nasal quality to speech.
- Mouth ulcer.
- Anesthesia, for example, from recent dental treatment.

*(See page 45)*

### ■ Common Cold

- Muffled or nasal quality to speech.

*(See page 466)*

### ■ Adenoids

- Muffled or nasal quality to speech.

*(See page 52)*

### ■ Stuttering

Tends to begin as a child begins to learn to talk, from two years onward.

### ■ Lisping and Rolling *R*s

Not necessarily a speech impairment, but a variation of normal. Common when children first learn to speak, and tends to disappear by the age of six. If marked or persistent, speech therapy may be appropriate. Indeed, early attention from a speech therapist can prevent speech disorders becoming permanent.

## POSSIBLE

### ■ Cleft Palate

*(See page 81)*

### ■ Neurological Disease

Any disease that can affect control of the tongue, soft palate, and related structures will give slurred and unclear speech. A stroke, motor neuron disease, multiple sclerosis, and Parkinson's disease are examples. Cerebellar disease, in particular, can give rise to a speech impediment.

### ■ Chronic Sinusitis

May give a muffled or nasal quality to speech. *(See page 49)*

### ■ Benign Tumors

Including nasal polyps, may give a muffled or nasal quality to speech. *(See page 50)*

## RARE

### ■ Malignant Tumors of Nose or Mouth

*(See Cancer of the Nose, page 46)*

## HOARSE VOICE OR NO VOICE

Severe cases of hoarseness may suffer complete loss of voice; mild cases merely a temporary thickening or roughening.

The causes can be divided into three main categories: those affecting the vocal cords themselves; those affecting the nerves supplying them; and those caused by other disease of the larynx. All cases of hoarseness lasting more than 10 days should be reported to a doctor.

*(See also Problems with Swallowing Plus Hoarse Voice on page 118)*

### PROBABLE

### ■ Smoking, Drinking, Excessive Talking or Shouting

Obvious and familiar when combined, but also capable of inflaming the vocal cords in isolation.

• Hoarseness.

• Sore throat.

• Settles with resting the voice in three to four days.

If you keep up these insults to your vocal cords, recovery may be slow, indeed you may suffer total loss of voice. Rest (not talking) is the only answer.

Excessive coughing can also damage the vocal cords.

## ■ Laryngitis or Tonsillitis

*(See pages 222 and 135)*

## ■ Common Cold

May occasionally involve the larynx, resulting in hoarseness.

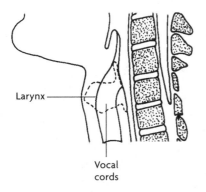

Larynx

Vocal cords

## POSSIBLE

## ■ Vocal Nodules

Also called singer's nodes. Typically in singers pitching their voice higher than their natural range.

• Progressive hoarseness.

The nodules often need to be removed by surgery.

## ■ Surgery

Surgery to the neck, particularly to the thyroid gland, may damage the recurrent laryngeal nerve. Recovery takes a few weeks but the hoarseness can be permanent. If so, there are methods of improving the speech.

After any operation where a breathing tube has been passed down the throat, slight hoarseness and a sore throat is usual.

## ■ Myxedema

Swelling around eyes and feet as a result of an underactive thyroid gland, plus highly distinctive, deep, gruff voice.

## ■ Epiglottitis

*(See page 229)*

## ■ Cancer of the Larynx

*(See page 121)*

## ■ Inhalation

Inhalation of smoke or chemicals can cause temporary hoarseness.

## RARE

## ■ Foreign Bodies

*(See page 49)*

## ■ Thoracic Aortic Aneurysm

The aorta is the main artery in the chest. An aneurysm is a swelling due to weakness of the wall. This can cause hoarseness by local pressure on the recurrent laryngeal nerve.

## ■ Cancer

Any malignant tumor in the chest, but especially on the esophagus or lung, may press on or invade the recurrent laryngeal nerve causing hoarseness. However, this symptom is usually one of the last to occur.

*(See Noticeable Blood Vessels on the Neck, page 145; Swollen Lymph Nodes in Neck, page 135; and Problems with Swallowing, below)*

## ■ After Radiotherapy

Radiotherapy is sometimes used to treat cancer of the larynx, leaving the patient hoarse.

## ■ Sarcoidosis

A disease (cause unknown) giving enlarged lymph nodes and deposits in various tissues, including the larynx, hence hoarseness.

## ■ Myasthenia Gravis

*(See page 19)*
*(See also Phlegm in the Throat, page 126)*

## CLEARING THE THROAT

*(See pages 120 to 121)*

## PROBLEMS WITH SWALLOWING

### POSSIBLE

## ■ Globus Hystericus

Often seen in young women with a history of anxiety-related illness: a certain belief that there is something stuck in the throat; sensation of choking. Requires full medical examination and often intensive investigation to exclude other causes. If all is normal, strong reassurance is all that is needed.

## ■ Esophagitis

*(See page 141)*

### RARE

## ■ Achalasia

A narrowing of the gullet at the lower end. Appears in young adults.
• Difficulty in swallowing.
• Regurgitation of undigested food into the mouth.
• Vomiting.
• Loss of weight.
• Occasionally, chest infections with fever.

■ **Congenital Atresia of the Esophagus**

At birth:
- All feeds regurgitated.
- Frothy saliva from mouth.
- Difficulty breathing while being fed.
- Episodes of cyanosis (blueness).
- Recurrent pneumonia, either from overspill into the lungs or a fistula (communication) between the esophagus and main windpipe.

■ **Cancer of the Esophagus and Cancer of the Stomach**

*(See pages 117 and 118)*

■ **Epiglottitis**

*(See page 229)*

■ **Neurological Disease**

Typically MND/Myasthenia gravis *(see page 19)*.

## PROBLEMS WITH SWALLOWING PLUS REGURGITATION OR VOMITING

**PROBABLE**

■ **Esophagitis**

Caused by stomach acid flowing back up into the gullet.
- Burning pain on swallowing.
- Food and fluid regurgitated.
- Bitter taste in mouth.
- Heartburn.
- Pain in middle of chest, at front or at back, or down arms.
- Food "sticks" behind breast bone.
- Aggravated by spicy foods and alcohol.

Relieved by antacids.

**POSSIBLE**

■ **Peptic Stricture**

A narrowing of the gullet caused by long-standing reflux esophagitis.

- Food regurgitated with fluid.
- Heartburn.
- Associated with weight loss after prolonged period.
- Chest infections associated with regurgitation.
- May be associated with hiatus hernia *(see page 235)*.

■ **Pharyngeal Pouch**

*(See page 132)*

**RARE**

■ **Cancer of the Esophagus**

Commonest in 50-plus age group.
- Difficulty in swallowing.
- Liquids swallowed more easily than solids.
- Some regurgitation of food.

- Rarely pain.
- Weight loss.
- Poor appetite.
- Fatigue.
- Anemia (particularly in women).
- Hoarse voice.
- Occasional chest infection with fever, due to regurgitation.

### ■ Cancer of the Stomach

Similar symptoms to esophageal cancer, but there may also be:

- Abdominal pain.
- Poor appetite, developing earlier.
- A feeling of fullness soon after eating very little.
- Symptoms of indigestion that persist, do not respond to usual treatment, or become more severe.
- Feeling bloated.

- A previous ulcer.
- Anemia.
- In later stages, occasional difficulty in swallowing.

### ■ Other Cancers

Secondary tumors or large primary tumors outside the esophagus, but within the chest, can compress the esophagus, giving rise to:

- Difficulty in swallowing.
- Weight loss.
- Poor appetite.
- Weakness.
- All in addition to the symptoms of the primary tumor.

### ■ Thoracic Aortic Aneurysm

*(See page 115)*

## PROBLEMS WITH SWALLOWING PLUS HOARSE VOICE

### PROBABLE

### ■ Laryngitis

*(See page 222)*

### POSSIBLE

### ■ Foreign Body (Such as a Bone) in Gullet

- Pain and discomfort on swallowing.
- Hoarseness.
- Feeling of "something in the throat."

Hoarseness which persists in the absence of other symptoms can be a sign either of laryngeal polyps or of cancer. Early treatment will significantly affect the outcome for the better. Seek your doctor's advice as early as possible.

## RARE

### ■ Myasthenia Gravis

A disorder causing weakness and tiring of the muscles.

- Weakness of muscles.
- Drooping eyelids.

- Double vision.
- Hoarse, weak voice.
- Difficulty in swallowing.
- Possibly weight loss.

### ■ Cancer of the Esophagus

*(See page 117)*

## PROBLEMS WITH SWALLOWING PLUS WEIGHT LOSS

This combination of symptoms is likely to be an indication of serious illness. Seek help soon, since early intervention will significantly improve your chances of recovery. Smoking and drinking to excess will increase the risk of esophageal problems and cancer of the stomach.

### PROBABLE

### ■ Esophageal Stricture

*(See Peptic Stricture, page 117.)* The symptoms are the same, but can be caused by, for instance, accidental or deliberate swallowing of toxic chemicals.

### ■ Cancer of the Esophagus

*(See page 117)*

### POSSIBLE

### ■ Benign Tumor of the Esophagus

Such as a fibroma, leiomyoma, or hemangioma.

- Intermittent difficulty in swallowing.

- Sensation of "something" in the gullet.
- Health otherwise good.
- Minimal weight loss, unless tumor is large.

### ■ Multiple Sclerosis

In addition to motor and sensory changes *(see page 326):*
- Difficulty in swallowing.
- Some risk of regurgitation of food into chest.
- Gradual weight loss.

### ■ Motor Neuron Disease

Progressive muscle weakness with:
- Difficulty in starting to swallow because of poor tongue muscle control.
- Risk of inhaling food or fluids.
- Gradual weight loss.

*(See also page 418)*

### ■ Parkinson's Disease

In addition to the tremor, mask-like face, and slowness of movement:

- Difficulty in starting to swallow.
- Occasional choking.
- Weight loss.

## Pseudobulbar and Bulbar Palsy

These conditions are usually set off by a stroke (pseudobulbar palsy) or motor neuron disease (bulbar palsy). They cause:
- Difficulty in speech.
- Difficulty in swallowing.
- Regurgitation of food into nose.
- If prolonged, weight loss.

### RARE

## Chagas' Disease

Common in South America. Caused by infection with *Trypanosoma cruzi*. Symptoms are similar to those of achalasia *(see page 116)*.

## Myasthenia Gravis

*(See page 19)*

## Scleroderma

A disease that can affect many organs and which will usually have been diagnosed already. Typically affects women in their 30s and 40s.
- Associated with pain because of esophagitis *(see page 121)*.
- Slow weight loss.

## Systemic Lupus Erythematosus

*(See page 476)*

## Cancer of the Stomach

*(See page 118)*

---

## PROBLEMS WITH SWALLOWING PLUS PAIN

### PROBABLE

## Tonsillitis

*(See page 135)*

## Pharyngitis

The pharynx lies behind the tonsils at the back of the mouth, above the voice box and gullet.
- Pain on swallowing.
- Back of throat is noticeably red.
- Possibly enlarged lymph nodes—similar to tonsillitis, but tonsils are not inflamed.

If you have had your tonsils removed, pharyngitis may develop in response to an infection which would otherwise have caused tonsillitis.

## Laryngitis

*(See page 222)*

## POSSIBLE

### ■ Candidiasis (Thrush)

- Discomfort making swallowing difficult.
- White patches seen at the back of the throat and sides of mouth.

Most often nowadays caused by overuse of inhaled steroids. Common in the immunosuppressed (including those with HIV) and the elderly.

### ■ Esophagitis

Similar to reflux esophagitis, but the main symptom is:

- Burning pain behind the breast bone within a few seconds of swallowing.

Plus:

- Spread of pain to the arms.
- Heartburn.
- Aggravated by spicy foods or alcohol.

### ■ Esophageal Spasm

Spasm of the muscles of the gullet.

- Chest pain initiated by eating or emotional stress (if severe, can be mistaken for a heart attack).
- The condition can be mild or severe.
- Pain varies in intensity during an attack.
- Can be painless.

- Intermittent difficulty in swallowing, often at the same time as the pain.

### ■ Ulcers of the Tongue and Mouth

*(See page 80)*

### ■ Glossitis

Swollen, painful tongue, occasional fever, sometimes associated with riboflavin deficiency.

### ■ Herpes Simplex

A viral infection causing pain and formation of fluid-filled spots or ulcers. May be present in mouth, throat, or esophagus.

- Severe pain associated with the herpes sore.
- Vesicles and intensely painful ulcers seen in mouth.
- Feeling very unwell.
- Fever.

## RARE

### ■ Cancer of the Esophagus

*(See page 117)*

### ■ Cancer of the Larynx

- Persistent hoarseness.
- Occasionally pain on swallowing because of spread or ulceration.

## PROBLEMS WITH SWALLOWING AND PAIN IN THE MOUTH

### PROBABLE

■ **Tonsillitis**

Tonsils at the back of the mouth, either side of the throat, become inflamed.

- Enlarged tonsils.
- Occasional white spots on tonsils.
- Reddening in the throat.
- Pain on swallowing.
- Occasionally, associated cough.
- Fever.
- Enlarged lymph glands in neck may be tender.

■ **Laryngitis**

Infection involving the larynx, the "voice box," in the neck.

- Hoarse voice, or difficulty in speaking at all.

- Fever.
- Pain on swallowing, but less severe than with tonsillitis.

### RARE

■ **Ludwig's Angina**

Severe infection of the floor of the mouth.

- Severe pain.
- Can cause breathing difficulty because of swollen upper airways.
- Pain on swallowing.

The condition is usually associated with poor oral hygiene, and problems with infected teeth or gums.

■ **Cancer of the Esophagus**

*(See page 117)*

## SWOLLEN THROAT

*(See Swollen Lymph Nodes in Neck, page 135)*

## LUMP IN THROAT

*(See Problems with Swallowing, page 116)*

## SORE THROAT

Common reasons for a sore throat are covered under *Problems with Swallowing Plus Pain, page 120.*

If you think you have this symptom in isolation, see *Swollen Lymph Nodes in Neck, page 135; Isolated Lumps and Swellings In or On Neck, page 130; Stiffness or Pain in Neck, page 132; Problems with Swallowing Plus Pain, page 120;* or *Ulcers in the Mouth, page 80.*

It is, however, most likely to occur along with fever (*see below*).

## SORE THROAT WITH FEVER

**PROBABLE**

■ Common Cold

*(See page 466)*

■ Tonsillitis

*(See page 122)*

■ Laryngitis

*(See page 122)*

### Smoking

Smokers are likely to suffer from exaggerated symptoms if they have any of the conditions listed here. They are also likely to take longer to recover than non-smokers and are at greater risk of developing complications, such as secondary infections of the ears or chest.

■ Pharyngitis

*(See page 120)*

**POSSIBLE**

■ Infectious Mononucleosis

"Glandular fever" *(see page 136).*

■ Dental Infections

*(See page 136)*

**RARE**

■ Glossitis

*(See page 121)*

■ Ludwig's Angina

*(See page 122)*

■ Adverse Drug Reaction

Sore throat, inflammation of the mucous membranes of the mouth, and fever are all possible symptoms of adverse drug reactions, especially if accompanied by a rash.

## ULCERS IN THE MOUTH

### PROBABLE

■ **Aphthous Ulcer**

• Small and multiple (or larger and solitary).

• Anywhere in mouth or on tongue, typically behind lower lip at the front.

• Extremely painful; aggravated by acid fruits.

• May be aggravated by sharp dentures or other dental problems.

• Often appears at times of stress.

Most heal after a few days, but larger ones take longer, though rarely more than 8 to 10 days. Treatments for aphthous ulcers are often unsatisfactory. Pain-relieving gel or tablets may be bought from a drug store. Most brands of toothpaste contain sodium lauryl sulfate (SLS) and sensitivity to this is sometimes the cause.

■ **Drugs**

The most common drug cause is nicorandil (an anti-angina treatment).

■ **Hematological**

Any cause of marrow suppression.

■ **Herpes Simplex**

*(See page 121)*

### POSSIBLE

■ **Erythema Multiforme**

Irregular red marks. May be associated with a reaction to drugs or an infection. Most common in children and young women.

• Itchy rash anywhere on body; not unlike measles rash.

• Pale-centered wheals, sometimes called "target lesions."

• Sore throat.

• Headache.

• Fever.

• Ulceration in the mouth and throat.

There is a severe form of the condition, called Stevens-Johnson syndrome.

### RARE

■ **Cancer of the Mouth or Throat**

May occur anywhere in mouth or throat. Tobacco users are at risk, especially pipe-smokers and tobacco-chewers.

Suspicion is aroused by:

• Long-standing, large ulcers (more than two weeks).

• Ulcer with irregular shape.

• Ulcers on surfaces of polyps.

• Ulcers with raised edges.

• Feeling unwell.

• Bad breath.

• Enlarged lymph nodes in neck.

## ■ Syphilis

Ulcers in the throat can mean primary, secondary, or tertiary syphilis. Ulcers are likely to be:
• Single.
• Shallow.
• Hard at the base.
• Painless.
• Non-bleeding.
   And they have:
• A raised, reddened margin.
• Enlarged lymph nodes may be present.

## ■ Pemphigus

A skin disease in which fluid-filled sacs appear on the skin at sites of pressure and trauma.
• Fluid-filled sacs in the mouth.
   These burst, forming:
• Ulcers which may remain for weeks.

## ■ Crohn's Disease

The following symptoms always accompany other signs of gastrointestinal disease.
• Aphthous-type ulcers (*see above*).
   Recurrent diarrhea, with or without weight loss, in an otherwise fit person who has aphthous ulcers suggests the possibility of Crohn's disease.

## ■ Celiac Disease

*(See page 144)*

## ■ Behçet's syndrome

Most common, though still rare, in some Middle Eastern countries.
• Recurrent major ulceration in mouth and throat.
   Followed by:
• Ulcers on the genitals.
• Eye inflammation and arthritis.

## ■ Leukemias/Myeloma

• Ulceration in the mouth.
• Persistent sore throats.
• Infections.
• Feeling unwell.
• Bruise easily.

*(See also page 497)*

## ■ Tuberculosis

• Small ulcers.
• Sore throat.
• Difficulty in swallowing.
• Excessive salivation.

*(See also page 224)*

## ■ Hematological (Blood) Disorders

Any cause of marrow suppression. Which, typically, you are always trying to clear.

## PHLEGM IN THE THROAT

### PROBABLE

■ **Vasomotor Rhinitis**

• More or less constant production of mucus in the nasal passages.

• Clear discharge from front of nose. The mucus also dribbles into the throat from the back of the nose (the two are connected). This last is known as post-nasal drip.

• Brought on by a change of environment or atmosphere.

• Difficulty in breathing through nostrils.

• Not associated with other symptoms of allergic rhinitis (*see below*).

> There is some evidence that modern living, with its sealed windows, central heating, and indoor life, has increased the volume of house dust generally, and that rhinitis is, as a consequence, much more common.

■ **Allergic Rhinitis**

You are likely to have a known allergy, typically to pollen, dust, or animals.

• Clear discharge from front of nose and into throat.

• Difficulty in breathing through the nostrils.

• Watery eyes.

• Sneezing.

• Wheezing.

A family history of asthma, eczema, or hay fever is often found in those with this condition.

■ **Chest Infection/Chronic Lung Sepsis**

Particularly in patients with chronic chest conditions, for example, bronchitis, cystic fibrosis, and bronchiectasis. Smokers are also a high-risk group.

• Persistent coughing up of green or yellow phlegm.

• Fever.

• Feeling unwell.

• Sometimes, difficulty in breathing.

Normally requires antibiotics.

### POSSIBLE

■ **Sinusitis**

Any of the nasal sinuses may become infected, causing local pain/discomfort.

• Persistent nasal discharge (green or yellow).

• Headache.

• Pain over affected sinus.

- Fever.
- Bad breath.

### ■ Nasal Polyps

Polyps are fleshy growths or tumors, almost never malignant. Often multiple.
- Can sometimes be seen by looking into nose.
- Obstruction in nose.
- Clear discharge occasionally.
- Loss of sense of smell.
- Often associated with allergies.

### RARE

### ■ Cancer of the Nasal Fossa or Nasopharynx

Most common in the elderly.
- Foul smelling and tasting nasal discharge.
- Persistent pain.
- Bad breath.
- A lump may be seen in the mouth or nose; or a facial swelling may develop.
- Toothache may develop.
- Bloodstained nasal discharge or sputum.

## WHITE SPOTS VISIBLE IN MOUTH AND THROAT

### PROBABLE

### ■ Milk

Especially in babies. Can easily be wiped off, leaving a healthy oral surface.

### ■ Candidiasis

Otherwise known as thrush or monilia. Most commonly seen in newborn babies or infants. (It has been known for parents to mistake thrush for milk on the inside of a baby's cheek; but the white patches are hard to remove and doing so will cause the baby some discomfort.)
- White patches in mouth (which, unlike milk, are hard to remove and cause discomfort).
- Associated reddening.
- Lips, tongue, and cheek may be painful.
- Patches may be dislodged, but not always easily.

Often associated with antibiotic therapy, general ill-health, and (more rarely) immunosuppression.

### ■ Tonsillitis

*(See page 135)*

### POSSIBLE

### ■ Koplik's Spots

A sure sign of measles *(see page 458)*.
- White spots inside the mouth opposite the molar teeth.

• Spots are about the size of a grain of salt with surrounding reddening.

Other symptoms of measles are:

• A red rash starting by the ears spreading over seven days to the body and limbs.

• Runny nose.

• Reddened eyes.

• Cough.

> Persistent white patches in the mouth can be a sign of serious illness, and should not be ignored. Consult your doctor if:
>
> • Patches persist.
>
> • They cannot be removed easily.

## ■ Lichen Planus

Irregular, small, shiny purplish lesions on the skin. Can occur all over the body, including the genital area. Very itchy.

• Most common in the middle-aged.

• Multiple, fine white lines on lips, tongue, and cheek.

• White spots in the same region.

• Sometimes ulcers between the spots and lines.

A small risk of progression to mouth cancer.

## ■ Leukoplakia

• White patches on the tongue or lining of the mouth.

• Cannot be scraped off.

• Occasionally disappear leaving a red base.

• Possibly localized hardening under the patch.

A not insignificant risk of progression to mouth cancer, so persistent white patches should never be ignored.

Associated with smoking (particularly pipe-smoking) and rubbing dentures. Also, it is increasingly found in people with AIDS.

## RARE

## ■ Keratosis Pharyngis

• Small white or creamy lumps seen on tonsil surface.

• Frequently no other symptoms.

Persistent, white patches in the mouth that persist can be a sign of serious illness, and should not be ignored.

Consult your doctor if:

• Patches persist.

• They cannot be removed easily.

Seeking professional help early is always worthwhile.

# THE NECK

## NOTICEABLE BLOOD VESSELS ON THE NECK

Newly developed, visible blood vessels are a sign of underlying disease that need careful investigation, and probably tests, before treatment can be started.

### PROBABLE

#### ■ Heart Failure

The pump fails to circulate blood adequately, typically after a heart attack. May be associated with one or more of the following:
• Prominent symmetrical veins on each side of the neck that distend more as the patient lies flat.
• The prominence varies with respiration and heartbeat.
• Shortness of breath worse on lying flat.
• Shortness of breath on walking.
• Bluish discoloration of face.
• Swelling of ankles and legs.

### POSSIBLE

#### ■ Malignant Tumor Within the Chest

Malignant tumors (primary or secondary) within the chest can compress the great veins inside the chest, giving rise to:
• Symmetrical prominent veins on head, neck, and upper chest unaffected by bodily position.
• Face may appear congested and reddened.
• The face, neck, and upper chest may be swollen.
• Breathing may be normal.

In addition, there may well be the following general symptoms of:
• Weight loss.
• Poor appetite.
• Weakness.
• Feeling unwell.

■ **Pericardial Effusion**

Fluid distends the sac around the heart. May be caused by infection, autoimmune disease, tumor, or after a heart attack and can cause:

- Shortness of breath when lying flat.
- Prominent neck veins (symmetrical).
- Tightness in the chest, varying with movement.
- Fever (with infection).
- Feeling unwell.

### RARE

■ **Benign Tumor Within the Chest**

Large benign tumors within the chest can compress the great veins inside the chest, giving rise to the same symptoms as malignant tumor(s) *(see page 129)*.

■ **Constrictive Pericarditis**

Increasing rigidity of the sac around the heart. Caused by tuberculosis or other infection or injury, often many years afterwards.

- Rapid pulse (sometimes irregular).
- Low blood pressure.
- Tiredness.
- Prominent neck veins—more prominent on breathing in.
- Fluid in the abdomen.
- Liver enlargement.

## ISOLATED LUMPS OR SWELLINGS IN OR ON NECK

Isolated lumps may be associated with a number of structures in the neck in addition to the lymph nodes *(see page 135)*. These include the skin and the salivary or thyroid glands. A few are present from birth.

### PROBABLE

■ **Boil**

A skin infection commonly originating in a hair follicle or follicles.

- Painful.
- Localized reddening.
- Skin warm to the touch.
- Localized swelling.

- A yellow center that may discharge pus.

■ **Sebaceous Cyst**

- Superficial.
- Painless (unless infected).
- Present for many years.
- Slowly increases in size.
- Has a central "punctum"—the opening to the blocked sweat gland that causes the cyst.

■ **Lipoma**

A benign fatty tumor that can be superficial or extend under the skin. Same characteristics as a sebaceous cyst, except:

- No punctum.

## POSSIBLE

### ■ Diffuse Thyroid Gland Enlargement

The thyroid gland lies on both sides of the neck, just below the laryngeal prominence or Adam's apple.

- Movement of swelling up and down on swallowing.
- Diffuse swelling—no separate lumps.
- No other symptoms.

Other causes of diffuse thyroid swelling can be divided into those causing excess thyroid hormone secretion and those causing an underactive thyroid *(see page 350 and page 351)*. Both require professional attention.

### ■ Isolated Thyroid Nodule—Benign

A localized lump within the thyroid, which can be benign or malignant *(see right)*.

- Can be felt either side of the neck, just below the laryngeal prominence or Adam's apple.
- Moves up and down on swallowing.

May be associated with signs of overactive or underactive thyroid.

### ■ Submandibular Duct Stone

Beneath the jaw, on each side of the tongue, are two salivary glands, the sub-mandibular glands. Stones may form in the ducts of the glands or the body of the gland, causing:

- Painful swelling (normally on one side).
- The swelling increases when eating.
- The swelling reduces between meals.
- Swelling can sometimes be felt in the mouth, under the tongue.

## RARE

### ■ Cervical Rib

*(See page 133)*

### ■ Diffuse Thyroid Gland Enlargement (Malignant Tumor)

Features of thyroid enlargement, plus:

- Irregular symmetric enlargement.
- Movement of swelling up and down on swallowing may be lost.
- Trachea (wind pipe) may be compressed, causing difficulty in breathing.

### ■ Isolated Thyroid Nodule— Malignant

A localized lump within the thyroid gland.

- Moves up and down on swallowing.
  May have no other symptoms, but can cause:
- Hoarseness.
- Pain.
- Drooping of one eyelid (Horner's syndrome).

### ■ Thyroglossal Cyst

• Lies in the middle of the neck at the front.
• Near the surface.
• Moves up if the tongue is stuck out.
• Painless.

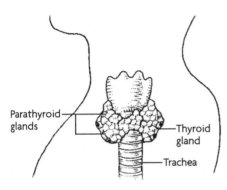

*The Thyroid*

Parathyroid glands
Thyroid gland
Trachea

### ■ Pharyngeal Pouch

A swelling on one side of the neck caused by a defect in the upper gullet.

• Varies in size.
• Causes variable difficulty in swallowing.
• Enlarges while eating or drinking.
• May "gurgle" as fluid empties from it.
• Old food may be regurgitated.
• Can be emptied by direct pressure on it.
• Not painful, but can be uncomfortable as it increases in size.

### ■ Sternomastoid Tumor

Present from birth—not a true tumor.

• Lump sited in the middle of the muscle at the side of the neck.
• The face is turned away from the side of the lesion.

### ■ Submandibular Tumor

May be benign or malignant.

• One-sided enlargement of gland.
• Progressive.
• May become painful.
• Lymph nodes may be involved.

---

## STIFFNESS OR PAIN IN NECK

### PROBABLE

### ■ Acute Stiff Neck

• Associated with sleeping in awkward position; also with exposure to cold.
• Pain on movement localized to neck.

• Neck movements limited by pain and muscle spasm.

### ■ Acute Neck Sprain

• Associated with sudden twisting/turning or bending.

- Extreme pain on any movement.
- Pain in upper back and head.
- Marked muscle spasm limiting neck movement.

### ■ Whiplash Injury

Typically present after a car crash (when hit from behind or from the front).
- Pain in neck and upper back.
- Neck held stiffly.
- Pain may have taken a few hours to develop after injury.
- Pain and stiffness may persist for weeks.
- May have pain and weakness in arms.
- Reduced range of neck movement.

### ■ Wryneck (Torticollis)

- Head pulled down on affected side.
- Chin points toward the opposite shoulder.
- The affected muscle is a solid band.
- Neck movements are considerably restricted.

Typically, the condition occurs on waking: suddenly you cannot move your neck freely. Wears off in a day or two.

## POSSIBLE

### ■ Cervical Spondylosis

Caused by degeneration of the lower cervical intervertebral discs. Sufferer is typically middle-aged.
- Pain in neck and back.

- Painful over neck.
- Worse on waking.
- Slight limitation of movement.

Occasionally:
- Pain in arms.
- Numbness in arms.
- Weakness in arms.

A scan of the neck might show a prolapsed lower cervical intervertebral disc.

### ■ Cervical Rib

Some people are born with an extra rib, or with a fibrous band, which constricts nerves and arteries in the neck. Symptoms may appear in the late twenties.
- May be a palpable lump in the neck.
- Neck is rarely painful.
- Pain behind collarbone.
- Pain on the inner side of the arm after or when carrying something such as groceries.
- Intermittent coldness and blueness of fingers.

### ■ Rheumatoid Arthritis

Patients with known rheumatoid arthritis may get degenerative changes in the neck.
- Pain is common.
- Range of movement is reduced.
- Weakness and sensory changes may be present in upper and occasionally lower limbs.

## RARE

### ■ Cervical Spine Infection

Tuberculous infection still occasionally occurs.

- Mild neck pain.
- Pain on any movement.
- Head may be held in hands.
- Stiffness, with reduced movement.
- Occasionally, there may be sudden paralysis as the spinal cord gets involved.

### ■ Meningitis

Infection of the lining of the brain and spinal cord. Usually, other marked symptoms, such as fever, will be present.

- Neck stiffness—inability to bend the neck forward because of pain and muscle spasm.
- Headache.
- Feeling unwell.
- Fever.
- Fine purple rash that does not blanch on pressure with a drinking glass.

If meningitis is suspected, call a doctor immediately.

### ■ Prolapsed Cervical Disc

May be caused by sudden movements and degeneration of the intervertebral discs. There is a sudden onset of symptoms, which may include:

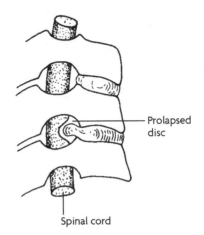

*Prolapsed Lower Cervical Disc*

- Neck pain and stiffness.
- Pain and altered sensation in the arms.
- Muscular spasm of the neck and upper back.
- Symptoms may resolve and then return.

### ■ Spinal Cord Tumors

Progressive onset of symptoms may include:

- Altered sensation in arms and legs.
- Areas of numbness.
- Weakness in arms and legs.
- Wasting of muscles.
- Ability to pass urine may be affected.

## SWOLLEN LYMPH NODES IN NECK

Most people have temporarily enlarged lymph nodes (also known simply as "glands") in the neck at some time. This is generally associated with infection or inflammation, either locally or of the whole body. Sometimes, just one is enlarged, giving a single swelling. Occasionally, recurring or persistent enlargement may indicate more serious underlying disorders.

Enlarged lymph nodes need to be distinguished from other lumps in the neck, such as enlarged salivary glands *(see Isolated Lumps or Swellings In or On Neck, page 130)*.

If enlarged lymph nodes persist in the neck for more than two weeks, and particularly if other symptoms are present, you must see your doctor.

### PROBABLE

#### ■ Common Cold

Or upper respiratory tract infection (URTI). These can occur alone or in combination:
• Tender lymph nodes enlarged symmetrically below ears and under jaw.
• Fever.
• Malaise.
• Sore throat.
• Cough.
• Runny nose.
• Earache.

Usually cures itself.

#### ■ Tonsillitis

• Tonsils enlarged
• Throat looks red.
• Tender lymph nodes enlarged below and behind jaw.
• Often enlarged more on one side than the other.
• White spots often apparent on tonsil surface (pus emerging from tonsil).
• Fever.
• Feeling unwell.

Requires antibiotics. Your doctor may take swabs from the tonsils, particularly if the surface is purulent. Frequent attacks

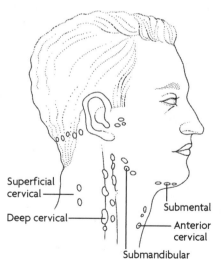

*Swollen Lymph Nodes in Neck*

may necessitate referral to a specialist throat surgeon.

### ■ Local Infection or Inflammation (Acne, Impetigo, Sebaceous Cyst)

• Nearest lymph nodes will be enlarged and may be painful.

• Pain and tenderness in scalp (look in hair).

• If a lump is present, it may be an infected sebaceous cyst.

• If an area is scaly/reddened/weeping/itchy, consider impetigo, dermatitis, eczema/psoriasis—see your doctor to distinguish which it is.

### ■ Dental Infection

Diseases of the gums or teeth may be associated with lymph node enlargement.

• Enlarged tender nodes, which tend to be those nearest the affected tooth.

• Toothache.

• Bleeding gums (gingivitis).

• Teeth with loose fillings.

• Dental abscess (painful tooth/gums and local swelling).

## Possible

### ■ Glandular Fever—Infectious Mononucleosis

Caused by infection with the Epstein-Barr virus and sometimes known as "kissing disease." A disease of children and young adults.

• Generalized lymph node enlargement and tenderness, but neck nodes, including those at the back of the head, may be most affected.

• Fever.

• Sore throat.

• Feeling unwell.

• Symptoms may last for a few days to a few weeks.

• Characteristic changes in the blood: your doctor may confirm the diagnosis with a blood test.

• Spleen may become enlarged in up to 50 percent of cases.

### ■ Toxoplasmosis

A parasite that infects 50 percent of us. Mostly cures itself in one to three weeks. Acquired by eating infected, raw, or lightly cooked meat (or through contact with cat feces). Only about 20 percent of people affected actually have symptoms.

• Fever.

• Enlarged lymph nodes—neck nodes predominant—which may also be tender.

• Feeling unwell.

Diagnosis is confirmed by a blood test or by removing a lymph node and examining it under a microscope.

If a pregnant mother develops toxoplasmosis, there is a risk of the baby being damaged. Brain and eyes are primarily affected. In many countries, there is routine screening for toxoplasmosis.

Avoiding toxoplasmosis in pregnancy:
- Never eat raw or uncooked meat.
- Wash all fruit, vegetables, and salads well.
- Do not empty cat litter trays. (If you must do so, wear protective gloves.)
- Wear gloves for gardening.

■ **Peritonsillar Abscess**

Similar signs to tonsillitis, but:
- Pain on opening mouth also present because abscess or "quinsy" has developed.

Requires surgical drainage.

■ **Epiglottitis**
- Very painful throat.
- Pain on swallowing.
- Breathing changes.
- Open mouth breathing.
- Lymph nodes may be enlarged.
- High fever.

Get medical help urgently.

**RARE**

■ **German Measles**

Rubella. Most common in children.
- Runny nose.
- Red rash, mainly on body.
- Enlarged, tender neck lymph nodes, particularly over the back of the scalp, just above the neck.
- In teenage and adult females, there may be pains in the joints of the hands.

The use of the measles-mumps-rubella (MMR) vaccine can eradicate this in a population.

■ **Tuberculosis**
- Isolated non-tender lymph node enlargement; most common in immigrants.
- Redness.
- Skin overlying node(s) breaks down.
- Intermittent fever.

Skin tests and blood tests, or biopsy of the node, confirms the diagnosis. Drug treatment is required.

■ **Cancer of the Mouth or Upper Respiratory Passages (including Larynx)**

All these cancers can cause enlarged lymph nodes, often as a result of the cancer spreading. These are diseases especially of smokers in the fifty-plus age range.
- Persistently enlarged but painless lymph nodes.
- Other lump developing in mouth/tongue or palate.
- Change in voice.
- Weight loss.
- Feeling unwell.
- Persistent pain in mouth or neck.
- Dentures not fitting.
- Anemia.

## ■ Cancer Elsewhere in the Body

• Enlarged painless lymph nodes above the collarbone may suggest spread of a tumor from within the chest or abdomen, but would normally be accompanied by other symptoms from those areas.

## ■ Leukemias

Some or all of the following in combination:

• Enlarged painless lymph nodes in the neck or elsewhere.
• Persistently feeling unwell.
• Pallor, due to anemia.
• Shortness of breath.
• Fatigue.
• Bruising.

## ■ Lymphomas

May have no symptoms apart from:

• Painless, generalized enlargement of lymph nodes.

Later stages include:

• Fever.
• Weight loss.
• Anemia.

## ■ HIV/ARC/AIDS

HIV (human immunodeficiency virus) tends to infect people for years without making them ill. Eventually, however, it causes ARC (AIDS-related complex) and finally full-blown AIDS (acquired immune deficiency syndrome). The symptoms listed below cover the whole range from ARC to AIDS.

• Enlarged lymph nodes.
• Fever.
• Feeling unwell.

Anyone in a high-risk group for HIV infection should report persistently enlarged lymph nodes to their doctor. Effectiveness of treatment depends on early diagnosis.

# ABDOMEN: DIGESTIVE SYSTEM

The abdominal cavity lies below the rib cage and above the pelvic bones. The terms tummy, stomach, and gut are often used, the latter two incorrectly since they are organs that lie within the abdominal cavity.

The abdomen contains the organs of digestion and absorption: part of the esophagus, the stomach, the small intestine (including the duodenum, jejunum, and ileum), and the large bowel (including the appendix, colon, and rectum). It also contains organs connected to the gut that supply the chemicals necessary for digestion: the liver, pancreas, gallbladder, and biliary tract.

The abdomen also contains organs covered in other sections of this book, including the kidneys, ureters, and bladder, which are concerned with excreting urine, and the adrenal glands, which are responsible for secreting hormones that control many of the body's functions. The spleen, which is essentially like a

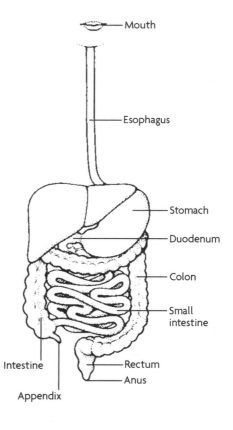

*Digestive System*

very large lymph gland, is located under the rib cage on the left side.

In men, there are also the prostate gland and the seminal vesicles, part of the reproductive system. In women, there are the uterus or womb, the fallopian tubes, and the ovaries. There are also many important blood vessels and nerves located here.

## VOMITING

Vomiting can be forceful or it can be passive, as when one regurgitates food into the mouth. Sometimes, bitter gastric or duodenal juices are vomited, sometimes undigested food, and sometimes blood (either fresh or old—sometimes called "coffee grounds" because of its appearance). In order to diagnose the underlying cause, you have to take precise note, however disagreeable, of the nature of the vomit. Excluded from this section are the all-too-familiar and obvious causes of vomiting: too much to drink, too much rich food to eat, and travel sickness.

Terminology: "Gastric contents" means typical vomit: partially digested and undigested food, pinkish yellow, frothy, foul-smelling. "Duodenal contents" means bile-stained (green), thin fluid, mixed with slime and clear secretions. "Fecal vomit" is exactly as the name suggests and is associated with a more severe or chronic vomiting situation where partially digested bowel contents are returned to the stomach and vomited.

### PROBABLE

#### ■ Gastroenteritis/Food Poisoning

Gastric or duodenal contents. Likely to be viral or can occur as part of food poisoning. Abdominal pain may be a feature.

Vomit is likely to contain partially digested and undigested food, and will look like "typical vomit" at first. After several vomits, clear, greenish-yellow liquid and slime.

*(See page 166)*

#### ■ Acute Gastritis

Gastric and duodenal contents with old blood, which appears as streaks of brown staining or looking like coffee granules. This is likely after a very heavy drinking bout. Abdominal pain might be a feature *(see page 171)*.

#### ■ Pregnancy

Gastric and duodenal contents. Other symptoms of pregnancy will be pronounced:

• Nausea, usually most marked on waking.

- Tendency to acid stomach and heartburn.

*(See also page 146)*

### ■ Migraine

Gastric and duodenal contents. Other migraine symptoms will be present *(see page 109)*.

### POSSIBLE

### ■ Peptic Ulcer

*(See page 169)* Gastric and duodenal contents.

### ■ Hiatus Hernia and Esophagitis

- A feeling akin to regurgitation.
- A feeling of acid in the lower throat; bilious taste.
- Symptoms of heartburn.
- If severe, vomiting undigested food; also, vomiting old (and sometimes fresh) blood.

### ■ Cancer of the Stomach

Vomiting can be a late feature of stomach cancer and may be present with other signs of cancer, such as malaise, marked weight loss, and anemia. Gastric and bowel contents.

- Likely to follow a progressive feeling of fullness after eating small quantities.

*(See also Stomach Disease, page 163)*

### ■ Intestinal Obstruction

- Pain in abdomen that comes and goes.

- No wind or feces passed rectally.
- Abdomen becomes distended.
- Bloated feeling.

Gastric and bowel contents, occasionally like diarrhea. *(See also page 166)*

### ■ Post-Gastrectomy Syndrome

*(See page 156)* Duodenal contents.

### ■ Pyloric Stenosis

The pylorus (from the Greek word for a "gate-keeper") is a muscular narrowing at the outlet of the stomach. Rarely, in newborn babies (invariably less than six weeks old), there is some overdevelopment of this muscle, which then blocks emptying of the stomach. Effortless and sometimes projectile vomiting of undigested milk develops within a few minutes of a feed. A very simple operation remedies the problem.

In adults, the gastric outlet can be narrowed by chronic scarring from an ulcer or from a cancer in this area. The vomit will be gastric contents (never bile stained) and can be quite spectacular as the stomach attempts to empty against the blockage.

### ■ Drugs

Many drugs have nausea and vomiting as side effects, including the opiates and many drugs used as chemotherapy agents for cancer.

## ■ Radiotherapy

Exposure to irradiation is a potent cause of nausea and vomiting. It typically comes on about four to eight hours after exposure and can limit a patient's ability to tolerate their treatment.

## ■ Diabetes

Uncontrolled diabetes, particularly insulin-dependent diabetes, can cause a dangerous situation with vomiting and rapid onset of dehydration. Sometimes, this can be the first presentation of diabetes.

## ■ Inner Ear Disease

Vertigo from vestibular neuronitis or benign paroxysmal positional vertigo (BPPV) can cause severe nausea and vomiting.

## RARE

## ■ Chronic Pancreatitis

*(See Diarrhea Plus Abdominal Pain, page 166)*
• Gastric contents.

## ■ Brain Tumor

*(See Brain section, page 405)*
• Gastric contents.

## ■ Brain Stem Stroke

A stroke in the brain stem can cause very severe vomiting, but other features are usually overwhelming.

## ■ Renal Failure

Acute or chronic.
• Mental confusion.
• Headache.
• Breath smelling of urine.
• Vomiting gastric contents.
• Coma.

## ■ Bulimia

*(See Anorexia Nervosa, page 437)*

## ■ Botulism

A dangerous but extremely rare form of food poisoning.
• Malaise.
• Nausea.
• Dizziness.
• Vomiting gastric and duodenal contents.
• Abdominal cramp and diarrhea.
• Breathing problems.
• Pupils wide open.
• Collapse leading to coma.

## ■ Cholera

*(See page 167)*

## ■ Bezoars

Occasionally, a fur ball can develop inside the stomach from constantly chewing on the hair. This gradually fills the cavity of the stomach and then any food consumed results in discomfort and sometimes vomiting.

## VOMITING BLOOD

*(See Abdominal Pain Plus Vomiting Blood, page 170)*

## VOMITING AND HEADACHE

*(See especially Migraine, page 109; see also Headache, page 108, and Headache with High Fever, page 111)*

## REGURGITATION

*(See Vomiting, page 140)*

## PROMINENT BLOOD VESSELS ON THE ABDOMEN

Unusually large surface veins sometimes develop on the skin of the abdomen. They may be a sign of an abnormality of underlying blood vessels and can be caused by blockage of vessels, pressure from some types of abdominal distension, or local pressure on veins from growths.

Other symptoms that may be present if any of these causes apply are:
• Leg swelling, sometimes one-sided.
• Lower abdominal wall veins most prominent.

• Caput medusae (Latin for "head of Medusa," one of the Gorgons in Greek mythology whose beautiful hair was changed into a head of serpents by the god Athena)—distended veins radiating out from the umbilicus.

Some conditions (all rare) that can cause these symptoms are acute pancreatitis *(see page 148)*, cirrhosis of the liver *(see page 149)*, malignant ascites *(see page 149)*, or ovarian cyst *(see page 149)*.

## GENERALIZED SWELLING OF THE ABDOMEN IN BABIES AND CHILDREN

**PROBABLE**

■ **Normal Variant**

The pot-bellied child is simply made that way, and because the tummy naturally bulges in childhood, it will not necessarily do so in adulthood.

### ■ Constipation

In some toddlers and children, there is a strong psychological element to constipation. It may well develop at potty training, when the child resists parental exhortation to pass stools, and it can develop into a lifelong habit.

Clothes may get soiled with feces—"apparent diarrhea"—and the underlying problem is a hard constipated stool, filling and blocking the rectum. This causes irritation and a constant urge to defecate. The irritation causes some "hurry" in the colon, resulting in a more liquid stool reaching the rectum before the fluid content has been reduced. This fluid stool then leaks past the blockage and escapes without conscious control.

Whatever you do, don't allow potty training to become a battleground between you and your child. A relaxed approach is usually best. All children will learn in time to control their bowels and bladder. Most problems are caused by overzealous caregivers pushing a child to be "clean" before he or she is ready. If you are in any doubt, get advice from your doctor.

*(See also Constipation, page 161)*

### POSSIBLE

### ■ Cystic Fibrosis

Most symptoms of this hereditary disease are caused by abnormal body secretions.
- Failure to thrive, but healthy appetite.
- Thin, with distended abdomen.
- Recurrent chest infections.
- Large amounts of smelly feces.
- Finger clubbing.
- Occasionally, the rectum may slip out through the anus (rectal prolapse).

### ■ Celiac Disease

Caused by an allergy to gluten, a component of wheat (in cereals, for example). Normally, the child will be underweight and will not grow as expected.
- Often, the child has a fair complexion.
- Child is unhappy.
- Appetite is poor.
- Muscles are wasted.
- Abdomen is distended.
- Occasional diarrhea and vomiting.

Treatment for celicac disease is a gluten-free diet for life, and a complete recovery can be expected.

### ■ Pre-Term Birth

Babies born pre-term may become constipated with bowel distension due to the presence of meconium, the greenish bowel contents present at birth. This stage usually passes quickly.

Prematurity is a measure of birth weight—less than 2,500 grams.

## RARE

### ■ Hirschsprung's Disease

Part of the bowel fails to develop proper-er nervous tissue and fails to work correctly, resulting in the progressive distension of the large bowel by feces. Large quantities may be retained. The abdomen may become massively swollen. Symptoms of constipation appear soon after birth, but the diagnosis is sometimes not made for years.

### ■ Kwashiorkor

Malnutrition caused by insufficient protein. All too common in underdeveloped countries, especially in poor, rural areas in the tropics.
- Unhappy child.
- Distended abdomen.
- Swelling of face and limbs.
- Dry, thin hair.
- Pigmented areas of skin.
- Occasional diarrhea.

## GENERALIZED SWELLING OF THE ABDOMEN

Described by doctors as distension. The common causes are obesity, wind, feces, fluid, or, in women, pregnancy. Doctors often find it difficult to decide whether there really is distension.

This section does not deal with isolated lumps or bumps felt in the abdomen and it excludes pregnancy. These aside, there are *many* causes of abdominal swelling; some, as one would expect, are harmless, and some suggest serious underlying disease.

It is important to consider whether symptoms associated with abdominal swelling are new and uncomfortable (such as pain and indigestion) or have built up slowly, possibly during a period when your personal circumstances al-

tered (for example, reduced exercise, "comfort eating," family crisis, or bereavement). Usually, it will be clear to you whether your symptoms are part of a long, even lifelong, history of abdominal discomfort or are new and therefore more likely to suggest an illness.

### PROBABLE

### ■ Obesity

An obvious and extremely common diagnosis, but worth considering in its own right. Fat does not just accumulate below the skin, it accumulates in the body cavities. Determine your correct weight for height and age, or ask your doctor what it should be. Any excess weight has to be stored somewhere.

## ■ Wind

Doctors call it flatus. Produced by the fermentation of food in the gut. Most of us are aware of those foods that cause the most wind.

## ■ Poor Muscle Tone

Many women develop protruding abdomens after childbirth. Often, intensive exercise is needed to get the abdominal wall muscles to revert to their original tone, and sometimes they never do. Men can also find that they acquire a "pot belly," either when they stop exercising or when they indulge in the steady consumption of beer.

## ■ Constipation

Most people have one bowel movement a day for most of their lives. Constipation is a term individuals may use if they believe they are not passing stools either easily or frequently enough. In fact, constipation should be divided into three types.

First, that in which hard, pellet-like or rock-like stools are passed, a common condition caused by change in diet and/ or lifestyle, often in younger people and in children.

Second, there are people who have bowel movements at long intervals—say, every week or fortnight. This has been their pattern for a long time, but they describe themselves as constipated. In fact, there is nothing essentially wrong: they are a variant of normal.

The third type is constipation of sudden onset, often in the elderly. Sometimes, it is impossible even to pass wind. This may suggest an underlying disorder, so report it to a doctor—it must be investigated.

Most people have regular bowel movements (even though they may be preoccupied, perhaps even obsessed, by variations). Often, bowel movements occur at about the same time every day. However, it is not necessarily abnormal not to have such a regular habit. What is always important is a *change from your usual pattern.* It is this that should be reported to your doctor.

## Possible

## ■ Pregnancy

Again, an apparently obvious diagnosis, but some women are taken unawares by pregnancy. Enough to say that an enlarging abdomen, missed periods, heartburn, fullness and discomfort of the breasts, with or without morning sickness, in a sexually active woman in the reproductive years are sound reasons for doing a home pregnancy test.

## ■ Irritable Bowel Syndrome

This is a remarkably common condition

in Western society, affecting most people to some extent from time to time. Sometimes, the symptoms are quite severe and unpleasant and cause a lot of concern to the individual, but examinations and tests are all normal. It is probably caused by abnormal motility of the gut. It tends to come and go and be related to anything that affects the gut's activity; for example, stress, change of diet, or unusual food. The typical picture is:

• Intermittent abdominal pain relieved by opening bowels.

• Variable bowel habit, fluctuating from loose frequent stools with urgency to constipation.

• Passage of mucus.

• Abdominal distension.

• Wind.

### ■ Diverticular Disease

A diverticulum is a small pouch on the wall of the large bowel. Along the length of the large bowel are three longitudinal muscles, and between these the wall of the bowel is relatively weaker. Chronic low-grade constipation results in the bowel having to squeeze harder to move the stool down and this increased pressure causes small pouches to develop through these weaker areas. Most people develop them as they get older, but only a few will get symptoms. These usually

arise if one of the diverticula becomes inflamed.

• Change of bowel habit.

• Steady or colicky abdominal pain, often on the left side.

• Abdominal distension.

• Pellet-like stools.

• Occasional passage of dark to bright red blood from the rectum.

If the inflammation becomes severe, with:

• Fever.

• Intense pain.

• A tender lump in the abdomen.

This condition is then called diverticulitis. It usually resolves with antibiotic treatment.

Decreasing the amount of food you eat allows the gut to rest and will also help. In the long term, it is important to maintain a high-fiber diet to enable the large bowel to function at a lower pressure, as the stool becomes softer.

### ■ Heart Failure

Severe untreated heart failure can result in the accumulation of fluid in the abdominal cavity in addition to several other symptoms. *(See page 210)*

### ■ Perforated Viscus

A hollow internal organ. The major symptom of this condition is pain, which will dominate any discomfort or swelling of the abdomen.

Any of the hollow organs within the abdominal cavity can become inflamed or damaged. If the inflammation or damage is severe enough, the wall of the organ—typically the stomach, small bowel, colon, or appendix—bursts. Gut contents leak into the abdominal cavity. This material contains organisms that can cause peritonitis (inflammation of the abdominal cavity) if treatment is delayed. This can be fatal.

The symptoms are similar whichever organ perforates, although initially the site of pain may be different. An inflamed appendix, a peptic ulcer, and a diverticulum may all burst.

- Sudden onset of severe pain.
- Fever.
- Very tender abdomen (muscles of the abdominal wall appear rigid).
- Pale, sweating face, sunken eyes.
- Eventually, distension of the abdomen caused by leakage of gas and contents from the gut.
- Shock may develop *(see page 420).*

### ■ Bowel Cancer

Includes cancer of the colon and rectum. This can block the intestine, either gradually or suddenly. Though a common symptom is a change in bowel habit (type or frequency of stool), swelling

(distension) of the abdomen may be caused by a buildup of food, fluid, feces, or wind. Other possible symptoms may include:

- Colicky, abdominal pain.
- Possibly intermittent symptoms.
- Slime or mucus in stool.
- Abnormal stools.
- Blood in stools.

## Rare

### ■ Acute Pancreatitis

Abdominal pain will be a major and primary symptom of this condition. It is inflammation of the pancreas, which lies at the back of the abdominal cavity and produces chemicals, known as enzymes, which help with digestion of food. If inflamed, the pancreas can actually start digesting your own innards. There are mild or very severe, and sometimes fatal, forms. People who drink excessive amounts of alcohol or who have a history of gallbladder disease are at increased risk. Features include:

- Continuous, central abdominal pain.
- Pain may radiate to the back.
- Vomiting.
- Malaise.
- Slight jaundice may appear a couple of days after the initial attack.
- Bruising/discoloration around the umbilicus or flanks after two to three days.

Some individuals who collapse for no apparent reason are later found to have pancreatitis.

## ■ Cirrhosis of the Liver

An irreversible degeneration of the liver that has many causes. Perhaps the most well-known is alcohol abuse. Features of advanced cirrhosis are:

• Malaise, weakness.
• Weight loss.
• Anorexia.
• Swelling of the ankles.
• Abdominal distension due to fluid in the abdominal cavity (ascites).
• Vomiting, sickness.
• Vomiting blood, blood in stools.
• Jaundice.
• Mental deterioration.
• Easy bruising.
• Red vascular marks on skin (spider nevi).
• Clubbing of the nails *(see page 302).*

In men:
• Enlargement of the breasts.
• Shrinkage of the testes.

Other causes of cirrhosis, of which there are several different types, include active chronic hepatitis, hemochromatosis, Wilson's disease, primary biliary cirrhosis, Budd-Chiari syndrome, and chronic cardiac failure.

In most cases, the individual is aware of the primary diagnosis before cirrhosis develops.

## ■ Malignant Ascites

Cancer of any organ within the abdominal cavity may lead to the formation of fluid in the abdominal cavity (ascites). In addition to the symptoms of the original cancer, individuals may develop:

• Tense, distended abdomen.
• Swelling of the ankles.
• Shortness of breath (due to pressure on the diaphragm).

## ■ Ovarian Cyst

Very occasionally, an enormous cyst may develop on an ovary, causing abdominal distension. It requires surgery.

## ■ Intestinal Obstruction

The intestine is a term for the stomach and the small and the large bowel. Blockage can occur for many reasons. The features are similar:

• Colicky, often central abdominal pain (site dependent on cause).
• Abdominal distension; if low, ileum or colon/rectum obstruction is likely.
• Vomiting may be an early feature of stomach or jejunal obstruction, later involving the ileum. It tends to be a late feature of colon obstruction.
• Constipation—no stools and often no wind.

• Loops of bowel may be seen undulating under the skin surface as they try to overcome the obstruction.

• Perforation may ultimately occur *(see Perforated Viscus, page 147)*.

Urgent medical attention is needed.

Causes include:

Hernia—Strangulated hernia (rupture) in groin may become painful and not be able to be pushed back.

Cancer—Other features of cancer may have been present earlier; for example, altered bowel habit (constipation/diarrhea), weight loss, anorexia, or anemia.

Inflammation—For example, Crohn's disease or diverticular disease. A fibrous internal band, sometimes referred to as adhesions, is common after abdominal surgery. The bowel gets twisted internally around fibrous tissue present from, or after, birth.

Volvulus—The bowel twists on itself, causing a blockage.

Gallstone—Occasionally, a gallstone passes into the bowel and gets jammed in the narrowest part (the end of the ileum).

## ■ Ulcerative Colitis

Chronic disease of the colon. Main features:

• Diarrhea.

• In acute attacks, blood, mucus, and pus are passed.

• Abdominal pain and fever in acute cases.

• As a complication of some cases, abdominal swelling.

## OVERALL SWELLING OF THE ABDOMEN PLUS DIARRHEA

### PROBABLE

■ Obesity

■ Wind

*(See page 146)*

### POSSIBLE

■ Constipation

Occasionally, someone, especially an elderly person, can become so constipated that other gut contents leak out of the rectum past the impacted mass of feces. This gives the impression of diarrhea.

■ Irritable Bowel Syndrome

■ Diverticular Disease

*(See page 147)*

■ Factitious Diarrhea

Some people take laxatives as a matter of habit and yet complain of diarrhea. They may be doing so in order to lose weight, but sometimes doctors are faced with people who cannot explain why they take laxatives so often, or they may deny it altogether. So this is worth considering for any individual who complains of diarrhea, yet is otherwise well. Some laxatives cause associated abdominal distension and discomfort.

### ■ Crohn's Disease

Tends to occur in young adults.
• Intermittent, colicky pain with or without diarrhea.
• With or without weight loss.

• Spontaneously resolves and relapses.
• Sometimes taken for a "grumbling appendix."
• Occasionally, intestinal obstruction due to narrowing of bowel.

Drug treatment and/or surgery may be needed.

### RARE

### ■ Bowel Cancer

*(See below)*

### ■ Ulcerative Colitis

*(See page 459)*

## OVERALL SWELLING OF THE ABDOMEN PLUS CONSTIPATION

### PROBABLE

### ■ Wind

### ■ Constipation

*(See pages 146 and 161)*

### POSSIBLE

### ■ Irritable Bowel Syndrome

### ■ Diverticular Disease

*(See page 147)*

### RARE

### ■ Bowel Cancer

Most bowel cancer originates in the rectum, colon, or cecum. It may present in many ways or be found incidentally on routine examination. It is possible to divide symptoms into right colon plus cecum and left colon plus rectum. *(See also Intestinal Obstruction, page 149)*

Right colon plus cecum:
• Vague lower abdominal pain.
• Pain may localize to right side.
• Mass in right side of abdomen.
• Change in bowel habit (often diarrhea, occasionally constipation).
• Anemia and associated symptoms *(see page 430)* due to slow blood loss.

Left colon plus rectum:
• Increasing constipation.
• Intermittent diarrhea.

- Colicky abdominal pain and distension.
- Blood present when passing stools.
- Mass in left side of abdomen.

Any persistent change in bowel habit in someone over fifty must be assessed by a doctor.

## QUICKLY FEELING FULL ON EATING

### ■ Post-Gastric Surgery

If surgery to remove a diseased stomach leaves only a small part behind, relatively small meals make you feel replete.

### ■ Stomach Cancer

*(See Stomach Disease, page 163)*
- Bezoar *(see page 142)*.
- General malaise.

## WORMS

There are four types of worm that most commonly affect humans. In developed countries, the only type of worm normally seen is the threadworm.

Threadworms are an extremely common infestation among schoolchildren. Most children will have them at some time. Typically, a child wakes with an itchy anus at night, as the female worm typically comes out onto the anus at night to lay her eggs. Small, white, thread-like worms can be seen on the skin of the anus and, less easily, in the stools.

Treatment is simple, with medicine that should normally be taken by all family members. The commonest source of threadworm infestation is another child with them, but the eggs can live in garden soil. Washing hands and scrubbing nails helps prevent infection or reinfection.

### PROBABLE

### ■ Threadworm
- Anal irritation.
- May prevent sleep.
- Worms observed in stools.

### POSSIBLE

### ■ Roundworms *(Ascaris lumbricoides)*
- May be no symptoms.
- Worm observed in stools.
- Occasionally, abdominal pain.
- Occasionally, the lungs become inflamed.
- Occasionally, an urticarial skin reaction develops *(see page 263)*.

### ■ Hookworms

- May cause chronic bleeding from small intestine.
- Anemia.
- Malaise.
- Diarrhea.

### ■ Tapeworms

- Abdominal discomfort.
- Increased appetite.
- Segments of worms seen in stools.

All types of worm infestation should be assessed and treated by a doctor.

## TAR-LIKE STOOLS

*(See Blood from the Back Passage, page 156)*

## PALE-COLORED FECES

Feces are normally colored brown by a mixture of the body's bile pigments and bacteria. Certain conditions hinder this pigmentation; and sometimes bile is excreted instead via urine, which then appears dark brown or orange. There may also be jaundice and sometimes itching.

Jaundice occurs when pigments that are normally excreted in bowel or urine as waste products build up in the body to such an extent that they color the eyes and skin with a yellow tinge.

### PROBABLE

### ■ Gallstones

*(See Cholecystitis, page 172)*

### ■ Hepatitis

Several different types of virus cause hepatitis. Some are more significant than others and so suspected hepatitis needs professional attention. In some cases, the disease is so mild it is assumed to be a cold or flu.

- Lethargy.
- Loss of appetite.
- Loss of desire for cigarettes and alcohol.
- Nausea.
- Joint pains.
- Variable rash.
- Right-sided upper abdominal pain.
- Fever.
- Diarrhea.

The pale stools, dark urine, and jaundice appear (if, indeed, they are going to) after a few days. In mild cases, jaundice may not be a feature.

## POSSIBLE

■ **Cancer of the Pancreas**

*(See Diseased Pancreas, page 164)*

■ **Chronic Pancreatitis**

*(See page 167)*

■ **Cirrhosis of the Liver**

*(See page 149)*

■ **Liver Tumors**

*(See Liver Disease, page 164)*

■ **Drugs**

Rarely, certain drugs can cause damage and swelling of the tiny bile ducts in the liver and cause jaundice with a picture similar to blockage of the main bile duct, with pale stools and jaundice.

## RARE

■ **Jaundice of Pregnancy**

Occurs in a small proportion of women. Normally harmless and appears in the final three months.

■ **Biliary Atresia**

Failure of the biliary tract to develop properly in a fetus.
• Jaundice a few days after birth.
• Itching.
• Retarded growth.
• Cirrhosis develops.
• Malabsorption.

Liver transplants offer hope.

■ **Sclerosing Cholangitis (Adult)**

For some unknown reason, the bile ducts grow fibrous and shrink.
• Progressive jaundice.
• Itching.
• Liver failure after a few years.

## VERY RARE

■ **Cancer of the Bile Ducts**

Causes jaundice with pale feces and dark urine, associated with other signs of cancer, such as weight loss.

## DIARRHEA

Can be difficult to define; perhaps the most useful criterion is whether the passage of stools is loose enough or frequent enough to be inconvenient.

Diarrhea may be watery, green-yellow, bloody (bright red, dark, or tarry), a nor-mal color, or mixed with mucus and pus. Strictly speaking, blood passed via the anus is not diarrhea, but as it is often difficult to tell it from liquid stools, it is also included under this heading.

## PROBABLE

### ■ Gastroenteritis

Loose, runny, watery. *(See page 166)*

### ■ Irritable Bowel Syndrome

Slightly loose normal stool. *(See page 146)*

### ■ Diverticular Disease

Normal stool, but may be blood-streaked or with dark blood mixed in. *(See page 147)*

## POSSIBLE

### ■ Factitious Diarrhea

Loose, but normal. *(See page 150)*

### ■ Crohn's Disease

Loose, but normal. *(See page 151)*

### ■ Ulcerative Colitis

Loose stools with blood, mucus, and pus. *(See page 459)*

### ■ Bowel Cancer

Loose, but normal, and may be blood-streaked. *(See page 148)*

### ■ Celiac Disease

Loose, pale, and bulky. *(See page 144)*

### ■ Chronic Pancreatitis

Loose, pale, bulky, smelly. *(See page 167)*

### ■ Bacillary Dysentery

Loose, bloody, with pus and mucus. *(See page 167)*

### ■ Sprue

Malabsorption that starts with an initial attack of diarrhea.

• Persistent diarrhea.
• Stools are bulky, pale, and fatty.
• Progressive weight loss.
• Anorexia.
• Anemia.
• Edema.
• Inflamed tongue.

Requires antibiotics.

### ■ Traveler's Diarrhea

Diarrhea after traveling in countries with poor standards of hygiene. Needs investigation if bloody, persistent, or the sufferer feels very unwell.

### ■ AIDS-Related Diarrhea

Patients with acquired immunodeficiency syndrome (AIDS) commonly have diarrhea and abdominal pain as symptoms. Investigations are needed to decide whether these symptoms are related to AIDS alone or to bacterial infection.

### ■ Hyperthyroidism

Loose, but normal. *(See page 350)*

■ **Kwashiorkor**

Loose, but normal. *(See page 129)*

■ **Post-Gastrectomy Syndrome**

After the removal of part of the stomach (a gastrectomy), diarrhea is a common complaint. Fortunately, since the introduction of modern ulcer-curing drugs, gastrectomy is no longer as common an operation as it once was.

■ **Drugs**

Many drugs (e.g., Metformin) cause diarrhea as a side effect. Discuss with your doctor.

**RARE**

■ **Carcinoid Syndrome**

*(See page 168)*

■ **Cholera**

Profuse, watery. *(See page 167)*

■ **Typhoid**

Loose, watery. *(See page 168)*

## BLOOD FROM THE BACK PASSAGE

This can appear in several forms: fresh, bright red; darkish, coming from the colon; or "tarry," coming from even higher up the gut, such as the duodenum. In general, any disease that can cause bleeding in the gut may produce either vomited blood and/or blood passed in stools.

**PROBABLE**

■ **Piles**

Medical term, hemorrhoids. These lumps are engorged veins from the lining of the rectum and are pushed out from the anal canal; a very common complaint.

• Bright red bleeding after defecation, seen in the toilet and on toilet paper.

• Pain is not a symptom of uncomplicated hemorrhoids.

• Fleshy lumps felt protruding intermittently from the anus after defecation, which can and should be encouraged back above the anal sphincter. However, some hemorrhoids remain permanently protruding.

Piles are normally caused by a diet that is abnormally low in roughage; stress, leading to changes in diet; or pregnancy, which puts pressure on the veins around the rectum. You can usually cure 90 percent of piles by increasing the amount of roughage in your diet, ideally by adding bran. Severe cases may need injection or, rarely, surgical treatment.

## ▪ Anal Fissure

*(See page 158)*

### POSSIBLE

### ▪ Polyps

Intestinal polyps (growths of the tissue lining the ileum), which are initially benign growths, may cause anemia or episodes of rectal bleeding. As they grow, the risk of cancerous change increases. *(See also Bowel Cancer, page 148)*

### ▪ Diverticular Disease

*(See page 147)*

### ▪ Bowel Cancer

*(See page 148)*

### ▪ Bleeding Peptic Ulcer

This can cause a black, tarry bowel movement, in association with other symptoms. Sometimes a black stool is the first and only sign of a significant episode of internal bleeding from the gut. The stool is black because the blood is altered by its passage through the gut. It is shiny black and has a distinctive unpleasant smell (the black stool that occurs with iron therapy does not have the same smell and is matte black).

### ▪ Drug-Induced

Certain drugs (particularly steroids and nonsteroidal anti-inflammatory drugs, or NSAIDs, including aspirin) may cause gastric bleeding. Initial symptoms may include vomiting blood or tarry stools.

### RARE

### ▪ Esophageal Varices

Delicate, distended veins in the lower end of the esophagus. They may be present with cirrhosis of the liver *(see page 149)*. Esophageal varices may cause massive vomiting of blood and also bleeding from the back passage or the appearance of black stools. This condition can be fatal because of sudden blood loss.

### ▪ Intussusception

This condition is extremely painful and a medical emergency. Intussusception is a bowel abnormality that tends to occur when the body tries to expel unwanted

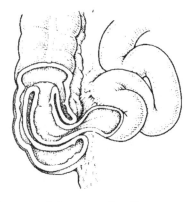

*Intussusception*

tissue such as polyps. (See illustration on page 158.)

In children, it is the most common form of bowel obstruction. Often, no underlying cause is found, but sometimes it can be caused by inflamed lymph nodes in the wall of the intestine or a condition known as a Meckel's diverticulum.

- Severe, colicky abdominal pain.
- Thighs and knees drawn up because of pain.
- Blood-stained stools and mucus are passed (though this is usually a late sign).
- Vomiting.
- Abdominal distension.

### ■ Jejunal Diverticula

Like the colon, the jejunum (a section of the small intestine) may develop multiple diverticula. *(See Diverticular Disease, page 147)*

- Tarry stools.
- Often pain free.
- Sometimes diarrhea due to altered digestion and absorption.

### ■ Meckel's Diverticulum

This is like an extra appendix but originates in the ileum (the last part of the small intestine). Very rarely, it can cause bleeding or an intussusception *(see page 157)*.

## PAIN AROUND ANUS OR IN RECTUM

### PROBABLE

### ■ Piles

*(See page 156)*

### ■ Anal Fissure

A small tear in the surface tissue of the anal canal, usually caused by the passage of hard feces. Sometimes this can be a feature of Crohn's disease, though it may have been caused by injury (perhaps during anal intercourse).

- Local pain, worse after passing a stool.
- Pain stops the individual from wanting to move their bowels, and they can become constipated.

- Occasional bleeding (bright red) may be noted (in toilet or on toilet paper).

Pain-relieving creams that allow anal muscle relaxation may help healing, which will often occur spontaneously.

### ■ Proctalgia Fugax

This odd condition is probably due to cramping of the muscles that internally support the anus. Brief episodes of intense, deep anal pain can occur without warning. Often relieved by reducing stress levels and ensuring a high-fiber diet.

## POSSIBLE

### ■ Anal Abscess

The anus or anal canal and rectum are common sites for infection, because of the moist environment and the many organisms present in feces.

All abscesses need surgical assessment and treatment.

• Localized throbbing pain (either around the anus or in the rectum).
• Local tender swelling.
• Reddening of the skin, if near the surface.
• Often fever.
• Often malaise.
• Often a fast pulse rate.

Possible underlying diseases that cause severe or recurrent abscesses are diabetes mellitus *(see page 180)* and Crohn's disease *(see page 151).*

## RARE

### ■ Fistula-in-Ano

A fistula may be the final result of an abscess that has burst through the skin and bowel, creating a false passage.

• Persistent fecal discharge on skin near anus.

## ITCHING ANUS

Itching is usually a sign of inflammation, infection, or infestation of the skin's surface. It can occur as a result of an underlying illness in the rest of the body, which makes the skin more vulnerable to this sensation in one particular area.

### ■ "Occupational Hazard"

The term is a euphemism for the fact that, by its nature, the anal area, moist and subject to infective organisms, is prone to infection and irritation. People who sit all day (particularly in well-contoured car seats) and who have stressful jobs are perhaps especially prone to this problem.

Regular washing and proper drying will reduce itching. On the other hand, overzealous washing and wiping can damage the skin surface, also causing minor irritation and itching. A mild steroid cream can be helpful; get a doctor's advice.

### ■ Threadworm

*(See page 152)*

### ■ Piles

*(See page 156)*

### ■ Yeast Infection

Because this area is continuously moist and damp, it is vulnerable to yeast and fungal infections such as thrush, which is caused by the yeast *Candida*. Simple antifungal creams can cure the condition. However, it may recur.

### ■ Low-Grade Infection

In children especially, a low-grade infection with a bowel organism *(Enterococcus faecalis)* can cause a chronic anal irritation and merits a swab and appropriate antibiotic treatment.

### POSSIBLE

### ■ Pruritus Ani

Some people scratch the anal region as a matter of habit or when tense. Constant scratching causes inflammation, cracking, itching, and discomfort.

### ■ Lichen Sclerosus et Atrophicus (LSA)

This condition is not rare, but is often missed. *(See Skin section)*

### ■ Anal Fissure

*(See page 158)* Individuals with anal fissures occasionally complain of local itching or irritation.

### ■ Fistula-in-Ano

*(See page 159)* Those with anal fistulas occasionally complain of local irritation and itching.

### ■ Pilonidal Sinus

A small hole underneath the skin between the buttocks, thought to be created by a hair growing into and under the skin. It can cause recurrent infection and itching.

### RARE

### ■ Diabetes Mellitus

*(See page 180)* Some diabetics complain of an itching perianal region, for which no other local cause is apparent.

### ■ Shingles

Rarely occurs in the anal region. Painful itching can precede the onset of this unpleasant blistering condition. When it involves this area, it is a medical priority.

## CHANGE IN BOWEL HABIT

*(See Constipation, page 161, and Diarrhea, page 154)* Any change in bowel habit that does not have a simple explanation, such as a sudden change in diet, should be reported to your doctor.

## CONSTIPATION

A diagnosis as well as a symptom. *(For details on constipation as a diagnosis, see page 146)*

### PROBABLE

■ **Inadequate Diet**

A diet too low in fluids and/or roughage will cause constipation.

■ **Pregnancy**

There are two main causes for constipation in pregnancy:
• Decreased movement of the gut.
• The pressure of the growing womb on the colon.

*(See page 146)*

■ **Anal Fissure**

*(See page 158)*

■ **Drug Side Effect**

Many painkillers, in particular codeine and morphine, contain substances that may cause constipation. Many other drugs may also cause constipation as a side effect.

### POSSIBLE

■ **Diverticular Disease**

*(See page 147)*

■ **Intestinal Obstruction**

*(See page 149)*

■ **Bowel Cancer**

*(See page 151)*

■ **Pre-term Birth**

*(See page 144)*

■ **Immobility**

Anyone relatively immobile or bedridden (for example, the elderly or anyone who has had a head injury, stroke, or progressive neurological disease) is prone to constipation.

### RARE

■ **Crohn's Disease**

*(See page 151)*

■ **Hirschsprung's Disease**

*(See page 129)*

## A SWELLING FELT WITHIN THE ABDOMEN

Any organ inside the abdomen can, if diseased, appear as a swelling, a lump, or a mass. You might notice this yourself or your doctor may do so at a routine examination. This is such a general symptom that we'll list only the principal possible causes here. You must a see a doctor if you suspect any of these problems. Pregnancy is excluded from the possibilities.

## PROBABLE

### ■ Inguinal and Femoral Hernias

Hernias are protrusions of bowel through weak spots in the muscular wall of the abdomen. Although not, strictly speaking, in the abdomen, they may be noticed as lumps in the groin. Inguinal hernias are very much more common than femoral hernias.

• May make a gurgling sound.
• Can be pushed back into the abdomen.
• May disappear at night, reappearing once you are up and about.
• In men, hernias may extend down into the scrotum.
• Hernias gradually enlarge.

Sometimes the bowel gets trapped in the hernia, causing intestinal obstruction *(see page 149)*. If this happens, the following may be noticed:

• The hernia becomes painful.
• It cannot be pushed back.
• Intermittent abdominal pain.
• Possibly vomiting.

Surgery may be needed.

### ■ Umbilical Hernia

Symptoms are the same as for inguinal and femoral hernias *(see above)*, but are less likely to obstruct the gut. They are most common in babies and infants, particularly in African Americans. They sometimes disappear as the abdominal muscles develop.

## POSSIBLE

### ■ Enlarged Bladder

Usually caused by an enlarged prostate *(see page 188)*.

• Mid-line swelling in the lower abdomen above the pubic bone.
• Constant pain.
• Inability to pass urine.
• Possibly dribbling of urine.

### ■ Aortic Aneurysm

Swelling of the body's main artery. It may burst without warning.

• Abdominal pain.
• A swelling in the middle of abdomen that pulsates in time with the heartbeat.
• Back pain.
• Sometimes, sudden collapse.

Often, the individual is unaware of the aneurysm until the sudden onset of severe pain.

### ■ Cancer of the Colon or Rectum

*(See Bowel Cancer, page 148)*

### ■ Enlarged Gallbladder

The gallbladder may become enlarged for two main reasons. If it is caused by infection:

- Upper right abdominal pain.
- May be a tender mass jutting below the right rib margin.
- Pain may be made worse by breathing in.
- Fever.
- Malaise.

If it is a tumor (of the pancreas, bile ducts, or gallbladder):

- Jaundice.
- Non-tender mass in right upper abdomen.
- Pale stools.
- Dark urine.
- Other signs of malignant disease may be present.

## ■ Problems of the Ovaries

Ovarian cysts *(page 149)* and cancer of the ovaries can produce abdominal swelling, which can be extreme.

## ■ Stomach Disease

Virtually the only reason for a palpably enlarged stomach in an adult is a tumor, although even in established cases (for example, stomach cancers), the enlarged stomach can only be felt in a minority of individuals. The pylorus may be felt occasionally in babies with hypertrophic pyloric stenosis *(see page 141)*. Other features of stomach cancer (rare under the age of forty-five) include:

- Anorexia.

- Indigestion and abdominal pain.
- Weight loss.
- Anemia.
- Upper abdominal midline mass.
- Occasionally vomiting, if the pylorus in blocked.
- Even more occasionally, vomiting blood.
- Sometimes the individual goes to a doctor complaining of jaundice and ascites *(see page 149)*, both the result of the tumor having already spread.
- Hypertrophic pyloric stenosis.
- Mostly in baby boys, the stomach outlet is blocked by thickened intestinal muscle.

## RARE

## ■ Appendicitis

Inflammation of the appendix. A lump is rarely a noticeable feature of appendicitis; however, if appendicitis is not diagnosed at an early stage, a lump may subsequently appear a few days later, which can be felt in the right side of the abdomen; called an appendix mass.

- Right-sided lower abdominal pain— often starts over the belly button, or umbilicus, and then moves down and to the right.
- Pain worse on pressing over appendix.
- There may be fever.
- Anorexia.

- Nausea and sometimes vomiting.
- Malaise.

## ■ Kidney Disease

Kidney enlargement may be noticed on the right or left sides of the abdomen and in the loin, and may be felt as a mass. Enlargement is caused by tumor, polycystic disease, or urinary obstruction *(see relevant entries in Digestive System and Urinary System sections)*.

Enlargement is one, not often very noticeable, symptom of these conditions.

## ■ Liver Disease

The liver lies under the right rib cage but extends across the midline. An individual may feel or see the enlargement as a mass moving in and out with respiration. The main reasons for enlargement are:

Cirrhosis *(see page 149)*.

Cancer—Several types of cancer can spread to the liver, including breast and lung. But they do not automatically do so; and in most cases, the cancer is already diagnosed and being treated. Occasionally, the liver is the original site of the tumor, known as a hepatoma; it can be treated surgically.

Infection—The liver may become infected by a number of organisms and liver abscesses may develop:

- Swinging fever.
- Sweating.

- Right upper abdominal pain.
- Enlarged, tender liver.
- Sometimes jaundice.
- Malaise.

Hydatid disease—Infection from a tapeworm; causes cysts to form in the liver:
- Often no symptoms.
- Occasionally, the liver is enlarged because of a big cyst.

## ■ Diseased Pancreas

The pancreas lies at the back of the abdomen and may enlarge through inflammation or malignant disease.

Cancer of the pancreas—Symptoms include:
- Abdominal pain.
- Wasting.
- Nausea.
- Jaundice.
- Pale stools.
- Dark urine.
- Occasional vomiting.

Pancreatitis—*(See page 148)* Acute pancreatitis sometimes develops a complication called a pseudocyst, a large cyst that may be felt as a mass in the middle of the abdomen.

## ■ Diseased Spleen

The spleen may be felt as a mass in the abdomen when enlarged two to three times its normal size. Its tip can be felt under the left rib margins. It may be enlarged by any viral infection (typically, glandular fever), but if it is noticed as a mass, the main causes would be:

Malaria *(see page 465).*

Kala-azar (visceral leishmaniasis)—An infection spread by sandflies:

- Fever.
- Sweating.
- Massive splenic enlargement.
- Liver enlargement.
- Lymph gland enlargement.
- Anemia.

Chronic myeloid leukemia:

- Anemia.

- Discomfort in abdomen due to large spleen.
- Night sweats.
- Fever.
- Loss of weight.
- Occasional generalized itchiness.

Myelofibrosis—Often in association with other illnesses such as cancer:

- Anemia.
- Weakness.
- Enlarged spleen.
- Gout.

### ■ Diseased Uterus

*(See Cancer of the Womb, page 341)*

## RIGID ABDOMEN

*(See Perforated Viscus, page 147)*

## TENDER ABDOMEN

*(See all symptoms under Abdominal Pain, pages 165–173 and 478–480)*

## CONSTANT VERY SEVERE PAIN IN THE ABDOMEN

As a main symptom, this will quite rightly send you straight to a doctor. Don't delay the visit. The causes listed here are not common, but they need immediate attention.

**POSSIBLE**

### ■ Perforated Viscus

*(See page 147)*

### ■ Mesenteric Vascular Occlusion

The blood supply to the gut is interrupted because of blockage in the gut's main blood vessels.

- Severe pain, starting suddenly.
- Bloody stools.
- Vomiting.
- Shock.
- Occasionally, abdominal distension.

**RARE**

■ **Acute Pancreatitis**

Occasionally, pancreatitis starts suddenly with very severe upper abdominal pain *(see page 148)*.

■ **Ruptured Aortic Aneurysm**

*(See page 162)*

## SEVERE BUT INTERMITTENT ABDOMINAL PAIN

This suggests a different set of causes to those of constant severe pain *(see above)*.

**PROBABLE**

■ **Kidney Stones**

- Early appendicitis *(see page 163)*.

**POSSIBLE**

■ **Intestinal Obstruction**

*(See page 149)*

■ **Biliary Colic**

Caused by gallstones temporarily blocking a bile duct.

- Intense pain lasting from minutes to hours.

- Pain is in upper abdomen and may pass to shoulder tip.
- Vomiting.
- Individual is pale and clammy.
- Possibly jaundice.
- Possibly fever or shivering.
- Very rarely, the pain from a heart attack can be present as abdominal colic.
- Uterine cramps (period pains).
- Ectopic pregnancy.
- Torsion of an ovarian cyst.
- Torsion of the testicle can present with abdominal pain as the nerve supply to the testicle is dragged down into the scrotum and therefore pain is referred to the central abdomen.

## DIARRHEA PLUS ABDOMINAL PAIN

**PROBABLE**

■ **Gastroenteritis**

Otherwise known as food poisoning.

Often caused by viral infections, but certain bacterial causes (such as *Campylobacter*) characteristically cause painful and sometimes bloody diarrhea. Very common. Episodes rarely last more than twenty-four to thirty-six hours and cure themselves.

- Abdominal pain.
- Vomiting.
- Watery diarrhea.
- Muscle/joint pains.
- Headache.
- Occasional fever.

## ■ Irritable Bowel Syndrome

*(See page 146)*

## POSSIBLE

## ■ Bowel Cancer

## ■ Crohn's Disease

## ■ Ulcerative Colitis

*(See page 459)*

## ■ Chronic Pancreatitis

Inflammation of the pancreas resulting in permanent and irreversible damage. Alcohol is commonly implicated; if you have the condition, you will have to stop drinking.

- Pain worsened by food and alcohol. Often very persistent.
- Malabsorption, due to lack of digestive enzymes, causes fatty diarrhea.
- Weight loss.
- Diabetes develops *(see page 180)*.
- Occasionally associated with jaundice, pale stools, and dark urine.

## ■ Bacillary Dysentery

Caused by person-to-person spread of a bacterium *(Shigella)*.

- Fever.
- Abdominal pain.
- Watery diarrhea.
- After one to three days, bloody diarrhea with mucus.

Most cases cure themselves, although antibiotics may help.

## RARE

## ■ Pernicious Anemia

The lining of the stomach stops producing acid and other essential substances. Occurs in people over thirty years of age.

- Anemia, slow onset.
- Sore tongue.
- Tingling and/or numbness of extremities (peripheral neuropathy).
- Fever.
- Abdominal pain.
- Diarrhea.
- Mild jaundice.

## ■ Cholera

Common in some underdeveloped countries. Caused by an organism *(Vibrio cholerae)* present in water, so it's a major problem when water supplies are contaminated.

- Initially, mild diarrhea.
- Then, large volumes of diarrhea.

- Vomiting.
- Abdominal pain.
- Thirst.
- Muscle cramps.
- Slight fever.

Treatment is aimed at minimizing dehydration.

## ■ Typhoid Fever

Caused by one of the *Salmonella* organisms. In the first week:

- Increasing fever.
- Abdominal pain.
- Headache.
- Cough.

In the second week:

- General malaise.
- Apathy.
- Fever.
- Abdominal distension.
- Diarrhea.
- "Rose" spots on abdomen.

Fatal in some cases, but antibiotics can change the course of the disease.

## ■ Post-Gastrectomy Syndrome

Gastrectomy is surgical removal of the stomach. After a meal, within two or three hours, there may be:

- Upper abdominal distension.
- Faintness.
- Weakness.
- Palpitations.
- Sweating.
- Diarrhea.

## ■ Carcinoid Syndrome

Carcinoid tumors may appear in any part of the gut. They cause many symptoms, due to the chemicals they secrete, including:

- Facial flushing.
- Explosive, watery diarrhea.
- Abdominal pain.
- Asthmatic wheeze.
- Pain in the abdomen and weight loss.
- Sweating.

## ABDOMINAL PAIN AND PROGRESSIVE LOSS OF WEIGHT

This combination needs to be taken seriously. Your doctor will consider the following possibilities. They are not listed in order of probability; diagnosis depends upon accompanying symptoms.

Crohn's disease *(see page 151)*.

Ulcerative colitis *(see page 459)*.

Chronic pancreatitis *(see page 167)*.

Cancer of the pancreas *(see page 181)*.

Cancer of the stomach *(see page 163)*.

Cancer of the bowel *(see page 151)*.

Spread of cancer to the liver *(see page 448)*.

## ABDOMINAL PAIN PLUS VOMITING

### PROBABLE

■ **Gastroenteritis**

*(See page 166)*

■ **Mesenteric Adenitis**

Often mistaken for appendicitis in children *(see page 163)*. This condition is caused by enlargement of lymph glands in the abdomen, usually caused by a viral infection with an adenovirus. Typically, there are common cold symptoms, plus:
• Pain and tenderness in the right lower abdomen; pain may also be present throughout the abdomen.
• Fever.
• Nausea and vomiting.

The adenitis settles of its own accord.

### POSSIBLE

■ **Peptic Ulcer**

The term covers ulcers of the stomach and duodenum. There is a wide range of symptoms, which vary considerably from person to person.
• Pain in the epigastrium (upper middle part of the abdomen).
• Pain is recurrent.
• Heartburn may be present.
• Pain may radiate to the back.
• Night waking because of pain is common.

• Possibly nausea and vomiting.
• Food can either improve or worsen the pain.

Ulcers can bleed, causing anemia and tarry stools or hematemesis *(see Blood from the Back Passage, page 156, and Abdominal Pain Plus Vomiting Blood, page 170)*.

They can also perforate *(see Perforated Viscus, page 147)*.

■ **Appendicitis**

*(See page 163)*

■ **Kidney Stones**

*(See page 184)*

■ **Ovarian Cyst**

Ovarian cysts may be attached to the ovary on a stalk. If the cyst rotates, it will tighten the stalk, causing severe pain.
• Sudden onset of lower abdominal pain.
• Vomiting.
• Cyst may bleed, causing pain and irritating the inside of the abdominal cavity.

May mimic appendicitis if on the right ovary.

■ **Salpingitis (Pyosalpinx)**

Abscess on a fallopian tube—one possibility in the wider picture of pelvic infection *(see page 296)*.

■ **Biliary Colic**

*(See page 166)*

■ **Stomach Cancer**

*(See Stomach Disease, page 163)*

### RARE

■ **Meckel's Diverticulum**

A diverticulum is an out-pouching or a little sac; this type occurs in the ileum.

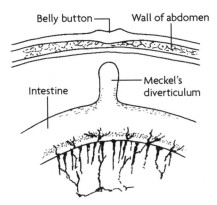

*Meckel's Diverticulum*

Symptoms mimic appendicitis if it becomes inflamed *(see page 163)* and may also cause:
- Anemia.
- Intestinal obstruction.
- Rectal bleeding.

■ **Acute Pancreatitis**

*(See page 148)*

■ **Intestinal Obstruction**

*(See page 149)*

■ **Porphyria**

A group of metabolic diseases. The following are the most common features:
- Intermittent abdominal pain.
- Vomiting.
- Constipation.
- Fever.
- Fast pulse.
- Neurological abnormalities.

Rarely, poisoning from various toxins (for example, arsenic) can cause this presentation.

## ABDOMINAL PAIN PLUS VOMITING BLOOD

A rare combination, but if you have both these symptoms, you must consult your doctor. Bleeding may continue even without vomiting, putting you in danger until the source is detected and the bleeding stopped.

### PROBABLE

■ **Mallory-Weiss Tear**

First noticed in studies of alcoholics. Any cause of severe, repeated vomiting can cause a small tear in the lining of the upper stomach or lower esophagus (gullet).

- Vomiting, often recurrent.
- Fresh blood may be vomited (hematemesis).
- Tarry stools.

Normally self-healing without further treatment, but admission to a hospital is usually recommended to control any further vomiting and stabilize any consequence of potentially severe blood loss.

### ■ Acute Gastritis

Inflammation of the lining of the stomach caused by food, drugs, alcohol, or infection.

- Indigestion.
- Occasionally, blood is vomited. This usually looks like coffee grounds as the blood is altered by the gastric juices.

### ■ Peptic Ulcer

*(See page 169)*

### ■ Drugs

Some drugs, particularly steroids and nonsteroidal anti-inflammatory drugs (NSAIDs), including aspirin, can cause gastric bleeding. This may be experienced as vomiting up blood or passing tarry stools (melena).

### POSSIBLE

### ■ Hiatus Hernia and Esophagitis

Inflammation of the gullet caused by reflux of stomach contents.

- Heartburn.
- Difficulty in swallowing.
- Bitter fluid comes into mouth ("waterbrash" or "repeating").
- Vomiting.
- Nausea.
- Occasional anemia.
- Occasionally, if very severe, may cause melena or hematemesis.

### RARE

### ■ Cancer of the Stomach

*(See Stomach Disease, page 163)*

---

## ABDOMINAL PAIN PLUS VOMITING AND FEVER

### PROBABLE

### ■ Gastroenteritis

*(See page 166)*

### ■ Urinary Tract Infection

*(See page 183)*

### POSSIBLE

### ■ Acute Pyelonephritis

*(See Kidney Infection, page 184)*

### ■ Pelvic Inflammatory Disease

*(See page 333)*

■ **Appendicitis**

*(See page 163)*

■ **Cholecystitis**

The gallbladder may become inflamed and infected because of gallstones, which form from fats, calcium, and pigment. Many people have them, but they often remain unnoticed unless the individual develops cholecystitis.

• Upper right abdominal pain.
• Tenderness just below the right rib margin.
• Pain may be made worse by breathing in.
• Fever.
• Malaise.
• Vomiting.
• Jaundice may develop if stones block the biliary tract.

See a doctor without delay.

### RARE

■ **Intestinal Obstruction**

■ **Acute Pancreatitis**

*(See page 148)*

■ **Meckel's Diverticulum**

*(See page 170)*

■ **Porphyria**

*(See page 170)*

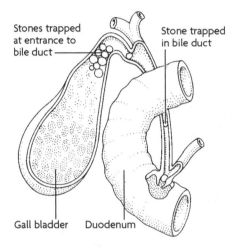

Stones trapped at entrance to bile duct

Stone trapped in bile duct

Gall bladder    Duodenum

*Gallbladder*

## ABDOMINAL PAIN, VOMITING, AND JAUNDICE

### PROBABLE

■ **Cholecystitis**

*(See above)*

■ **Biliary Colic**

*(See page 166)*

### POSSIBLE

■ **Acute Pancreatitis**

*(See page 148)*

## RARE

- Cancer of the Pancreas

*(See page 164)*

- Cancer of the Stomach

*(See Stomach Disease, page 163)*

---

## APPARENT CONSTIPATION ALTERNATING WITH DIARRHEA

This is a possible combination, but it is best to explore the possibilities in detail by reading individual entries *(see Constipation, page 161, Diarrhea, page 154, and Change in Bowel Habit, page 160).*

---

## CONSTIPATION AND ABDOMINAL PAIN

To explore the full possibilities, read Constipation *(page 161)* and Abdominal Pain *(pages 165–173).*

---

## INDIGESTION

Indigestion, heartburn, dyspepsia—these terms tend to be used interchangeably for a variety of symptoms of upper abdominal pain, flatulence, belching, acid in the mouth (waterbrash), and nausea.

Occasional mild indigestion, which is treatable with over-the-counter remedies, is of little significance. It becomes an important symptom when it recurs frequently or becomes more persistent than usual. It is a sign of change in your normal pattern of tolerance to food and carries a clear message—seek medical advice.

## PROBABLE

- Non-Ulcer Dyspepsia

A term used to describe a group of symptoms such as:

- Upper abdominal pain.
- Nausea.
- Flatulence and belching when there is no evidence of an ulcer after special tests.

- Hiatus Hernia and Esophagitis

*(See page 141)*

- Peptic Ulcer

*(See page 169)*

■ **Pregnancy**
*(See page 140)*

**POSSIBLE**

■ **Gallstones**
*(See Cholecystitus, page 172)*

■ **Ischemic Heart Disease**
Sometimes angina (heart pain) is misinterpreted by the person as indigestion. If the pain is not immediately relieved by an antacid or is aggravated by exertion, this possibility must be considered.

**RARE**

■ **Cancer of the Stomach**
*(See Stomach Disease, page 163)*

■ **Cancer of the Esophagus**

■ **Achalasia**

■ **Chronic Pancreatitis**
*(See page 167)*

## CRAMPING PAINS IN THE ABDOMEN

*(See all combinations of symptoms under Abdominal Pain, pages 165–173)*

## LOSS OF APPETITE

*(See page 482)*

## FLATULENCE OR BELCHING

*(See Indigestion, page 173)*

## DIARRHEA, BLOODY

*(See Diarrhea, page 154, and Blood From the Back Passage, page 156)*

## DIARRHEA PLUS VOMITING

*(See Diarrhea, page 154, and Vomiting, page 140; also, Gastroenteritis, page 166)*

## STOMACHACHE

*(See all combinations of symptoms under Abdominal Pain, pages 165–173)*

## NAUSEA

*(See Vomiting, page 140)*

## DYSPEPSIA

*(See Indigestion, page 173)*

## HEARTBURN

*(See Indigestion, page 173)*

# ABDOMEN: URINARY SYSTEM

## INCONTINENCE

Lack of control over the act of urination so that accidental or unplanned leakage occurs. Any irritation or inflammation may predispose to some degree of leakage. Age often worsens these problems. Millions of people worldwide have some degree of incontinence of feces and urine.

### PROBABLE

■ **Enlarged Prostate**

*(See page 188)*

■ **Bladder Neck Obstruction**

*(See page 188)*

■ **Urinary Tract Infection**

*(See page 183)* Especially common in the elderly.

■ **Irritable Bladder**

*(See page 189)*

■ **Stress Incontinence**

Often in women who have had a pregnancy.

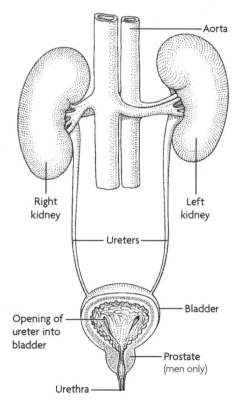

Aorta

Right
kidney

Left
kidney

Ureters

Bladder

Opening of
ureter into
bladder

Prostate
(men only)

Urethra

*Urinary System*

- Leakage of urine when coughing, laughing, sneezing, or exercising.
- Leakage when straining.

## POSSIBLE

### ■ Cystocele and Rectocele

These two conditions are common in women who also suffer from stress incontinence *(see above)*. They are caused by weakness of the vaginal wall, which allows the bladder (cystocele) or rectum (rectocele) to bulge into the vagina. This distortion of anatomy (often felt as a lump) can cause leakage of urine.

### ■ Prolapse

The structures that keep the womb in place deteriorate after giving birth and with age. In some women, this allows the womb to prolapse—to drop down into the vagina—where it may often be seen or felt.

- Red lump at vagina.
- Sometimes bleeds.
- Discharge may be present.
- Associated with urinary leakage.
- May be pushed back internally.
- Comes back out on straining, coughing, or sneezing.

### ■ Stroke

Anyone who has suffered a stroke may develop incontinence or difficulty in urination.

Sometimes the bladder distends with urine, but because of lack of sensation no pain is felt, although the individual may appear restless and sweaty. Some overflow incontinence may develop.

### ■ Epilepsy

In major epileptic fits *(see page 452)*, symptoms include:

- Jerking movements.
- Tongue biting.
- Urinary incontinence (the entire bladder empties spontaneously during the fit).

### ■ Multiple Sclerosis

*(See page 326)* Early symptoms reported to a doctor can include:

- Weakness, numbness, and "pins and needles" sensation in a limb(s).
- Heaviness in a limb(s).
- "Jumpy" legs.
- Muscular spasms.
- Blurred vision.
- Hesitancy, frequency, incontinence, and retention of urine may all be present.
- Altered sensation in limbs and trunk.

## RARE

These diseases can be associated with very sudden loss of bladder control, together with other symptoms.

### ■ Spinal Cord Injury

• Weakness of the limbs below the level of damage.

• Sensory loss below the level of damage.

• Loss of bladder control, usually resulting in retention of urine.

Urgent medical attention is required.

### ■ Cauda Equina Syndrome

Damage to the lowest part of the spinal cord. Can be caused by bone damage, tumor, or a slipped disc.

• Back pain.

• Loss of sensation in the lower back and around the buttocks and anus.

• Leg weakness.

• Loss of bladder control.

Urgent medical attention is required.

## NEED TO URINATE URGENTLY OR OFTEN

This symptom usually suggests that the bladder itself is irritated. The most common cause is urinary bladder infection *(cystitis, see page 183)*.

*(See also Problems with Urinating, page 188)*

## URINATING TOO MUCH OR TOO OFTEN

The obvious cause is drinking too much tea, coffee, or alcohol. These all stimulate the production of urine and can make you want to urinate during the night.

### PROBABLE

### ■ Urinary Tract Infection

*(See page 183)* Causes frequent urination and discomfort on urination, rather than excessive volume.

### POSSIBLE

### ■ Enlarged Prostate

*(See page 188)* Causes frequent urination rather than excessive volume.

### ■ Diuretics

A range of drugs given to reduce high blood pressure or to treat heart failure. Their intended effect is to increase the amount of urine passed in order to reduce the amount of fluid in the system and so lessen tension in the blood vessels. Some people taking these drugs find that they need to get up at night in order to urinate.

## ■ Diabetes Mellitus

*(See page 160)* New cases may suddenly experience:
- Increased volume of urine (polyuria).
- Increased thirst (polydipsia).
- Rapid weight loss.
- Malaise.
- Other symptoms such as vomiting, muscle cramps, or abdominal pain.

If untreated, coma and death may follow. In older people, diabetes may have few other symptoms and is often discovered simply on routine testing of urine or blood for sugar.

## RARE

## ■ Diabetes Insipidus

*(See page 493)* Don't confuse this with diabetes mellitus *(see above)*. It may arise spontaneously, after injury to the head (typically, after surgery or an accident), because of brain tumors, or due to infection. The main symptom is:
- Enormous volumes of urine—about 9 pints (5 liters) passed daily.

## ■ Chronic Kidney Failure

Any disease resulting in kidney failure can cause excess urine at some stage *(see Inability to Urinate, page 191)*.

## ■ Aldosteronism

You may hear this described as Conn's syndrome, which is one form of the disease. Caused by a tumor of the adrenal gland. The blood chemistry becomes abnormal with excessive amounts of the hormone aldosterone being produced, leading to:
- Muscle weakness.
- Excessive urination.
- Excessive thirst.
- High blood pressure.

## ■ Hypercalcemia

High levels of calcium in the blood may be caused by a number of conditions and diseases, including abnormalities of the parathyroid glands, excess vitamin D, sarcoidosis (a rare illness of body tissues leading to the deposit of material, described as sarcoid, in various sites in the body), malignant bone tumors (primary or secondary), and thyrotoxicosis (an illness caused by having too much thyroid hormone).

The symptoms of excess calcium in the blood are:
- Anorexia.
- Nausea.
- Vomiting.
- Thirst.
- Polyuria (passing urine more often than normal).
- Constipation.
- Muscle fatigue.

## URINE LOOKS DARK

### PROBABLE

#### ■ Concentrated Urine

If you have spent a long time in a hot atmosphere or if you have been very active physically, without also increasing your fluid intake, you may notice that your urine is a dark yellow color and that it is passed in small amounts. In the absence of other symptoms, this is normal. By increasing your fluid intake, or by avoiding the heat or exercise, urine will be back to normal within twenty-four hours.

### POSSIBLE

#### ■ Hepatitis

Inflammation of the liver. There are several different types; some, particularly hepatitis B and C, are more serious than the others. If you suspect hepatitis, you must see a doctor. General symptoms may include:
- Fever.
- Malaise.
- Anorexia.
- Muscle and joint pains.
- Jaundice.
- Dark urine; it can be dark yellow, orange, or brown.
- Stools may become pale.

#### ■ Foods or Drugs

Several foods and drugs can cause discoloration of different hues. Examples are:
- Orange—rhubarb, senna.
- Red—beetroot, blackberries.
- Green/blue—methylene blue dye.
- Some drugs used in the treatment of tuberculosis (TB) may also cause discoloration.

After stopping the food or drug, urine should be back to normal within about twenty-four hours.

### RARE

#### ■ Cancer of the Pancreas

A malignant tumor of the pancreas can block the bile ducts. This means that yellow bile is passed out in the urine.
- Jaundice.
- Dark yellow, orange, or brown urine.
- Pale stools.
- Abdominal and back pain.
- Weight loss, anorexia.

#### ■ Hemoglobinuria

In contrast to hematuria (which is the medical term for blood in the urine) hemoglobinuria means broken down red blood cells in the urine. It is caused by several different diseases or conditions and the urine is often more brown than red. It appears in association with illnesses and diseases such as hemolytic anemia, thrombocytopenic purpura, cardiac disease (for example, after valve replacement), malaria, and septicemia.

Discolored urine is unlikely to be the first or only symptom of these conditions, and in most cases the individual will already be under a doctor's care.

### ■ Crush Syndrome
*(See page 192)*

### ■ Melanoma

A melanoma is a form of skin cancer *(see page 248)*. In some advanced cases, the pigment melanin gets into the urine and colors it dark brown or black.

### ■ Alkaptonuria

This is an example of an inborn error of metabolism. In other words, the body fails to deal correctly with certain chemicals (in this case, tyrosine) in the blood; they are then excreted in urine, which becomes progressively darker if left standing.

## BLOOD IN URINE

The significance of blood in the urine varies greatly from the simple and easily treated to the severe and life-threatening. It should never be ignored as a symptom. If recurring, its significance increases. Again, do not ignore. Red blood cells in the urine (hematuria) may come from any part of the urinary tract—the kidneys, the ureters (which connect the kidneys to the bladder), the bladder, or the urethra. Blood may also appear in urine because of generalized disease.

It may become apparent in several ways. The urine may appear the color of blood (frank hematuria) or in smaller quantities it may only color it pinkish, or give it a smoky or cloudy appearance. Occasionally, clots of blood are passed with minimal coloring of the rest of the urine. Also, blood may appear only at the beginning or end of urination.

The male and female urinary tracts differ in that the male has a prostate gland and two seminal vesicles. In females of child-bearing age, menstrual loss of blood may sometimes be mistaken for blood in the urine. In these cases, the bloody discoloration disappears as the period ends.

Blood in the urine should always be taken seriously, especially in children. Investigation will be required. While an adult may commonly suffer an infection causing blood to appear in the urine, this is not acceptable in children. Any urine infection in a child is an unusual event and may be the first sign of an abnormality in the structure of the urinary tract. Rarely, accompanying swelling in the abdomen may be due to Wilms' tumor, a malignant tumor of the kidney seen in children, usually up to the age of three.

Some foods, particularly beetroot, can discolor the urine.

## PROBABLE

### ■ Cystitis

Inflammation of the bladder lining, giving symptoms of urine infection.

- Frequent passing of urine.
- Burning or scalding as you urinate.
- Bursting to go but little result.
- Having to rush to pass urine with urgency.
- Dull ache in lower abdomen; may persist or worsen after urination.
- Fever; backache.
- Dark, cloudy, or blood-stained urine.

Mild cases may clear without the use of antibiotics.

### ■ Urinary Tract Infection

Symptoms as for cystitis; in addition, there may be more severe symptoms such as:

- High fever.

- Pain in the back, loin, groin, or front of abdomen.
- Vomiting, nausea.
- Sweating.

Will require antibiotics.

Increasingly, the bacteria causing urinary infections (and cystitis) do not respond to commonly prescribed antibiotics. This is known as bacterial resistance.

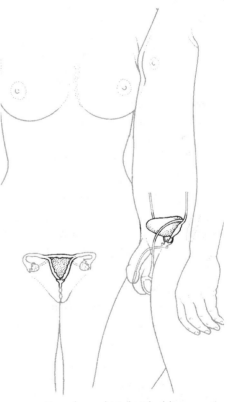

*Female and Male Bladder*

Hence, the importance, where possible, of sending a urine culture test to the laboratory before treatment starts.

## ■ Kidney Infection

Medical term for this is pyelonephritis. In this instance, the urine reveals infection, but in addition the kidney itself is affected. Symptoms as for cystitis, plus:

• Severe fever.
• Loin pain.
• Tenderness and sensitivity in the loin and side of abdomen.
• General feeling of being unwell.

Cystitis symptoms may not be marked, particularly in the early stages, when the symptoms may be confined largely to the upper abdomen; for example:

• Pain, vomiting, nausea.
• Rigors (shivering).

Severe and advanced cases (acute nephritis) will show diminished urine output, swelling of the face and ankles, headache, and other symptoms as above.

Treatment is with antibiotics, sometimes intravenously.

If you find symptoms persist after, or during, treatment with antibiotics, seek the result of your urine culture test. It will reveal which antibiotics can kill the bacteria. You will hear this referred to as a test to reveal bacterial sensitivity.

## POSSIBLE

### ■ Kidney Stones

• Extremely severe pain, coming and going in unbearable waves, localized to one side over the kidney area (loin and extreme side of abdomen).
• Vomiting.
• Sweating.

Typically, pain spreads from the back, around the side, to the front of the abdomen and from there to the scrotum/groin area.

### ■ Prostatitis

Affects men only.

• Fever.
• Pain in the rectal area behind scrotum.
• Difficulty in passing urine.
• Sensation of passing hot urine.

### ■ Benign Tumors of Bladder/Kidney

Benign tumors of the urinary tract may cause bleeding. Symptoms may include:

• Painless hematuria (blood in urine), sometimes copious.
• General health is otherwise sound.
• Occasional obstruction of the passage of urine, due to blood clot.
• Anemia (if there has been unrecognized bleeding for some time).

Urological assessment is required.

## ■ Enlarged Prostate

Affects men only. Difficulty in:
• Passing urine.
• Starting/stopping stream.
• Holding on to pass urine later, preventing dribbling.

Inability to pass urine (retention of urine) requires medical intervention and catheterization.

## ■ Cancer of the Prostate

*(See Enlarged Prostate above)* Diagnosis is frequently made during operative intervention for enlarged prostate symptoms. Now some authorities suggest screening for cancer of the prostate with a blood test, PSA (prostate specific antigen). For this, consult your doctor for counseling. After about eighty years of age, nearly every male has cancer of the prostate. It lies dormant in the gland, seldom causing severe problems at that age.

## ■ Chronic Nephritis

• Nocturnal passage of large quantities of urine.
• Anemia.
• Swelling.
• Shortness of breath.

## ■ Injury

Injuries to the lower chest or pelvis (such as a blow or a stab wound) may damage underlying structures. If you have any blood in your urine after such an injury, whether in large or small quantities, you will need a full medical assessment in order to rule out serious damage to the urinary, or any other, system.

## ■ Exercise

It is now widely recognized that certain types of prolonged, repeated exercise—in particular, marathon running—may cause transient appearances of blood in the urine.

## RARE

## ■ Cancer of the Bladder/Kidney

Simple tests such as urine cytology, to examine the cell content of urine, can reveal the presence of malignant cells.
    Most common in adults over fifty.
• Painless hematuria (blood in urine).
• Pain in the loin.
• Swelling in loin or abdomen.
• Occasionally, bone pain, due to spread of the tumor.
• Fever.
• Loss of weight.
• Anemia.

## ■ Wilms' Tumor (Children)

The child has:
• One-sided, abdominal swelling.
• Painless blood in urine.

- Loss of appetite.
- Anemia.
- Pain in late stages only.

Modern drugs and medical techniques have revolutionized the treatment of this condition. Early diagnosis is important.

### ■ Endocarditis

Inflammation of the inner layer of the heart. Multiple symptoms appear and the affected individual will be very ill. Symptoms include:

- Rash.
- Joint pains.
- Finger clubbing *(see page 302)*.
- Fever.
- Chest pain.

### ■ Anticoagulant Therapy

Individuals who are taking anticoagulants (blood-thinning medications) may notice blood in their urine. They should consult their doctor, who will probably recommend reducing the dose of the drug.

### ■ Bilharzia

Schistosomiasis. Caused by a parasitic organism that inhabits water. Common in Africa, the West Indies, South America, and Japan.

- Blood in urine.
- Pain on passing urine.
- Frequent passing of urine.

Cancer of the bladder can develop, as well as liver damage.

## BLOOD IN URINE PLUS PAIN WHEN URINATING

The Probable causes are urinary tract infection, cystitis, and kidney stone.

The Possible causes are acute pyelonephritis and prostatitis.

The Rare cause is bilharzia.
*(All are covered under Blood in Urine, page 182)*

## KIDNEY PAIN

The kidneys are situated at the side of the abdomen, toward the back. This area is known as the kidney or loin area. The most likely cause of pain in this area is infection. There are also a number of other possible causes *(see Blood in Urine, page 182, and Blood in Urine Plus Pain When Urinating, see above)*.

## PAIN WHEN URINATING

Pain when passing urine is almost always a sign of cystitis or urinary infection. Rarely, it can be one of the symptoms caused by a kidney stone or venereal infection such as NSU *(see Non-Specific Urethritis, page 189)*. Also, the conditions listed under Blood in Urine *(page 182)* may all cause pain on passing urine as an early symptom, prior to the appearance of blood in the urine.

## URINE LOOKS CLOUDY

A number of body products, but mainly blood, pus cells, and microorganisms, can have this effect. Other symptoms may well be noticed at the same time. Urine that is concentrated but normal often goes cloudy if left standing. Cloudy appearance does not always signify illness.

### PROBABLE

■ **Urinary Tract Infection**
*(See page 183)*

■ **Cystitis**
*(See page 187)*

■ **Kidney Stones**
*(See Blood in Urine, page 182)*

### POSSIBLE

■ **Acute Pyelonephritis**
*(See page 191)*

■ **Prostatitis**
*(See Blood in Urine, page 182)*

■ **Gonorrhea**
A sexually transmitted disease. It often has no symptoms in women, although vaginal discharge, pelvic inflammatory disease, and pain on passing urine may be experienced.

If a man has genital symptoms (and he may not), there will be:
• Urethral discharge.
• Discomfort on passing urine.
• Cloudy urine.
• Reddening and pain around the glans of the penis and urethra.
• Enlarged lymph nodes in the groin.

### RARE

■ **Bilharzia**
*(See page 186)*

## PROBLEMS WITH URINATING

These include such symptoms as hesitancy or difficulty in starting to urinate, poor urine stream, and dribbling. The underlying causes tend to be either obstruction to the passage of urine or structural abnormalities of the urinary tract. Pain on urinating due to other causes, such as infection or neurological defects, may also affect urination.

### PROBABLE

#### ■ Enlarged Prostate (Men)

The gland can be enlarged as a result of benign or malignant growth. Symptoms may be similar in both cases:
• Difficulty or hesitancy when starting to urinate.
• Poor stream.
• Terminal dribbling.
• Feeling as though the bladder has not emptied.
• Need to urinate during the night (nocturia).
• Sudden desire to pass urine.
• Some blood in the urine.
• Sometimes, leakage of urine (overflow incontinence).
• Later in the disease, acute obstruction occurs with inability to pass urine at all. Severe abdominal pain develops because of the distended bladder. In some cases,

the obstruction develops so slowly that the bladder compensates by enlarging over a period of weeks or months. There is minimal discomfort and the urine frequently leaks out, without the individual being able to control it. The bladder does not empty properly, remaining distended, which is often seen as abdominal swelling. This type of urine loss is called overflow incontinence. Medical assessment is always needed.

Cancer of the prostate may also cause:
• Back pain.
• Bone pain.

#### ■ Bladder Neck Obstruction

Symptoms similar to an enlarged prostate, but occurring in a younger age group and, occasionally, in women. Caused by overgrowth of the bladder muscle at its outlet to the urethra.

#### ■ Urinary Tract Infection

*(See page 183)*

#### ■ Gonorrhea

*(See page 187)*

#### ■ Non-Specific Urethritis

A common sexually transmitted disease caused by *Chlamydia*. Often, there are no symptoms. If there are symptoms, men will have:

• Discomfort or itch on passing urine, making it difficult to urinate.

• Discharge (white, yellow) from penis.

Women will have:

• Pain/burning on passing urine.

• Occasional vaginal discharge.

The womb and fallopian tubes can be infected *(see also Pelvic Inflammatory Disease, page 333)*.

## NON-SPECIFIC URETHRITIS (NSU)

It is very important to have this disease treated. You and your sexual partner must receive treatment since, even with a total absence of symptoms, *Chlamydia* may be present. Untreated chlamydial infections can cause infertility.

### POSSIBLE

#### ■ Irritable Bladder

A term encompassing different symptoms caused by irritation of sensory or motor nerves to the bladder. Other causes (such as infection) must be excluded first. Special tests are needed to confirm the diagnosis. Symptoms can be one or more of the following:

• Frequent desire to pass urine (for example, every thirty minutes).

• Pain over the bladder.

• Difficulty in passing urine (small volumes) and the bladder still feels full.

• Sometimes, retention of urine occurs.

• Occasionally, leakage of urine.

#### ■ Urethral Stricture

Urethral stricture is a narrowing of the outflow passage from the bladder. It is more common in men than women and may be caused by previous infection (perhaps gonorrhea), surgery, or damage by an instrument or a catheter (typically during delivery of a baby). Symptoms are progressive:

• Poor stream.

• Spraying of urine.

• Needing to strain hard to empty the bladder.

#### ■ Prostatitis

*(See page 184)*

#### ■ Kidney Stones

*(See page 184)*

#### ■ Drugs

*(See page 191)*

**RARE**

■ **Urethral Tumors**

Benign or malignant tumors may cause progressive obstruction of the urethra in men and women, leading to:
• Need to strain harder than usual to pass urine.

■ **Spinal Cord Damage**
*(See page 402)*

■ **Neurological Disease**
*(See page 376)*

■ **Stroke**
*(See Incontinence, page 177)*

## URINE DRIBBLES

Meaning either a poor stream or dripping when trying to stop the flow of urine. Can be a form of incontinence.

The following can all be occasional causes of dribbling *(see detailed coverage under Problems with Urinating, page 188).*

**PROBABLE**

■ **Enlarged Prostate**

*(See page 188)*

■ **Bladder Neck Obstruction**

*(See page 188)*

■ **Urinary Tract Infection**
*(See page 183)*

**POSSIBLE**

■ **Urethral Stricture**
*(See page 189)*

■ **Prostatitis**
*(See page 184)*

**RARE**

■ **Urethral Tumors**
*(See page 190)*

## URINATING AT NIGHT

You may often have had to get up during the night to pass urine, especially if you had anything to drink within a few hours of going to bed. It is only abnormal if it develops as a new symptom or if the number of times you get up increases significantly.

The most common causes are an en-

larged prostate gland (in men) and bladder irritability (in women). Drugs are another important cause. Diuretics can often be taken once daily, in the morning, to minimize this difficulty.

*(See also Problems with Urinating, page 188, and Urinating Too Much or Too Often, page 179)*

## INABILITY TO URINATE

The medical term is anuria, and it is a serious problem. Don't confuse it with passing small volumes of concentrated urine infrequently, as in hot atmospheres or after strenuous exercise.

Urination can be arrested for three main reasons: obstruction in the urethra, failure of the bladder muscle to contract, or both kidneys may stop producing urine because they are diseased or are affected by disease elsewhere.

The first two cases are described as retention of urine. In all three cases, but particularly in the last, there may be a period of hours or days when the volume of urine gradually diminishes.

In the case of obstruction, there will be severe pain because of an increasingly distended bladder. Failure to excrete urine results in a buildup of toxic chemicals in the blood—and so it is, of course, a medical emergency.

### PROBABLE

#### ■ Enlarged Prostate

The most common reason (in men only) for a sudden inability to pass urine is an enlarged prostate gland, causing an obstruction to the outlet from the bladder. You will feel pain as the bladder distends *(see page 188)*.

All the other causes in this section are much less common.

#### ■ Kidney Stone

*(See page 184)* If a stone lodges in the urethra or at the neck of the bladder, it will block the passage of urine. In addition to urine failure:

• Pain because of distended bladder.

In men, pain may radiate to the tip of the penis.

#### ■ Urethral Stricture

*(See page 189)*

### POSSIBLE

#### ■ Surgery or Injury

Any event that causes uncontrolled blood loss, and thus low blood pressure, can damage the kidneys and prevent them from working. The elderly, and those with chronically raised blood pressure, are vulnerable to this type of kidney damage.

#### ■ Drugs

A number of drugs may unexpectedly cause retention of urine, particularly in patients with prostatic disease. Examples are amitriptyline and imipramine.

#### ■ Pyelonephritis

*(See Kidney Infection, page 184)* In severe untreated cases, the kidneys may be so badly damaged that they stop working. No urine is produced and the patient gets more and more sick, with:

- Weak pulse.
- Fever.
- Rigors.
- Vomiting.

### ■ Malignant Tumors

Any malignant tumor of organs in or near the pelvis can involve parts of the urinary tract, blocking the urethra, ureters, bladder, or kidneys. Cancers of the colon, uterus, ovaries, bladder, and prostate can all have this effect. But it is very rare for anuria to be the first symptom, and the diagnosis has usually been made long before.

### ■ Shock

*(See also page 420)* If shock is untreated or untreatable, the kidneys fail to produce urine and gradually urine output tails off to nothing. A grave condition.

### ■ Septicemia

Infection of the bloodstream and whole body from any cause. It can lead to shock *(see page 420),* which, if untreated or severe, results in acute kidney failure. Possibly fatal.

### RARE

### ■ Injury

Direct injury to the urethra (particularly in men) occurs typically in car accidents where the pelvis has been fractured. Because of the damage, urine cannot pass. This is a medical emergency that in most cases is promptly treated because the patient is already in the hospital.

Very occasionally, a kick to the male scrotum or crotch may damage the urethra or, indeed, the spinal cord.

### ■ Spinal Cord Damage

### ■ Neurological Disease

*(See page 474)*

### ■ Poisoning

A number of substances may directly damage the kidneys, causing kidney failure. These include mercury, arsenic, and bismuth.

### ■ Blood Transfusion

If a patient is given blood that is incompatible with his or her own, the result may damage the kidneys and cause kidney failure. This is one reason why such care is taken when giving blood, and why it is only given when needed.

### ■ Crush Syndrome

Damaged leg muscles, sustained in a crushing injury to the lower limbs, causes toxins to enter the bloodstream, resulting in direct damage to the kidneys.

Discolored urine may be a symptom. The longer the limb is crushed, the greater the risk.

# THE HEART

The heart is a superb pump: it gives years of service, responding automatically to all the varied demands of growth, activity, and stress, so that we are rarely aware of its action.

How does the heart work? Two major systems, both electrical, control the heart's activity; there is also a built-in mechanism that increases the heart's muscular effort in response to high demand.

Emotion and stress are communicated to the heart by a branch of the nervous system called the autonomic system. It is this system that, for example, sets the heart beating faster when you notice a bull in the next meadow, and continues to increase both its speed and power when you realize there is no fence between you and the bull.

Within the heart itself, there are two electrical pacemakers that control the rate of heartbeats. The main one, the sinoatrial node, normally sets the rate, transmitting a regular firing signal down an electrical pathway to the second pacemaker, a relay station called the atrioventricular node. From there, the signal to beat is transmitted to the rest of the heart by other electrical tracts.

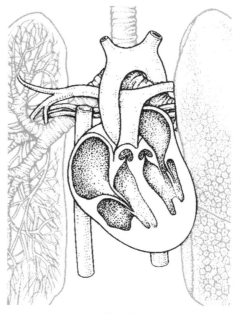

*Heart*

The atrioventricular node may also act as a pacemaker should the sinoatrial node fail for some reason.

Clearly, there are many opportunities for malfunction in this system. If there is a problem, heart rhythms may be too fast, too slow, or irregular. These irregularities are felt in various ways, perhaps a thumping in the chest or a fluttering sensation, but sometimes only skilled examination can detect a problem. This section analyzes the possibilities.

It is important to realize that occasional rhythm disorders are common and are not necessarily a sign of disease. It is remarkable that there are not more of them, considering that an average heart will be making some 3 billion heartbeats during a seventy-year lifetime. Where irregularities decrease the pumping efficiency of the heart significantly, faint-ness, dizziness, or, at worst, collapse may follow.

It is worth remembering that the diagnosis of heart irregularities, palpitations, and similar disorders can be a highly technical matter. Tremendous advances in research have been made in recent years. The sources of electrical malfunction can now be traced to individual sections of wiring in the heart, in some cases, allowing precise surgery to control the fault.

We've journeyed from seeing the heart as something that can break to thinking of it as a mechanism that would do credit to a Grand Prix Formula One computerized fuel management system. As with so many other systems in our bodies, with a more precise understanding has come admiration of the sophistication of an activity we take for granted.

## HEART MAKES EXTRA BEATS

This is a common symptom with an interesting explanation. What happens is that the heart beats twice in rapid succession, but the extra beat goes unnoticed. However, the next beat of the heart is delayed by a fraction of a second and it is this slight delay that you may be aware of. During the delay, blood continues to fill the heart, bringing into play an automatic mechanism that makes the heart beat more forcefully the more full it gets. The next beat after the delay is, therefore, extra powerful and is felt as a thump in the chest.

### PROBABLE

■ **Unexplained**

In the young or early middle-aged.
- Happens occasionally.
- Otherwise sound health.

- The extra beat causes no other symptoms: no faintness or chest pain.

## ■ Too Much Coffee or Tea

The small amounts of caffeine in these drinks is responsible for the "lift" they provide. Taken in excess—and what constitutes excess is an individual matter— the caffeine will cause:

- Rapid heart rate.
- Extra beats.
- Tremor.
- Anxiety.
- Increased output of urine.

Treatment is simply to reduce intake.

## ■ Alcohol

Alcohol has a direct effect on the heart. This increases with time and excessive use and can lead, in rare cases, to heart failure.

## ■ Cigarette Smoking

Nicotine has a stimulant effect on the heart, increasing its rate and output. Extra beats are one reflection of this.

## ■ Fever

Heart rate rises by about ten beats per 0.5 degree centigrade rise in temperature and increases the chance of extra beats. Some infections, as well as causing fever, can irritate the heart.

## POSSIBLE

### ■ Anxiety

Anxiety has its effect via the autonomic nervous system, increasing the resting rate of the heart and the chances of extra beats. Other well-known features include:

- Tension in neck and shoulders.
- Constant feeling of pressure in the head.
- Excess sweating, tremor.
- Constantly feeling that something dreadful is about to happen.

### ■ Indigestion

It is uncertain how indigestion affects the heart. Probably it results from a reflex action in those nerves that serve both the digestive system and the heart, though there may be direct irritation of the heart by a distended stomach. The features of indigestion are familiar.

- Bloating, belching.
- Acid, burning sensation after meals.
- Discomfort felt behind breast bone.

## RARE

### ■ Complications of Heart Attack

Extra beats are common in the days after a heart attack, often producing few symptoms. They have a different origin from benign extra beats, arising instead from spontaneous beating of the ventricles, the main pumping chambers of the heart. It is usual to continuously monitor the heart's electrical activity in the days after a heart attack looking for just such ventricular extra beats. They can be a warning of the sudden, uncontrolled activity of the ventricles, which causes collapse and possibly sudden death.

### ■ Excess Digoxin

Digoxin is a drug used to treat heart failure and some irregular pulses. In excess, it causes:

- Nausea and vomiting.
- Very slow pulse with extra beats.
- Fatigue.
- Red or green hallucinations.
- Abdominal pains.

Mild cases can be corrected by temporarily dropping digoxin. Severe cases need intensive treatment in a hospital.

### ■ Rheumatic Carditis

Fortunately, this once-common disease in children is now a rarity in the developed world, but it is still prevalent elsewhere.

- Begins two to three weeks after a bad sore throat.
- Joint pains; stiffness flitting from limb to limb.
- Fever.
- Rashes rapidly coming and going.
- Rapid pulse, extra beats.
- Sudden, fidgety movements.

There is danger of permanent damage to the heart valves, leading later to heart disease.

## HEART BEATS IRREGULARLY

People's sensitivity to their heartbeat varies. Some will feel that a very rapid but regular heart rhythm is an irregularity, while others are able to focus precisely on the rhythm. A doctor will listen to the heartbeat through a stethoscope while feeling the pulse at the wrist; this often allows a simple rhythm to be diagnosed. Where there is doubt, an electrocardiogram (ECG) of the heart is needed.

### POSSIBLE

### ■ Sinus Arrhythmia

Careful observation of your own pulse will reveal a change in rhythm as you breathe. The autonomic pathways slow the heart as you breathe out and let it run faster as you breathe in. In some people, this is particularly noticeable and may cause alarm. It is not a disease but an exaggeration of a normal reflex. The reflex is especially noticeable in children.

- Otherwise well.
- Clear relationship to breathing.
- Rhythm changes by about ten beats per minute faster or slower.

### ■ Sick Sinus Syndrome

The sinoatrial node is the trigger in the heart that fires the electrical signal that causes the heart to beat. So vital is this area of the heart that it has its own blood supply, but with age that blood supply can become diseased, resulting in erratic functioning of the trigger.

- Pulse may vary between very fast or very slow.
- Symptoms vary from none at all to fainting to loss of consciousness.

Treatment is usually a pacemaker.

### ■ Extra Beats

Extra beats happening frequently will give the impression of an irregular heartbeat. It is difficult to diagnose this situation without an electrocardiogram (ECG). Treatment aims to cure the underlying cause. *(See Heart Makes Extra Beats, page 194)*

### RARE

### ■ Pulmonary Embolus

A blood clot blocking the circulation to part of the lung and usually arising from a clot in a vein in the calf.

- Sudden feeling of pressure in the chest.
- Breathlessness.
- Possibly sharp chest pain and coughing blood.
- Heart rhythms varying from fast but regular to irregular.

## PALPITATIONS (INCLUDING RAPID REGULAR HEART RATE)

Strictly speaking, "palpitations" simply means an awareness of the beating of the heart, but most people use it to mean not just awareness of the heart but an awareness of some abnormality in the beat. So, this symptom is subdivided into: (1) an awareness of a rapid but regular heartbeat; (2) rapid and irregular heartbeat; and (3) irregular heartbeats. Extra heartbeats *(See Heart Makes Extra Beats, page 194)* may also cause palpitations. There is much overlap between causes, so it is best to check in all relevant sections.

## RAPID BUT REGULAR HEART RATE

### PROBABLE

■ **Fever**

Heart rate rises by ten beats per minute per 0.5 degree centigrade rise in temperature, so that very high fevers will be accompanied by correspondingly high pulse rates. There is no specific treatment. Relief comes with the disappearance of fever.

■ **Exercise**

Any but the gentlest exercise will cause a modest rise in heart rate as the heart responds to the increased demand from the muscles and the lungs for larger quantities of oxygen-rich blood. Pulse rates above 120–146 per minute should be viewed with suspicion as a sign of overexertion, under-fitness, or some combination of the two. Chest pain appearing on exertion should always be checked.

■ **Emotion**

Heart rate increases with excitement or acute emotional turmoil through the mechanism of the autonomic nervous system. Accompanying features include:
• Dry mouth.
• Rapid breathing.
• Tremor.

Such a response is normal in many circumstances such as fear, sexual arousal, and sudden emotional shock. It is part of a coordinated system that prepares the body for exertion and to cope with stress. The response becomes abnormal if the individual begins to suffer from chronic anxiety, keeping his or her body in a constant state of increased arousal.

■ **Paroxysmal Tachycardia**

A term used to cover otherwise unexplained episodes of rapid heartbeat. There may be underlying causes, such as an excess of stimulants (coffee, alcohol, cigarettes) *(see Heart Makes Extra Beats, page 194)*, heart disease *(see page 201)*, or electrical conduction disorders *(see page 199)*.

Investigation involves wearing a recording device to capture the rapid rhythm so that its nature can be analyzed. Treatment can then be directed appropriately.
• Abrupt onset of rapid heart rate.
• Entirely regular rhythm.
• If rate is fast enough, faintness or light-headedness.
• Stops as abruptly as it began.

Occasionally, the rhythm is so fast or so prolonged that the heart becomes exhausted, causing breathlessness. This requires medical intervention to correct the rhythm.

## POSSIBLE

### ■ Pregnancy

There is a slight but sustained rise in heart rate during pregnancy, by about ten beats per minute. So, if your usual rate is seventy beats per minute, it can be expected to rise to eighty per minute. In this way, the heart copes with the demands of the growing womb, placenta, and baby.

### ■ Anemia

In an anemic state, there is less capacity to transport oxygen around the body. The heart compensates by increasing its speed of pumping. This will only be a noticeable feature in cases of severe anemia. Other symptoms are:

- Pallor.
- Slight breathlessness.
- Fatigue.

Anemia alone is not a complete diagnosis. Further investigation is needed to find the cause.

### ■ Heart Failure

The early symptoms can be quite undramatic.

- Tiredness.
- Breathlessness on modest exertion.
- Increased heart rate.
- Swelling of ankles.
- Breathlessness while lying flat.

Further tests are needed to determine the reason for the heart failure *(see also page 212).*

### ■ Hyperthyroidism

An overactive thyroid gland can cause extra beats or a sustained rapid pulse *(see page 202).*

### ■ Drugs

There are several over-the-counter drugs that can cause rapid heart rates in a few individuals, including cold remedies containing pseudoephedrine or phenylpropanolamine. Certain anti-asthmatic drugs such as salbutamol may have a similar effect.

## RARE

### ■ Electrical Conduction Disorders

These can be thought of as short circuits in the heart that disrupt the usually smooth control of heartbeat. Though relatively rare, there is much interest in these conditions for the light they shed on the electrical circuitry of the heart. There are surgical treatments available to cut the abnormal electrical circuits responsible for the disorder; otherwise, they are controlled by medication. One of the least rare of these rare conditions is the Wolff-Parkinson-White syndrome, which strikes most commonly in young adults:

- Recurrent bursts of rapid heart rate.
- Characteristic changes on the electrocardiogram (ECG).

### ■ Beri-beri

A deficiency of thiamine (vitamin $B_1$), common in Third World countries, where polished rice (which is low in thiamine) is a staple diet. In the developed world, it occurs not infrequently in alcoholics, who have diets deficient in vitamins.

- Tender muscles.
- Rapid, bounding pulse.
- Often swollen ankles.
- Dementia, unsteady gait.

Rapid recovery is possible if it is recognized and treated early enough.

### ■ Bleeding

Serious external bleeding is obvious, but internal bleeding can continue for several hours with few symptoms apart from:

- Increases in pulse rate.
- Thirst.
- Faintness on standing.

    Eventually there will be:
- Pallor.
- Cold extremities.

- Confusion, collapse.

### ■ Myocarditis

Inflammation of the heart muscle due to a variety of causes, most of which are infections. Some possibilities are viral illnesses, influenza, trypanosomiasis (a parasitic infection), or diphtheria.

- Sudden onset of a feverish illness.
- Breathlessness; swelling of ankles.
- Breathlessness when lying flat.
- Rapid pulse.

The diagnosis requires blood tests, ECG recordings, and, in difficult cases, biopsy of heart muscle.

### ■ Cardiomyopathy

A wide group of disorders where there is a non-inflammatory disturbance of the heart muscle. Many cases are congenital (it can run in families), related to alcoholism, or due to coronary artery disease.

- Heart failure, tiredness, breathlessness.
- In young people, fainting episodes during exercise.
- Rapid heart rates that may be both regular and irregular.

Diagnosis is by ECG and heart biopsy. These disorders need drug treatment to reduce the risk of sudden serious heart rhythm disturbance.

## RAPID, IRREGULAR HEARTBEATS

Most such rhythms are either atrial fibrillations or atrial flutters. Atrial fibrillation is extremely common in older people. It may be the result of diseased coronary arteries, but frequently there are no other symptoms and life expectancy is little changed. The condition occasionally occurs in bursts in young people, when it is known as paroxysmal atrial fibrillation.

The basic defect is uncontrolled contraction of the atria, the small antechambers where blood first arrives in the heart. In fibrillation, the atria beat at rates upwards of 400 per minute, every one of those contractions sending off to the ventricles, the main pumping chambers, a signal to beat. Fortunately, only a fraction of these signals get through, but still enough to give a heart rate of between 100–150 beats per minute. The resulting heart rhythm is totally irregular, as felt at the pulse or as heard over the heart.

Not surprisingly, atrial fibrillation reduces the pumping efficiency of the heart and therefore causes breathlessness and swollen ankles. It also carries a small risk of sending off a blood clot, which may cause a stroke or block arteries in the limbs. It is usual to treat fibrillation with drugs, to both slow the rhythm and strengthen the heart. Consideration would be given to reducing clotting of the blood by giving the anticoagulant warfarin.

Atrial flutter is a less common condition in which the atria beat at a regular rate of between 240–360 beats per minute. This is still too fast to trigger regular contractions of the ventricles, which beat at half or a quarter of the atrial rate (90–180 beats per minute). Though, strictly speaking, this is a *regular* rapid heart rhythm, frequently the rate keeps changing abruptly, going from 180 to 120 to 90 and back again, giving an impression of irregularity. Atrial flutter is a symptom of serious heart disease and needs hospital treatment. Episodes lasting longer than a few minutes can exhaust the heart, sending the individual into rapid heart failure, of which increasing breathlessness is a symptom.

The causes below relate mainly to atrial fibrillation.

### PROBABLE

■ **Ischemic Heart Disease**

Blockage or "furring up" of the blood supply to the heart. This may produce no symptoms other than fibrillation, but frequently there will also be angina *(see page 234)*.

## ■ Hyperthyroidism

Atrial fibrillation may be the only sign of an overactive thyroid gland, especially in the elderly. Thus, it is routine to check for this condition, whose other symptoms include:

- Sweating.
- Tremor.
- Increased appetite.
- Protruding eyes.
- Weight loss.

### POSSIBLE

## ■ Mitral Stenosis

The mitral valve separates the left ventricle from the left atrium. Stenosis means that the valve has become narrowed and stiff. The most common reason for this used to be rheumatic fever, which is now rare in developed countries; the process of aging is the usual reason nowadays. The condition gradually strains the heart, eventually causing heart failure.

- History of rheumatic fever years before.
- Mildest symptoms are just fibrillation.
- As the condition worsens, breathlessness, cough with bloodstained phlegm.
- Eventually, swelling of ankles.
- There may be a permanent purple flush over the cheek bones.

Drugs are used to treat mild cases, with surgery to the valve being reserved for more severe cases.

## ■ Alcohol Abuse

Long-term alcohol abuse weakens the muscle of the heart, allowing various rhythm disorders to result.

## ■ Complications of Heart Attack

In the hours and days after a heart attack, the injured heart can produce a variety of disordered rhythms. The most worrying are ventricular tachycardias, where the ventricles go off into bursts of rapid beating that have the potential to turn into totally irregular, life-threatening beating. Monitoring and dealing with these ventricular rhythms is one major reason for observation in a coronary care unit after a heart attack.

- Rapid thumping in the chest.
- Faintness.
- As the condition worsens, loss of consciousness.

### RARE

## ■ Pneumonia

This severe chest infection can occasionally set off atrial fibrillation, which disappears after recovery. *(See page 216)*

## ■ Endocarditis

An infection of the valves of the heart that usually attacks valves that are already abnormal, for example, after rheumatic fever. Fibrillation is just one of a variety of symptoms.

- Night sweats.
- Malaise.
- Clubbed fingernails.
- Splinter-like lines under the nails.
- Anemia.

Aggressive long-term antibiotic treatment is needed to eradicate the infection.

### ■ Pericarditis

Constriction of the heart by fluid or by fibrous material can give rise to fibrillation.

*(See Pericardial Effusion, page 221)*

### ■ Atrial Septal Defect

There is a hole between the right and left sides of the baby's heart while it is in the womb. This hole should close at birth, but occasionally it remains open. Symptoms can take years to develop or a murmur may be detected on examination.

- Increased susceptibility to chest infections.
- Breathlessness.
- Palpitations including fibrillation are common.

## HEART BEATS SLOWLY

By convention, this is taken as a rate of less than sixty beats per minute. Frequently, it is an incidental finding in someone without symptoms, but very slow rates (below forty beats per minute) are likely to cause dizziness, fainting, and, in the elderly, confusion. There are two main causes of very slow rates. The pacemaker of the heart may be sending out a slow rhythm or there is a block to the pacemaker rhythm so that the ventricles beat at a much slower rate than the signals sent from the pacemaker. An electrocardiogram (ECG) is needed to diagnose these conditions properly.

### PROBABLE

### ■ Fitness

A slow pulse is common in athletes and others who perform regular physical exercise.

### ■ Drug-Induced

Digoxin is a drug that causes a very slow pulse if given in excess. Another widely used class of drugs called beta-blockers slows the pulse to around sixty beats per minute, but this is an intentional effect and is a sign of correct dosage. Beta-blockers are used to treat high blood pressure and angina. Beta-blockers are important in the treatment of heart disease. Sometimes they are used to quell the symptoms of anxiety; due to their ability to stop palpitations and sweats, they are frequently taken by musicians and actors before performances.

## ■ Heart Block

Heart block comes from disease of the conducting pathways that transmit the pacemaker signal to the rest of the heart. The ventricles have their own pacemaker, which triggers them at 30–40 beats per minute, so there may be no dramatic symptoms even with complete heart block. The usual reason for this problem is aging or poor blood supply to the heart; it can also happen after a heart attack. Symptoms, in increasing order of severity, include:

• None at all, but noticed on an electrocardiogram (ECG).
• Awareness of a slow, thudding heartbeat.
• Tiredness.
• Dizzy spells.
• Recurrent abrupt loss of consciousness.

Treatment is with an artificial pacemaker to maintain regular contraction.

## POSSIBLE

### ■ Hypothyroidism

An underactive thyroid gland, whose other symptoms include:

• Coarse dry skin.
• Sensitivity to cold.
• Slow thought, tiredness.
• Gruff voice.

Treatment with thyroid hormone has to be lifelong.

## ■ Sick Sinus Syndrome

Caused by the effects of aging on the pacemaking area of the heart. This can cause rhythms from slow to fast and any combination in between.

• Palpitations.
• Dizzy spells.
• Tiredness.

*(See also page 197)*

## ■ Congenital

Some people are born with a slow pulse, but doctors would be prudent to search for other signs of heart disease, such as heart murmurs or abnormal electrocardiogram (ECG) traces.

## RARE

### ■ Cardiomyopathy

A general term for diseases of the heart muscle. The effect is to cause the rapid appearance of heart failure with either slow or rapid heart rates. *(See also page 200)*

# THE CHEST AND LUNGS

## BREATHING PROBLEMS

We breathe in order to provide the body's cells with the oxygen essential to their function and to get rid of carbon dioxide, which is produced as a waste product of metabolism. It is no surprise that breathing is affected by all sorts of bodily disorders, often from the lungs or heart.

Breathing also helps to regulate the body's acid-alkaline balance. Because the brain controls breathing, disease and also drugs can affect those parts of the brain that, day in and day out, keep us breathing.

This section begins with causes of sudden breathlessness, then continues with breathlessness appearing over relatively long periods. Causes tend to overlap, so

you will see the same diagnoses coming up repeatedly. We make no apology for this as breathlessness is an alarming symptom and some repetition is helpful.

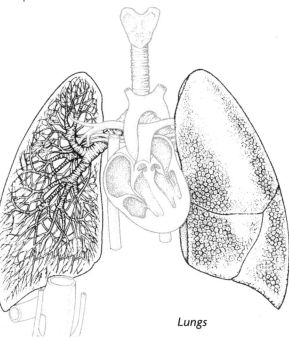

*Lungs*

205

# Heimlich Maneuver

The Heimlich Maneuver is named after the American physician (Henry Jay Heimlich) who has promoted this simple, life-saving procedure. It is to be used on someone who is choking as a result of inhaling food or other solid objects and is unable to clear the object.

- Stand behind the person choking.
- Extend your arms in a hug around their upper abdomen.
- With clenched fists make a hard, fast squeeze just under the breast bone.

The maneuver forces a blast of air out of the lungs, sufficient to dislodge something stuck in the upper airway. For full details, see any modern manual of first aid.

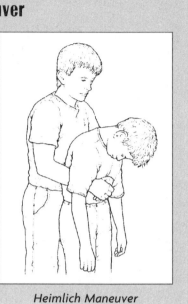

*Heimlich Maneuver*

## RASPING, SNORING BREATHING

Also described as stertorous breathing. It is only occasionally a symptom of disease, usually just a nuisance.

Snoring is the result of vibration of the soft palate, which is at the back of the roof of the mouth. The cure is simply a matter of trying out different sleeping postures or changing the number or firmness of your pillows. Reducing alcohol intake may help, as well as losing weight, if you are overweight.

**PROBABLE**

- Snoring

*(See left)*

**POSSIBLE**

- Adenoids

Adenoids are pads of tissue at the back of the nose, similar to tonsils. They are probably intended to counter infection, which might enter through the mouth and nose. In childhood, adenoids can grow so large that they obstruct nasal breathing. The child exhibits:

- Nasal speech.
- Snoring.
- Mouth breathing.
- Recurrent ear infections.

Treatment is occasionally surgical removal of the adenoids, if there is no sign of a natural decrease in their size and breathing is significantly affected.

### ■ Sleep Apnea

In sleep apnea, the breathing is obstructed, often at the back of the throat and surrounding structures. This typically occurs in adults, particularly men who are overweight or have a size 17" collar size or greater. The adult exhibits:

- Snoring.
- Periods when they seem to stop breathing, which then restarts with a loud chortling noise.

- Waking unrefreshed in the morning and feeling tired during the day.
- Tendency to fall asleep during the day or even while they are driving a car.

Treatment is weight loss where required, and, if the sleep apnea is severe, wearing a special mask while sleeping that keeps the airway passages open. Occasionally, surgery can help.

### ■ Stroke

A blood clot or bleeding in the brain causing:

- One-sided paralysis.
- Coma.
- Stertorous breathing, typically if the individual goes into a deep coma.

### ■ Alcoholic Stupor

Drinking to the point of collapse frequently gives this symptom.

## HOARSE, WHEEZY INTAKE OF BREATH

This is probably a stridor caused by a foreign body *(see Asphyxia, page 228)*.

## CHEST ABNORMALLY SHAPED

### PROBABLE

### ■ Congenital

Twists of the spine can gradually produce a misshapen chest. These can some-times be treated if spotted early enough.

- Seen from behind, the spine is curved.
- Curve becomes more prominent on bending forward.

Another congenital abnormality gives a funnel-shaped chest with a depressed breastbone. This too can be corrected by surgery, which is recommended if there is a risk of the depression pressing on the heart, but usually no treatment is needed.

## POSSIBLE

### ■ Chronic Obstructive Airway Diseases

A general term covering chronic bronchitis and emphysema. The continual effort of breathing in these conditions can eventually, in adult life, cause a barrel-shaped chest.

*(See page 215)*

## RARE

### ■ Asthma

Chronic, severe asthma that is inade-

quately treated can result in a young adult who has:
• A broad, over-inflated chest.
• Prominent rib margins.
• Prominent breastbone, which gives a pointed appearance to the front of the chest.

The reason is thought to be years of extra effort by the muscles between the ribs, which have to work harder in asthma. They gradually pull the lower ribs into a prominent shape. This is seen less and less as asthma treatment improves.

### ■ Rickets

This disease, due to lack of vitamin D, can give rise to unsightly prominent joints where the ribs join the breast bone. Now a rarity in developed countries.

## BREATHLESSNESS, RAPID ONSET

Considered here are attacks of breathlessness that happen rapidly, yet fall short of abrupt suffocation or asphyxia. There should be little difficulty in recognizing the seriousness of the situation, except perhaps with babies and children, where you should be alert to drowsiness and breathlessness that interferes with feeding.

## PROBABLE

### ■ Asthma

This common illness is more of a nuisance than a disability for most asthmatics most of the time. However, asthma can turn suddenly and unpredictably into a life-threatening condition.

Muscle surrounds the airways right

down into the lungs. Asthma results from excessive constriction of that muscle, which narrows the airways and increases the effort required to shift air into the lungs. As a cause of chronic breathlessness, asthma is covered in detail under Breathlessness and Wheeze *(see page 214)*, where the common features of asthma are described. Severe, acute asthma is a potential killer. There is danger for the known asthmatic who underestimates the severity of an attack or for someone whose first attack of asthma is severe, unrecognized, and who has no standard treatment at hand. Signs suggesting asthma is getting out of control and that prompt medical attention is needed are:

• Poor response to usual asthma medication.

• Too breathless to talk in full sentences.

• The chest continually feels "tighter."

• Sweating, breathlessness, rapid pulse.

• Neck muscles strain in an attempt to increase breathing.

• As attack worsens, cyanosis (lips going blue), tiredness, pallor, drowsiness, confusion, coma. Call 911 if this were to happen and take ten puffs of your inhaler medication.

• Deterioration can take several hours or just a few minutes.

■ **Bronchiolitis**

This is an infantile equivalent of asthma. It is a winter disease, caused by a particular virus. It occurs in epidemics.

• Initially, the baby is snuffly, with a slight cough indistinguishable from a common cold.

• Wheezing begins and worsens over a few hours.

• Breathing produces a crackling sound, also felt through the chest.

• Breathlessness interferes with feeding.

• Breathing becomes rapid, often with grunting.

• At worst, pallor, cyanosis of lips.

First aid: put the child in a steamy atmosphere, which sometimes can improve things, and seek advice from a doctor. Occasionally, the child needs oxygen treatment in a hospital. Babies with this condition have an increased chance of being asthmatic later in life.

Children whose parents smoke are three times more likely to enter the hospital in their first year with a chest condition than infants of nonsmokers.

■ **Croup**

This is a viral infection affecting children between ages six months and three years. The child typically has symptoms of a temperature and a cold along with:

• Hoarse voice.

- Intermittent barking cough, often worse at night.
- Wheeze that occurs when the child breathes in (stridor).
- Breathing difficulties.

First aid: keep child as calm as possible and seek advice from a doctor.

## ■ Chest Infection

A severe chest infection or pneumonia can rapidly progress to difficulty in breathing.

- Wet cough, with colored phlegm.
- High temperature.
- Flaring nostrils.
- Rapid breathing.
- Pain over the affected part of the chest, particularly when breathing in.
- Cyanosis (blue color) of lips and tongue.
- Sometimes bloodstained phlegm.
- Confusion.

This is more likely in the elderly or in those who are debilitated for other reasons.

## POSSIBLE

## ■ Heart Failure

Predominantly a disease occurring later in life. There is often a history of heart trouble, perhaps heart attack, or high blood pressure.

- Early symptoms are tiredness, breathlessness on exertion.
- Swelling of ankles.
- Breathlessness worse on attempting to lie flat.
- Need to stack up pillows in order to sleep.
- In more advanced cases, waking from sleep with a feeling of suffocation.
- Copious, frothy, pinkish phlegm.
- Relief gained from sitting upright for a few minutes.

This situation may need urgent medical help if it occurs severely.

## ■ Pulmonary Embolus

This is where a blood clot lodges in the lung. It often arises from a clot that has already formed in a leg (deep vein thrombosis or DVT). It is more likely if someone has been on a long plane journey, is on the oral contraceptive pill, or has been immobile in bed in the hospital or at home for a while.

- Breathlessness.
- Pain on breathing in.
- Coughing up some blood.

This situation needs prompt advice from a doctor.

## ■ Acute or Chronic Bronchitis

A chest infection can be the minor, extra stress that pushes the individual with chronic bronchitis into severe breathing problems. The already limited effort that someone can put into breathing becomes too little to expel waste carbon dioxide or to take in fresh oxygen. The result is the equivalent of suffocation over a short period.

- Severe headache.
- Warm, blue hands; rapid pulse; twitching of muscles.
- Agitation, confusion worsening to coma.

This situation needs urgent help.

### RARE

#### ■ Allergic Alveolitis

The alveoli are the sacs in the lung where carbon dioxide is exchanged for oxygen. An allergic reaction causes inflammation in these sacs. The consequent swelling interferes with efficient gas transfer. The most common cause is an allergy to moldy hay, known as farmer's lung, and is widespread in areas of non-mechanized farming.

- Breathlessness, wheezing within a few hours of exposure.
- Fever, cough, and malaise; joint pains.
- Symptoms take a few days to disappear.

The chronic condition shows:

- Recurrent difficulty in breathing.
- Clubbed (highly curved) fingernails.

Treatment is to avoid exposure to the cause of the allergy.

## BREATHLESSNESS OVER DAYS, WEEKS, OR MONTHS

This type of breathlessness does not have particularly prominent secondary symptoms, at least not at first. And there are no hard and fast distinctions between all the conditions that share these symptoms, so read this section before drawing any conclusions.

Breathlessness that sets in over only a few days or weeks clearly needs investigation. Breathlessness that appears more gradually can be more puzzling. It should be judged in relation to your usual level of exercise: if your principal form of physical activity is opening the garage door, do not be too surprised at your breathlessness if you have to change a tire. Remember also that your ability to cope with sudden effort can decline completely unnoticed as long as you are still able to perform your regular activities. For example, shopping trips and gentle strolls may present no problem, but you may be alarmed at how breathless you become climbing stairs. This does not in itself suggest disease, just being out of shape.

But there is a pitfall in this: while it is natural to limit exertion to the level you know you can tolerate, that level may actually be abnormally low. The best guide is to compare yourself with others of your age and general fitness. If you are the one who has to rest halfway round a golf course, you may have a problem.

Bear this in mind before you jump to any conclusions. Ask yourself a few questions. How long has it been since you last did any exercise that made you sweat? Have you gained weight recently? Do you smoke heavily? Honest answers to these questions may be illuminating.

To improve your fitness, aim to achieve shortness of breath and sweating over a period of twenty minutes, at least three times a week. If you have a heart problem, seek advice from your doctor first.

There are other, everyday circumstances in which breathlessness is normal. Excitement, fear, and anger all generate a high breathing rates and may make you feel breathless. Only after you have excluded all these possibilities is it reasonable to wonder whether your breathlessness is a symptom of illness.

## PROBABLE

### ■ Coronary Artery Disease

This is where the arteries to the heart become furred up, reducing blood flow to the heart and so reducing the ability of the heart to deliver blood efficiently.

- Breathlessness may be the only symptom.
- Angina (chest pain) on exertion.
- When more advanced, the symptoms of heart failure (see below).

The diagnosis is made by a combination of exercise electrocardiogram (ECG) and angiography of the heart, where a dye is injected to show the arteries. Usually treated with an operation to open up the artery with an implanted tube called a stent or with coronary artery bypass grafting.

### ■ Heart Failure

Mainly a problem for older people. The symptoms of heart failure can mistakenly be put down to aging unless a dramatic or sudden deterioration occurs. There will often be a history of high blood pressure, angina, or heart attack. Early symptoms are:

- Tiredness, decreased tolerance of exercise.
- Swelling of ankles.
- Loss of appetite.
- Later, breathlessness while lying flat in bed.
- Sleeping on stacked up pillows.
- Breathlessness wakes you at night, with a frothy cough; symptoms pass after sitting upright for a while.

In the elderly, tiredness can be the only symptom of heart failure. Modern treatment has greatly improved the outlook for people with heart failure.

## ◼ Psychological

A possibility in a younger person. Friends or colleagues may notice overbreathing—often the individual leads a stressful life.
- Describes an inability to breathe in deeply enough.
- Otherwise, sound health.

Reassurance, and thorough investigations, revealing nothing, generally help these cases.

## POSSIBLE

## ◼ Chronic Obstructive Pulmonary Disease

Previously known as chronic bronchitis or emphysema *(see page 215)*.
- Breathlessness, often with wheeze.
- Usually in smokers.
- Breathing improved by anti-asthmatic aerosols.

The diagnosis needs confirmation by respiratory function tests.
*(See also page 438)*

## ◼ Pregnancy

A common feature of middle-to-late pregnancy, when the womb is enlarged and presses against the diaphragm.

## ◼ Anemia

Blood carries oxygen around the body, so that if the volume of blood in one's body drops significantly, breathlessness ensues, together with:
- Tiredness, easy fatigue.
- Pallor on the undersurfaces of eyelids, nail beds.

Symptoms of the disorder that causes the anemia may also be apparent, for example, blood loss or poor diet. Simple investigations should quickly confirm the diagnosis.

## ◼ Lung Effusion

The lungs react to irritation in the same way that the skin reacts to a minor burn. Tissue fluid seeps out, collecting in a pool at the base of the lungs. If this pool grows large enough, it compresses the lung above, reducing its ability to function and causing breathlessness. There are no specific symptoms to indicate an effusion: it has to be detected by medical examination or chest x-ray.

There is nearly always some predisposing condition. The most common are severe heart failure, pneumonia, pulmonary embolus, and lung cancer. These cause symptoms considered under Heart Failure *(page 199)*.

## ◼ Lung Cancer

A tumor may block off a major airway,

thereby putting out of action all or part of a lung, and causing breathlessness.

## RARE

### ■ Skeletal Abnormalities

Gross distortions of the chest wall cause the ribs to squash the lungs and heart so that their expansion is restricted. These deformities are called kyphosis or kypho-scoliosis (see *page 295*).

### ■ Occupational Lung Disease

A group of occupational lung diseases caused by years of exposure to dust. Common ones are silicosis (miners, pottery workers), pneumoconiosis (coal miners), and asbestosis. The symptoms are:
• Progressive breathlessness on exertion.
• Cough.

Dust control and masks reduce the risks for workers in hazardous industries.

### ■ Mountain Sickness

The direct effect of the lack of oxygen at altitudes of about 8,000 feet or higher. The young and fit are at risk just as much as the unfit or elderly; in fact, possibly more at risk because the young will be climbing faster. This is a dangerous condition. Early symptoms are:
• Breathlessness.
• Headache, tiredness.

If ignored, these will progress to:
• Profuse bloodstained cough.
• Nausea, confusion.
• Coma.

All cases need descent to lower altitudes; serious cases may also require resuscitation.

### ■ Fibrosing Alveolitis

The final stage of allergic alveolitis *(see page 211)* or sometimes of unknown origin.
• Chronic breathlessness.
• Clubbed fingernails *(see page 302)*.
• Cough, cyanosis.

## BREATHLESSNESS AND WHEEZE

Excluding acute chest infection *(see page 210)*, this extremely common combination points to narrowing of the airways, producing obstructed air flow. Often, there is an allergic factor: many asthmatics, sensitive to dust and fumes, exhibit these symptoms for hours, even days, on end.

### PROBABLE

### ■ Asthma

Some 10 percent of the population suffer

from asthma, and the number is believed to be rising. The classic features are:

- Recurrent breathlessness.
- Wheeze and cough.
- In children, persistent nighttime cough.
- Common colds that regularly go to the chest.

Doctors are often disinclined to label a child as asthmatic until there is no doubt, as it can be a disservice to the child. Helpful treatment is available.

*(See also page 208)*

## ■ Chronic Bronchitis

Chronic obstructive airways disease. Believed to result from years of exposure to fumes, chemicals, and smoke, of which cigarette smoke is the main avoidable culprit. The prime features are the gradual manifestation of:

- Increasingly persistent cough.
- Wheeze.
- Breathlessness.
- Large amounts of phlegm ("smoker's cough").

Chronic bronchitis does not have the same reputation as lung cancer, yet quality of life can be considerably reduced. Perpetual breathlessness, in severe cases, is every bit as miserable as the final stages of cancer. Stopping smoking is vital to slow the damage to the lungs.

## POSSIBLE

### ■ Occupational Asthma

This includes many conditions associated with specific industries, in particular those producing flax, sisal, hemp, or cotton, animal substances, certain metals, chemicals, and organic dusts.

- "Monday morning breathlessness" on re-exposure to the agent causing the allergy.
- Wheeze, breathlessness.
- Improvement over weekends and holidays when not exposed.

## RARE

### ■ Drug Reaction

The drugs in widest use that can produce this reaction are beta-blockers (used to control high blood pressure or angina), aspirin and similar antirheumatic drugs, and a few anticancer drugs such as methotrexate may also be responsible.

### ■ Aspergillosis

An infection caused by a fungus called *Aspergillus,* commonly found in rotting and decaying vegetation. For most people, *Aspergillus* is harmless. If the lungs are damaged by previous infection (such as tuberculosis) or asthma, the fungus may cause the following symptoms:

- Recurrent wheeze, cough.
- Feverish episodes.

The diagnosis is determined by blood tests and allergy testing.

## BREATHLESSNESS AND COUGH

### PROBABLE

■ **Chest Infection**

Recognized by the combination of:

• Cough with yellow or green phlegm.
• Fever, modest degree of malaise.
• Breathlessness plus wheeze.

All these symptoms appear in only a couple of days, often preceded by a sore throat and a common cold.

Antibiotic treatment is usual for these common and not very serious infections.

### POSSIBLE

■ **Chronic Bronchitis**

The strict medical definition is a cough productive of phlegm for at least three months of the year for at least two consecutive years. It is well known that smokers and workers in dusty environments risk developing the condition. The excessive production of phlegm amounts to an exaggeration of the lungs' defense mechanism against infection and dust: the gooey mucus traps the foreign matter, which the lungs then try to expel by coughing. In permanent overdrive, the lungs begin losing their efficiency. Individuals are at risk of frequent chest infections and, in the long run, progressive shortness of breath.

Though the disease cannot be re-versed, further deterioration can be delayed by giving up smoking and by avoiding dust and fumes.

■ **Pneumonia**

A serious chest infection, usually of rapid onset, with:

• High fever, chills.
• Rapid breathing and cough.
• Phlegm may be rust-colored or obviously contain blood.
• Aching or severe sharp pain in the chest.

Occasionally, especially in the elderly, pneumonia exhibits less clear-cut symptoms and is suggested by abrupt weakness and fever. Aggressive antibiotic therapy means that pneumonia is no longer the feared killer it once was, though it is still a worry in the elderly or those with preexisting problems, such as heart disease, chronic bronchitis, and diabetes.

*(See also page 180)*

### RARE

■ **Bronchiectasis**

In this disease, once far more common than it is today, the lung structure breaks down, making the lungs susceptible to pockets of chronic infection.

• Initially, frequent chest infections.

- Constant production of large amounts of colored phlegm.
- Phlegm often bloodstained.
- As it worsens, breathlessness, clubbed (highly curved) fingernails.
- Poor growth in children; fatigue.

## ■ Lung Cancer

This diagnosis must be considered not only for a cough with breathlessness but for any persistent breathing problem. Adult smokers are particularly vulnerable. *(See page 226)*

## ■ Tuberculosis

Now uncommon in developed countries, except in the poor, those with HIV/AIDS, immigrants from the Third World, and those who neglect themselves, such as alcoholics. The usual features are:

- Malaise, weight loss.
- Cough, often bloodstained.
- Breathlessness resulting from complications.

Treatment, though prolonged, cures the disease.

## BREATHLESSNESS AND FEELING TIRED/EXHAUSTED

Though lung disease is usually the cause of breathlessness, it can arise from subtle changes in the condition of the heart, blood, or metabolism. Fatigue will then be a prominent symptom, before breathlessness is noticeable. Breathlessness in these situations may result from an imbalance between acid and alkaline chemicals in the body. Major disturbances of regular body functions, such as diabetes and kidney failure, generates excess acid that the body tries to reduce by blowing off more carbon dioxide with heavy, deep breathing.

Remember that prolonged or severe breathlessness, for any reason, will eventually cause fatigue simply through exhaustion and a chronic lack of oxygen.

### PROBABLE

## ■ Anemia

Blood carries oxygen around the body so that if the volume of blood drops significantly, breathlessness ensues, together with:

- Tiredness, easy fatigue.
- Pallor, particularly the undersurfaces of eyelids or nail beds.

Symptoms of the disorder that causes the anemia may be evident, for example, blood loss from heavy periods, poor diet. Simple investigations indicate the diagnosis. *(See page 433)*

## ■ Heart Failure

Breathlessness is a frequent symptom in

the middle-aged; in the elderly, an early indication of heart failure can be unusual tiredness. Once this is recognized, look for other symptoms of heart failure:

- Swollen ankles.
- Breathlessness when lying flat.

*(See also page 212)*

## POSSIBLE

### ■ Heart Disease

Disturbance of heartbeat, with rhythms either too fast or too slow, felt as a flutter in the chest, or as palpitations. These are inefficient rhythms producing breathlessness with fatigue *(see page 217)*. Other forms of heart disease, such as valve problems, cause breathlessness by decreasing the efficiency of the heart. Those with a history of rheumatic fever may find this a problem. In general, these disorders can only be detected by medical examination.

*(See also Coronary Artery Disease under Breathlessness Over Days, Weeks, or Months, page 211)*

## RARE

### ■ Diabetic Complications

Diabetes is a condition that produces a high blood sugar level. The early symptoms are:

- Passing large amounts of urine.
- Thirst.
- Weight loss.

In young people, onset tends to be rapid, over a couple of weeks. In older people, it may go unnoticed, apart from slightly increased urine output and a vague sense of tiredness.

Diabetes affecting children and young adults is often caused by a lack of insulin, the hormone needed by the body's cells to make use of sugar. Thus, there are high levels of sugar in the bloodstream, yet the cells are unable to use it. But life must go on and the cells' metabolism turns to alternative means of generating energy. The trouble with these is their tendency to generate large amounts of acidic waste products. The body tries to compensate by blowing off large amounts of carbon dioxide, hence heavy breathing.

Meanwhile, sugar in the bloodstream spills out through the kidneys, dragging water with it. The final result is a dangerous state called diabetic ketoacidosis, and it is a major medical emergency.

- Dehydration, dry mouth, intense thirst.
- Deep, sighing breathing.
- Sweet smell on breath.
- Confusion, nausea.

Rapid treatment is life-saving. Known diabetics may fall into this state during other stressful illnesses.

### ■ Kidney Failure

Early symptoms are only:

- Increased passage of urine.
- Tiredness.

Blood tests at this stage allow diagnosis and consequent changes in diet, which may give years of reasonable health. If eventually the kidneys fail, there is an array of symptoms, including:

- Tiredness, developing into confusion.
- Deep, gasping breathing.
- Dry, furred tongue.
- Nausea, hiccups.
- Itching, anemia.

The development of kidney transplantation has revolutionized the treatment of this condition.

## BREATHLESSNESS AND CHEST PAIN

Symptoms of this kind are often caused by serious disruption of the output from the heart or by lung malfunction. If breathlessness is the most prominent symptom, see Asphyxia *(page 228)* or Breathlessness, Rapid Onset *(page 208),* as well as reading this section. If chest pain is most prominent, look at the sections on heartbeat. In view of the importance of these symptoms, some of the information found there is repeated here.

### PROBABLE

### ■ Chest Infection

The gradual appearance of fever, cough, and phlegm is often accompanied by a slight ache over both lungs. *(See page 210)*

### ■ Heart Attack

*(See also page 231)*

In a middle-aged person, suspect a heart attack if there is:

- Sudden central chest pain.
- Sweating.
- Pain radiating up to the jaws or into the left arm.
- Breathlessness.

These are the classic symptoms, but in quite a few cases the heart attack is "silent," meaning that chest pain is not the most obvious feature or may be absent. Instead, a heart attack may be suspected on the basis of:

- Sudden onset of breathlessness as a new symptom.
- Sudden worsening of existing breathlessness.

• Symptoms of heart failure: swollen ankles, breathlessness when lying flat, breathlessness during the night, tiredness.

Recently, there have been major advances in treatment, so that early recognition of the problem means a much improved chance of recovery. It is, therefore, essential to establish the diagnosis as soon as possible. Heart attacks are most common in older people, but are possible at any age, so always take dramatic chest pain seriously.

### ■ Pleurisy

The pleurae are the thin membranes that surround the lungs. They become inflamed for a variety of reasons, particularly infection, when you can feel a typical pain.
• Knife-like pain over a small area of the chest.
• Pain worse on breathing in.
• Breathlessness as a consequence of avoiding deep breathing.

Pleurisy commonly accompanies a chest infection. In this case, it sets in gradually over a few hours. A pneumothorax *(see right)* causes sudden pleuritic pain as can a pulmonary embolus *(see right)*.

Treatment aims both to relieve the pain and to cure the underlying condition.

### ■ Pneumothorax

Collapse of part of a lung, sometimes the whole lung. Quite common and needing appropriate treatment. However, pneumothorax is rarely life-threatening, though the pain may be disabling.

## POSSIBLE

### ■ Pneumonia

Suggested by a combination of:
• High fever.
• Rapid breathing.
• Painful cough.

*(See also page 216)*

### ■ Pulmonary Embolus

A blood clot that lodges in the blood supply to a lung. Sudden breathlessness follows the reduction in the lung's efficiency. Pain in the chest is not always a symptom, but will certainly be felt if the affected part of the lung begins to die from lack of oxygen. *(See page 227)*

### ■ Lung Cancer

This diagnosis should always be borne in mind when unusual breathlessness and chest pain are the symptoms in elderly individuals, particularly those who smoke. *(See page 226)*

### ■ Irregular Heartbeat

Very rapid or very slow heart rates can cause chest pain, with breathlessness a result of low output from the heart. *(See sections on heartbeat, pages 194–204)*

## RARE

### ■ Pericardial Effusion

The heart is surrounded by a lining that can become inflamed. This is known as pericarditis. Pericardial effusion is when the fluid released from inflammation collects around the heart, interfering with its ability to pump blood effectively. Most often, this condition follows a viral infection. Other causes may include heart attack, bacterial infections, inflammatory disorders such as rheumatoid arthritis, and occasionally trauma.

• At first, the sharp central chest pain of pericarditis.

• Pain seems to radiate to shoulders.

• Often relieved by bending forward; worse when lying down.

• Breathlessness, worsening as fluid builds up.

• Fever may be present, particularly if pericarditis has been caused by an infection.

This is not an easy diagnosis, but may be the reason for breathlessness after certain diseases. X-rays and irregular readings recorded by electrocardiogram (ECG) machines may suggest the diagnosis, but it is confirmed with an ultrasound examination of the heart.

### ■ Heart Tamponade

This is the most severe effect of a pericardial effusion *(see left)*. The condition may begin with pericarditis or perhaps an injury to the heart, such as a stab wound. Fluid or blood gathers around the heart until it is squashed and unable to pump. There are no straightforward or obvious symptoms apart from rapidly increasing breathlessness after the illness or injury that caused the pericarditis; occasionally, distended veins in the neck may also be observed.

Treatment is to urgently drain off the fluid.

## COUGH

Cough is generally a reflex action of irritated lungs or voice box, or lungs trying to expel phlegm or a foreign body. Most coughs are easily recognizable for the minor problem they are, but sometimes need to be taken more seriously because of duration, pain, or associated symptoms. In the very young and the elderly, coughs can be a sign of more serious illness and need more attention.

## DRY COUGH WITHOUT PHLEGM

Few of us pass a year without suffering this sort of cough. It nearly always reflects minor irritation of the lungs rather than more serious disease. It passes in a week or so of using simple remedies, such as aspirin or plenty of fluids, and avoiding dry atmospheres.

If there are other symptoms of illness, such as raised temperature lasting more than forty-eight hours, or if the cough becomes chronic, it would be sensible to see a doctor.

### PROBABLE

### ■ Common Cold

Cough, commonly accompanied by other common cold symptoms, such as:
• Rapid onset of sneezing and aches.

Usually cures itself.

### ■ Irritant Atmosphere

• Dry, dusty conditions.
• Cough is relieved in normal atmosphere.
• Not otherwise ill.

### ■ Postnasal Drip

Secretions from the nose or from the sinuses run to the back of throat and provoke cough. Treatment is aimed at the underlying condition, the most common

being chronic sinusitis, hay fever, and (in children) adenoid trouble.

### POSSIBLE

### ■ Laryngitis

A common winter illness causing many of the symptoms of the common cold, but also:
• Raw feeling in the throat.
• Hoarseness or loss of voice.
• Often develops into chest infection.

### ■ Tracheitis

Rather similar to laryngitis, but:
• Raw feeling more in lower neck/upper chest.
• Often "goes to the chest."
• Rasping feeling behind breastbone.

### ■ Asthma

One of the most common causes of chronic cough at all ages. The diagnosis, often difficult to make because cough can be caused by so many factors, is suggested by:
• Recurrent wheeze and breathlessness, particularly after exertion.

However:
• A frequent, dry, nighttime cough may be the first symptom, especially in children.

- Close relative(s) are very often asthmatic, too.
- Associated with eczema and hay fever.

### ■ Drug Side Effect

An unpredictable side effect of so-called angiotensin-converting enzyme (ACE) inhibitor drugs, increasingly used to treat high blood pressure and other heart conditions.

### ■ Acid Reflux

Severe acid reflux (heartburn) can spill up from the gullet and into the larynx, causing a cough.

### ■ Habit

- Not otherwise unwell.
- Worsens if attention given, goes when distracted.
- Worse if nervous.

### ■ Whooping Cough

The severe form of whooping cough, causing paroxysms of cough to the point of breathlessness followed by a whoop as air is breathed in, is now extremely rare thanks to immunization. A milder form, causing a prolonged cough in older children or occasionally in adults, is now increasingly recognized, but resolves on its own, though it may take three to four months to do so.

### RARE

### ■ Lung Cancer

*(See page 226)*

### ■ Tumor or Infection of Larynx

- Persistent hoarseness, pain in neck, enlarged glands in neck. *(See page 85)*

---

## COUGH PLUS PHLEGM

Most likely to be caused by a minor infection of the lungs, which in most people will resolve rapidly. Those with other preexisting serious conditions, such as heart disease or diabetes, may need antibiotics to control the infection.

### PROBABLE

### ■ Common Cold

- After first few days, a "wet" cough with colored phlegm, but otherwise feeling well.

### ■ Acute Bronchitis

- Cough, phlegm, and wheeze.
- Feeling mildly unwell.
- Some breathlessness.

### ■ Chest Infection

- Copious cough, phlegm, fever.

- Sweats and feeling unwell.
- Onset over a day or two.
- May be accompanied by pleurisy, a knife-like pain between the ribs when breathing in.

## POSSIBLE

### ■ Chronic Bronchitis

Cough, phlegm, and wheeze for weeks on end, possibly for most of the year. A disease especially of smokers, those with long-term exposure to dusty atmospheres, and of people who live in damp, northern climates. Don't dismiss the morning "smoker's cough"—this is your lungs telling you that they are being killed by fumes; their reaction is to push out large amounts of phlegm.
- Frequent episodes of bronchitis, summer and winter.
- Chronic cough.
- Breathlessness eventually becomes a constant feature.

It is essential to give up smoking. This helps to some degree, no matter how late you stop.

### ■ Pneumonia

A serious infection of part or all of one lung. You feel very ill.
- Rapid onset.
- Breathlessness or fast breathing.
- General aching, tiredness, cough.

- Sweats, sometimes drenching, especially at night.
- Pain over affected part of lung.

## RARE

### ■ Bronchiectasis

A disease in which the structure of the lungs breaks down, reducing their efficiency.
- Gradual appearance of chronic cough, with copious phlegm.
- Bad breath.

Chest x-ray needed to confirm diagnosis.

### ■ Tuberculosis

- Chronic fatigue, malaise, weight loss, anorexia *(see page 446)*.

Groups especially at risk are those with HIV/AIDS, those with low incomes who live in poor/overcrowded housing, immigrants, and alcoholics.

### ■ Lung Abscess

*(See under Cough Plus Bloody Phlegm)*

### ■ Inhaled Foreign Body

Typically in children. A child can (unnoticed) inhale a peanut or similar small object. A coughing fit probably follows, which the parent overlooks. Chest infection plus typical symptoms then develop and never really clear. If these symptoms are neglected, the child becomes listless and run-down after several weeks. Inhaling a foreign body sometimes creates stridor *(see Asphyxia, page 228)*.

### ■ Pneumoconiosis

A group of diseases in which the lungs become stiffer and stiffer, unable to expand properly.

• Associated with dusty industries such as coal mining.

• Cough, breathlessness, and wheeze is progressive over months and years.

• Finger clubbing *(see page 302)*.

### ■ Cystic Fibrosis

A childhood disease caused by inherited genetic abnormality.

• Repeated chest infections, failure to grow.

• Diarrhea, weight loss.

In some places, babies are screened for this at birth.

### ■ AIDS

Groups especially at risk are intravenous drug users, homosexuals, bisexuals, and heterosexuals with multiple partners, especially those from countries where HIV is more common.

• Weeks of malaise, weight loss, fatigue, fevers.

Diagnosis confirmed by blood tests. Sputum culture will show unusual organisms.

## COUGH PLUS BLOODY PHLEGM

A symptom that should not be ignored. In older people (over fifty) and especially in smokers, it calls for careful investigation. In younger people, there is more likely to be a relatively innocent cause. Even so, they should have an immediate checkup.

Remember that many cases of cough plus bloody phlegm are eventually diagnosed as "cause unknown"—and the symptom simply goes away.

### PROBABLE

### ■ Chest Infection

• Yellowish or greenish phlegm that contains streaks or blobs of blood, possibly red, possibly rust-colored. Not an uncommon symptom.

• Mildly unwell with raised temperature and aches.

### POSSIBLE

### ■ Pneumonia

*(See page 224)* The infection causes so

much inflammation that blood oozes into the lungs, where it mixes with phlegm.

### ■ Lung Cancer

There is now little doubt that smoking causes most cases of lung cancer, one of the most common forms of cancer. Smokers in particular, and especially smokers in the fifty-plus age range, should be alert to the early warning signs because the sooner the disease is diagnosed, the better the results of treatment.

None of these symptoms on their own is absolutely diagnostic of lung cancer, indeed they often prove to be false alarms. However, this is a situation when being overly cautious is to be encouraged, particularly if you are in the risk group. Combinations of two or more symptoms should arouse increased suspicion.

• A persistent cough, whether dry or with phlegm. Smokers get used to the "smoker's cough," making it all the more important to be aware if the cough worsens. An early lung tumor causes this symptom by irritating the lining of the air passages.

• Frequent or unusually persistent chest infections. This can mean that a small tumor is acting as a focus for repeated infection.

• Coughing blood. Even small amounts mixed with phlegm should be investigated and all the more so if the cough produces pure blood. A small tumor can have this effect by oozing blood from its surface.

• Breathlessness—because a tumor may cause collapse of part of a lung.

• Persistent pain or ache in the chest, which may be due to inflammation from a tumor.

• Loss of appetite and weight. For reasons not clearly understood, many cancers cause loss of weight and appetite before the cancer has otherwise shown itself.

Ninety-five percent of lung cancer cases are due to smoking. It is increasingly thought that the remaining 5 percent may largely be caused by secondhand smoke.

### ■ Bronchiectasis
*(See page 224)*

### ■ Cause Unknown

Despite thorough investigation, in some cases the cause remains unknown.

### RARE

### ■ Heart Failure

• Gradual onset of breathlessness, swollen ankles, inability to lie flat.

• Frothy pink sputum, rather than pure blood.

■ **Mitral Stenosis**

• History of rheumatic fever *(see page 202)*.

• Gradual development of breathlessness, fatigue, dilated veins on cheekbones (giving a flushed appearance), breathlessness when lying flat.

## COUGH, BLOODY PHLEGM, AND CHEST PAIN

Pain in the lungs points to inflammation or injury of the pleura, the thin outer "skin" that covers the lungs. Inflammation of the pleura frequently accompanies chest infections, when it is called pleurisy.

### PROBABLE

■ **Chest Infection**

*(See page 210)*

### POSSIBLE

■ **Pneumonia**

*(See page 216)* The phlegm is typically rust-colored (that is, bloodstained) rather than containing pure blood and is otherwise green or yellow due to the underlying infection.

■ **Pulmonary Embolus**

This is a blood clot blocking blood flow to part of a lung. Symptoms may range from mild to knife-like chest pain to collapse. Increased risk after surgery, in the obese, in those recovering from a heart attack, in women on the contraceptive pill, and during pregnancy.

• Coughing blood.
• Pain worse on breathing in.
• If the embolus is large, faintness and sweating, collapse.
• A swollen calf suggests a leg thrombosis *(see page 317)* as the source of the pulmonary embolus.

■ **Chest Injury**

Caused by an injury severe enough to damage the lungs directly, or to break a rib, which then punctures a lung.

• Knife-like pains.
• Worse on breathing in.

### RARE

■ **Lung Cancer with Secondary Spread to Bones**

In the later stages of lung cancer, a patient might experience this combination of symptoms. Cancer of the lung can spread to other parts of the body, for example, the bones. If a rib is involved, there will be persistent chest pain (especially at night), a specific tender spot on the rib, and other signs of the disease *(see page 226)*.

## ASPHYXIA (SUFFOCATION)

Obstruction to the flow of air through the mouth, down the trachea, or into the lungs. Always look for some simple reversible cause, typically something stuck in the throat. The symptoms of asphyxia are:

• Rapid or abrupt onset.
• Sudden cough, choking, and spluttering.
• Rapid cyanosis (bluish coloring) of lips, tongue.
• Panic.
• Stridor, a low- to middle-pitched sound from the larynx, mainly on breathing in. It is also caused by viral infection *(see Croup, page 209).*

Of course, your first move, if you suspect something trapped in the throat, will be to try to dislodge it using the Heimlich Maneuver *(see page 206).* Then, call for help and, if you know how, give artificial respiration until help arrives. Usually, these situations call for emergency attention as quickly as possible.

### PROBABLE

#### ■ Foreign Body

A piece of meat or a similar chunk of firm food is the usual culprit in adults. In children, foods such as peanuts can be to blame, but consider also small toys, pen caps, beads. The prime signs are:

• Choking.
• Acute stridor (noisy, hoarse, "wheezing" intake of breath).
• Clutching at throat.

If the foreign body gets past the larynx and makes its way down into the lungs, the coughing and stridor will pass. In the lungs, it will act as a focus for chronic infection or even a lung abscess. Cough and recurrent infection after a choking fit should be viewed with suspicion because of this possibility.

#### ■ Swelling of Larynx

An acute, severe allergic reaction causes widespread swelling of soft tissues, including the larynx. Call for an ambulance immediately.

Commonest after insect stings or injections. Some people are hypersensitive to specific foods: nuts are commonly to blame.

• Swelling of lips, limbs, and throat
• Acute wheezing.
• Collapse.

#### ■ Laryngotracheitis

A simple laryngitis may occasionally develop into severe swelling. Children whose airways are narrow, and will become obstructed on modest swelling of the soft tissues, are most at risk *(see Croup, page 209).*

- Hoarseness developing into stridor *(see page 207).*
- Labored breathing, cyanosis (bluish tinge to skin, especially lips).

## Possible

### ■ Pneumothorax

Lungs are similar to balloons in some ways, and, just like a balloon, sometimes part of a lung bursts and collapses. Small collapses go unnoticed. Large ones will cause noticeable symptoms, and if air continues to leak out from the puncture into the chest, rapid breathlessness will become a problem.

- Sudden, knife-like chest pain.
- Worse on breathing in.
- Breathlessness worsening over a few minutes.

Treatment of a large pneumothorax will require emergency treatment in the hospital: a needle will be inserted through the chest wall to let out the air compressed inside the chest.

## Rare

### ■ Epiglottitis

The epiglottis lies just out of sight at the very back of the throat. Infection can cause it to swell until it obstructs the back of the throat. This is an illness found in young children, whose airways are still narrow. It is uncommon now in most developed countries where children are vaccinated against the causative bacteria, *H. influenzae* type B (Hib).

- Begins as a simple sore throat.
- Child develops a very high temperature.
- Begins to drool saliva because swallowing is painful.
- Labored breathing, cyanosis.

If you suspect that your child has epiglottitis, it is important *not* to try to peer down the throat as that can cause complete obstruction. An examination should only be performed in the hospital, where an emergency tracheostomy can be undertaken if necessary.

### ■ Diphtheria

A terrible illness that routine vaccination has virtually eliminated from developed countries. A membrane forms at the back of the throat, which obstructs breathing. In addition, the germ responsible produces toxic substances that affect the heart and nervous system.

- Begins as a simple sore throat.
- A gray membrane forms at the back of the throat.
- Dramatic enlargement of lymph nodes in the neck.

- Breathlessness, cyanosis.

### ■ Tracheoesophageal Fistula

An abnormality of newborn babies. During embryonic life, the airways and the gullet develop in close proximity to each other. If the trachea opens into the gullet rather than the back of the mouth, food will travel straight from the gullet into the lungs.

- Cough, asphyxia each time the baby feeds.

- Chest infection develops rapidly.

Once recognized, the problem is cured by surgery.

### ■ Tumors and Cysts

Although these diseases of the larynx or thyroid gland grow quite slowly, they can rapidly increase in size if they start to bleed. The swelling causes obstruction.

The diagnosis might be considered in an adult who is known to have a growth and who suddenly becomes breathless.

## CHEST PAIN

Though chest pain is commonly and understandably taken as a sign of heart disease, there are many other causes to be considered, not all of them involving the heart. So many vital structures pass through the chest that the list of possibilities is long. There are the gullet, the great vessels coming from the heart, and the windpipe and the airways going down into the lungs. Pain may stem from the ribs themselves, the muscles between the ribs, or from the nerves. The lungs can ache and inflammation from within the abdomen may give rise to pain in the chest. And certainly, some chest pains, particularly perhaps in born worriers, are psychological. Finally, there are pains that remain totally unexplained, even after extensive investigation.

That said, sudden severe chest pain must be taken seriously and needs urgent medical assessment to exclude a heart attack. Advances in the treatment of heart attacks require that medical attention be given within a very few hours of the attack. It is therefore all the more important to get help as soon as possible. It is one area of medicine where doctors, given a classic picture, will back their hunches and treat first, diagnose later, even if immediate test results are negative.

This section is divided as follows: a heart attack, sudden chest pain, and persistent or recurrent chest pain.

## CHEST PAIN FROM A HEART ATTACK

Everyone should be aware of the classic symptoms of a heart attack because early treatment is vital.

- Sudden, severe central chest pain.
- Begins at rest.
- Worse on exertion.
- Pain is crushing, vice-like, gripping.
- May radiate up to the jaws or down the arms, usually the left arm.
- Breathlessness.
- Sweating.
- Cyanosis (blueness) of lips.

A heart attack occurs when the blood supply to part of the heart is blocked. Pain comes from the heart muscle in much the same way that cramp occurs in other muscles in different circumstances.

For many years, the treatment was to deal with the complications that can arise, such as heart failure or rhythm disorders *(see page 196)*. Nowadays, treatment aims to limit the amount of damage to the heart that occurs during the attack, but this calls for treatment within hours or less. This makes it all the more important to get an early diagnosis in the hospital.

Not all heart attacks will show all of the previous features. Pain is not always a prominent feature, especially in the elderly; sometimes there is just:

- Sudden onset of tiredness.
- Irregular pulse.
- Heart failure, with breathlessness and swollen ankles.

In these circumstances, much can still be done to help.

Keep this picture in mind when referring to the sections dealing with other causes of chest pain. Your doctor does.

## SUDDEN CHEST PAIN, POSSIBLY A HEART ATTACK

Sudden chest pain is always worrying, but just how worrying depends on associated features. The classical symptoms of a heart attack have been given *(see above)*, but subtleties may help sway the diagnosis. Did the pain come on very suddenly or over a few minutes? Is breathlessness a feature? Do you feel ill? Does movement make a difference? Were there previous symptoms?

Diagnostic possibilities are different at different ages. Heart disease would not be the first diagnosis for a young person, whereas in an older person it is often difficult to rule out heart disease completely, so tests will commonly be ordered even if the symptoms are not completely typical. It is generally safest for a layperson to regard severe chest pain in an adult as a disorder of the heart until proven otherwise.

Doctors will make additional judgments based on the individual's overall condition, including skin color, pulse, blood pressure, or signs of heart disease, such as fluid in the lungs or abnormal heart rhythms. An electrocardiogram (ECG) recording of the heart can be helpful, as are blood tests, but these take time—so doctors will often make a diagnosis based on history and examination while awaiting the outcome of these investigations.

## PROBABLE

### ■ Heart Attack

*(See page 231)* Should be suspected on the basis of:
- Sudden onset of severe, central chest pain.
- Onset at rest.
- Prolonged and crushing in nature.

## POSSIBLE

### ■ Esophagitis

Inflammation of the gullet can be extremely painful, with many features resembling a heart attack:

- Central chest pain.
- Spreads up to neck and down arms.
- Sweating.

Can be difficult to distinguish from heart pain. There may be a previous history of:
- Indigestion, belching.
- Burning pain after eating food.
- Taking drugs that irritate the gullet, such as aspirin.
- Relief with antacids.

However, if occurring for the first time in the middle-aged or elderly, heart disease must be carefully considered.

### ■ Nerve Irritation

Nerves run in bands between the ribs, encircling the chest. It is quite common for one of these nerves to become irritated, causing pain.
- Sharp chest pain.
- Radiates from the back toward the front of the chest.
- Worse on movement.
- No breathlessness or sweating.
- Pain comes and goes from minute to minute.
- Often one small part of the chest wall is tender.

This condition can be dramatic when it appears but it is entirely benign, needing no more than painkillers and rest.

## Peptic Ulcer

Ulceration in the stomach or upper small intestine (duodenum). The pain from a peptic ulcer tends to be:
- Confined to the upper abdomen ("pit of stomach" or solar plexus).
- Burning in nature.
- Worse at night.
- Appears to go through into the back.
- Preceded by weeks or months of indigestion.
- Possibly blood in vomit.
- Upper abdominal pain on pressure.

Treatment is totally different from that for a heart attack, consisting of intensive anti-acid treatment.

One in ten people will have an ulcer at some time in their lives. This condition used to be most common in men, but now it is almost as common in women. Smoking, family history, infection with a bacteria *(H. pylori),* and taking certain anti-inflammatory painkillers (aspirin, ibuprofen) all increase the risk of developing a peptic ulcer.

## Pneumothorax

Sudden collapse of part of a lung.
- Sudden, knife-like chest pain.
- Localized, usually to the side of the chest, not central.
- Breathlessness is a possibility.

## RARE

## Pulmonary Embolus

A blood clot lodging in the lungs, causing:
- Sudden pressure in chest.
- Discomfort rather than pain.
- Pain, if present, is knife-like.
- Breathlessness.
- Sudden cough with bloodstained phlegm.

Pulmonary embolus is associated with thrombosis of leg veins, giving a painful swollen calf. It can occur after surgical operations.

## Dissecting Aortic Aneurysm

The aorta is the great artery that carries blood away from the heart. If diseased, the walls can weaken, bulge, and eventually start to leak. In the days or weeks before this stage, there may be warning signs, such as:
- Vague upper chest pain.
- Pulsation (feeling of strong, throbbing pulse) in the upper chest.
- Breathlessness through obstruction of part of the lung.
- Hoarseness.

If the aneurysm begins to leak, there will be:
- Pain similar to heart attack.

- Possibly vomiting blood.
- Collapse through blood loss.

This condition is very difficult to distinguish from a heart attack by examination alone. The diagnosis is usually made as a result of a chest x-ray. Surgery is possible, depending on the site of the leakage. Frequently fatal.

## ■ Pericarditis

Inflammation of the lining around the heart, giving rise to:
- Sharp, central chest pain.
- Pain worse on movement.
- Pain worse on breathing.

Pericarditis may be caused by a viral infection. It can usually be treated and a full recovery is usual.

## ■ Pancreatitis

The pancreas lies at the back of the upper abdomen. It is the gland that produces insulin and other substances that digest food. If the pancreas becomes inflamed, these substances are released and start to "digest" the internal organs with which they come into contact. Inflammation of the pancreas is most common in alcoholics or in those with gallstones. The very severe pain of pancreatitis can appear to spread up into the chest.
- Pain radiates into the back.
- Nausea and vomiting.

There will be upper abdominal tenderness on examination. This is a serious condition that calls for intensive treatment in the hospital.

## RECURRENT OR PERSISTENT CHEST PAIN

This means symptoms that come and go over days, weeks, or months. Again, the possibilities depend on the person's age, previous medical history, and any associated features of disease.

Recurrent chest pain is common and is not always explainable. In young people, the reason often remains obscure, even after intensive investigation.

### PROBABLE

## ■ Angina

Angina is pain arising from the heart. The reason is nearly always coronary artery disease; that is, "furring up" of the blood vessels that carry blood to the heart itself. This causes a partial blockage of blood flow, and gives no symptoms until you exert yourself. Then, the heart's increased demand for blood cannot be met, resulting in angina:

- Central chest pain.
- Often radiates to the neck or down the left arm.
- Comes on with exertion.
- Goes after only a few minutes of rest.
- Worse in cold weather, after meals, or with emotional stress.

It is common to investigate angina with x-rays that highlight the blood flow around the heart, a technique known as angiography. The information gathered from this test will help the doctor to decide whether to replace the blood vessels to the heart, done in an operation known as coronary artery bypass grafting.

Angina is an important warning sign of heart disease, but in itself it is not usually dangerous and is *not* a warning of an imminent heart attack. However, angina should be investigated. It is often treated very effectively by angioplasty (where the blocked heart vessel is stretched with a balloon and often a stent is put inside the vessel to keep it open) or sometimes with surgery (heart bypass). If your angina is getting much worse, then you should contact your doctor urgently. If it is occurring at rest and not relieved by your medications, then after fifteen minutes of this you should call an ambulance.

### ■ Hiatus Hernia

A common condition in which part of the stomach moves up into the chest. As a result, the diaphragm—which normally creates a valve-type mechanism—allows gastric acid to cause pain in the upper part of the stomach and the gullet.

Symptoms may be noticed for the first time during pregnancy, or be made worse by it; this is also so if you are obese.

- Pain worse on lying flat or bending over.
- Pain that is burning or searing in nature.
- Pain may appear to radiate up to the neck.
- Burping or belching.
- Relieved by antacids.

Treatment varies from simply avoiding tight clothing and raising the head of the bed, to a range of drugs or, occasionally, an operation to tighten up the muscles. Modern medications, especially drugs called proton pump inhibitors, are extremely effective at relieving the symptoms of a hiatus hernia.

### POSSIBLE

### ■ Costochondritis

Where the ribs meet the breastbone, there are joints made up of cartilage, which can become inflamed. This may occur after injury, out of the blue, or sometimes in epidemics of a viral infection called pleurodynia or Bornholm disease (named after the Baltic island where an epidemic was documented).

- Onset over a few hours.
- Aching on either side of the breastbone.
- Individual joints may be swollen and tender.
- Worse on breathing or with changes of posture.
- Sometimes a mild fever.

This condition is not dangerous, but may be extremely painful and alarming at the start and can last for several weeks.

## ■ Da Costa's Syndrome

A kind of cardiac neurosis: a psychological problem of anxiety showing itself as:

- Recurrent pains over the heart.
- Breathlessness out of proportion to effort.
- Nervousness.
- Palpitations.

There is no doubt that individuals are genuinely distressed by their symptoms, which are treated by psychological support once heart disease has been ruled out.

## ■ Heart Rhythm Disorders

Very rapid or very slow heart rates can bring on angina, even in individuals with no other heart disease.

- Palpitations.

- Breathlessness.
- Abrupt onset, abrupt finish.

*(See pages 196–197)*

## ■ Lung Disease

Many disorders can give rise to chest pain, which may be mistaken for heart disease, including severe infections and cancer. *(See pages 209–210)*

## ■ Gallbladder Disease

Lying high up on the right side of the abdomen, a diseased gallbladder can give rise to pain that appears to be in the chest. It is most common in middle-aged women. There is usually little difficulty in distinguishing this as a cause.

- Pain builds up over a few minutes.
- Lasts for several hours.
- Pain and tenderness mainly under the ribs on the right side.
- May appear to radiate into the chest or to the tip of the shoulder.
- Nausea, vomiting is common.
- Restlessness.

A first attack may be puzzling, but usually a pattern emerges: pain provoked by certain foods, especially fatty ones, with episodes of niggling pain between major attacks. The usual reason is gallstones, for which there is a variety of treatments, mainly surgical.

## RARE

### ■ Aortic Valve Disease

This valve controls blood flow between the heart and the aorta, the major artery from the heart. The valve can become stiff and inefficient—this is known as aortic stenosis, usually a result of aging, though rheumatic heart disease was once a common cause.

Occasionally, children are born with an abnormal valve. As the valve is so stiff, the heart has to beat harder to force blood out and this puts a strain on it. For years, there may be no symptoms, but with increasing stiffness, there will be some combination of:

- Angina.
- Heart rhythm irregularities.
- Breathlessness.
- Fainting on exertion.

The condition produces a characteristic heart murmur that a doctor can detect. The treatment is by heart valve replace-ment, though other treatments are used in childhood or in the elderly and infirm.

### ■ Severe Anemia

It is unusual for anemia to become so severe without other symptoms, but it does happen occasionally, especially with pernicious anemia. This starves the heart of oxygen, and angina is the result.

- Pallor or yellowish tinge in pernicious anemia.
- Sore tongue.
- Tiredness, breathlessness.

Most forms of anemia respond rapidly to treatment.

### ■ Aortic Aneurysm

In the days or weeks before this ruptures, there may be intermittent chest pain. *(See page 481)*

### ■ Pericarditis

May account for several days of chest pain. *(See page 234)*

# THE SKIN

The skin is the largest organ in the body, although it is spread out very thinly. The fact that it can be examined so easily is especially useful for making a diagnosis. Changes in the skin are sometimes helpful in diagnosing underlying diseases affecting other systems in the body.

Many people are, understandably, reticent when it comes to discussing or showing changes in their skin, particularly in those areas normally hidden by clothes. Doctors *never* regard such changes as embarrassing—they think of them *only* as essential clues to diagnosis.

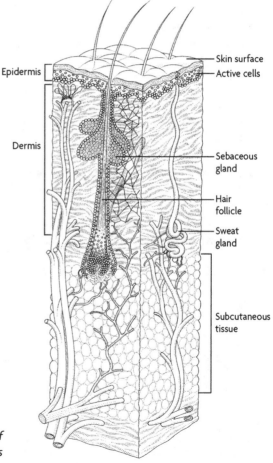

Epidermis

Dermis

Skin surface

Active cells

Sebaceous gland

Hair follicle

Sweat gland

Subcutaneous tissue

*Cross-section of Skin Layers*

239

# RASHES

Rashes are analyzed here in four key types, with cross-references to pages where they are covered in detail.

## RASHES DEVELOPING BLISTERS

■ Chicken Pox
*(See page 245)*

■ Impetigo
*(See page 243)*

■ Eczema
*(See page 242)*

■ Pustular Psoriasis
*(See under Psoriasis, page 246)*

■ Herpes Simplex
*(See page 243)*

■ Dermatitis Herpetiformis
*(See page 244)*

■ Herpes Zoster
*(See Shingles, page 243)*

## RASHES OF RED/PURPLE OR BLACK/DARK SPOTS

*(See Bleeding "Under" the Skin, page 259)*

## RASHES EXTENDING OVER MOST OF THE BODY

■ Chicken Pox
*(See page 245)*

■ Measles
*(See page 458)*

■ Dermatitis Herpetiformis
*(See page 244)*

■ Porphyria Cutanea Tarda
*(See page 244)*

■ Drug Reactions
*(See under Blue—General, page 250)*

■ Psoriasis
*(See page 246)*

■ Eczema
*(See page 242)*

■ Scalded Skin Syndrome
*(See page 244)*

■ German Measles
Rubella. *(See page 137)*

■ Tinea Versicolor
*(See page 253)*

■ **Urticaria**

*(See page 263)*

■ **Vitamin A Deficiency**

*(See Hard Skin, page 262)*

■ **Vitiligo**

*(See page 253)*

■ **Viral Infections**

*(See page 253; also, Papilloma or Wart, page 257)*

Smallpox is now considered to be eradicated worldwide.

## RASHES IN A LOCALIZED AREA

*(See section covering that part of body)*

## WHITEHEADS

*(See Blackheads and Whiteheads/Acne, below)*

## PIMPLES

*(See Blackheads and Whiteheads/Acne, below)*

## BLACKHEADS AND WHITEHEADS/ACNE

Most people have a number of blackheads at any one time and they are not necessarily a sign of any skin abnormality. They will develop whenever the skin's pores become blocked. If longstanding, or infected, they may become whiteheads, or even become acne vulgaris, commonly known as acne, teenage pimples, or "zits." The cause of acne is unclear, but changes in hormone levels after puberty and a sensitivity of the sebaceous glands to these hormone levels, resulting in excess grease production, are important. A bacteria known as *Propionibacterium acnes* has a fundamental role and is unique to mankind. Diet plays less of a role than was once thought. The changes acne makes to the skin are the visible effects of infection and inflammation.

■ **Acne Vulgaris**

• Starts at puberty.

• Blackheads—pinpricks of black matter and grease—can be seen blocking the entrance to sebaceous glands. Otherwise known as open comedones. The black is normal surface skin cells trapped in the grease that is too thick; it is not dirt.

• Most commonly affects the face, upper chest, and back.

• Skin may appear greasy.

• Skin bacteria infect the blocked duct and gland, causing local redness, pain, and swelling (papules).

• Pus develops, forming pustules (whiteheads).

• This process can continue for years.

If untreated, it can scar the skin. Modern treatments may improve matters considerably. The cornerstone of treatment is using agents (such as topical retinoids) that unblock the grease pores around hair follicles. If the acne is widespread, treatment by mouth is appropriate, and if severe, for example, with scarring, referral to a specialist for isotretinoin should be considered.

## BLISTERS

Collections of fluid trapped between different layers of skin. They come in different shapes and sizes: larger than 0.2 inches (5 mm), they are described here as bullae; smaller, as vesicles.

### PROBABLE

■ **Injury**

Extremes of heat or cold, friction, caustic chemicals, certain plants and some animals, jellyfish, and insect bites can all cause blisters.

• Localized to the site of injury.

• Surrounding skin may be reddened.

■ **Eczema**

• Often most marked in the skin flexures, for example, the creases at the elbows or behind the knees.

• Itching.

• Redness.

• Raised red areas.

• Vesicles.

• Weeping.

• Scaling.

• Crusting.

The vesicles of eczema, though, are often not seen as they are thin-walled and close to the surface. Furthermore, like all blistering conditions, the skin is very itchy and therefore scratched, which tears the vesicles open. Eczema on the soles of the feet or palms of the hands will produce tense blisters that persist as the overlying skin in these sites is very thick.

### ■ Herpes Simplex

This can causes blisters anywhere on the body. They are known as cold sores and occur around the mouth most commonly. The first infection with herpes simplex virus is usually very minor, but can occasionally be very nasty, causing hemorrhagic sores, particularly in and around the mouth. After the first infection, recurrences may occur at times of debility or after exposure to hot sun or the cold.

• Skin is locally irritable; tingling sensation.

• Then reddening and painful.

• Small lumps appear and go on to form vesicles.

• The vesicles burst and crust over.

• The whole cycle takes ten to fourteen days to subside.

*(See also Lips—Cracked, Sores, or Patches, page 77)*

### ■ Impetigo

A skin infection that is passed on easily by contact.

• Red spots that blister.

• A honey-colored infected discharge that forms crusts.

• Common around the mouth, face, and ears.

*(See also page 97)*

## POSSIBLE

### ■ Chicken Pox

*(See page 245)*

### ■ Shingles

Herpes zoster. Arises when the chicken pox virus is reactivated after lying dormant for years in the nerves of the area affected.

• Initially, an itchy, localized area of skin on half of the body.

• Pain develops.

• Reddening occurs; small lumps appear.

• Vesicles form.

• Crusting, followed by healing, sometimes taking up to a month.

• Pain (post-herpetic neuralgia) may be persistent and difficult to treat.

### ■ Erythema Multiforme

*(See page 80)* Vesicles and bullae may occur with this disease, which arises from an infection or a reaction to a drug or other medicine.

## RARE

### ■ Pemphigoid

In the elderly.

• Sudden onset of bullae on limbs and trunk. They may arise from reddened or swollen skin.

• Bullae may be filled with blood-stained fluid.

Requires aggressive treatment, often with steroids.

### ■ Psoriasis (Pustular)

*(See page 246)*

### ■ Dermatitis Herpetiformis

A very rare autoimmune disease.

• Itchy rash on the extensor (outer) aspect of elbows, knees, and buttocks.

• Multiple intensely itchy, small blisters appear in these areas.

• Almost always associated with celiac disease *(see page 144)*. Treatment of the celiac disease with a gluten-free diet usually controls the skin condition, but sometimes drug therapy (with dapsone, for example) is necessary.

### ■ Pemphigus Vulgaris

A very rare but serious condition affecting people usually over the age of fifty.

• Crops of widespread blisters called bullae on the skin and mucous membranes, often starting in the mouth.

• The blisters are very thin-walled and so tear easily, leaving weeping, reddened, and painful skin, which may become infected.

It cannot be cured, but treatment with steroids and antibiotics considerably improves matters and it usually eventually "burns itself out."

### ■ Porphyria Cutanea Tarda

• Associated with liver damage, often alcohol induced.

• Exposed skin blisters, scars, and becomes pigmented, after exposure to ultraviolet light.

Treatment includes giving up alcohol.

### ■ Epidermolysis Bullosa

Several exceedingly rare types of this inherited disease exist.

• Bullae develop after minimal injury—typically, minor friction—and become infected.

### ■ Scalded Skin Syndrome

Caused by infection in children and drug sensitivities in adults.

• Sudden onset of malaise.

• Raised temperature.

• Widespread redness.

• Multiple vesicles and bullae.

• Vesicles and bullae join, causing large areas of skin to lift off, like a severe scald.

May be fatal.

## SCARRED OR PITTED SKIN

In theory, any repeated inflammation or disease process will leave the skin scarred and pitted. In practice, the most common culprit is acne, the universal plague of adolescence *(see page 244)*. The worst cases leave permanent marks on the face and shoulders.

## SCALY SKIN

True scaling is limited to just a few conditions and diseases. Excluding the most common of them, dandruff *(see page 272)*, this leaves the following.

### PROBABLE

■ **Fungal Infections**
*(See page 258)*

■ **Eczema**
*(See page 242)*

### POSSIBLE

■ **Psoriasis**
*(See page 246)*

### RARE

■ **Pellagra**
Vitamin $B_3$ (niacin) deficiency.
• Dementia.
• Severe diarrhea.
• Scaly changes (dermatitis) of exposed skin.

■ **Ichthyosis**
*(See page 268)* If the skin surface is damaged and fluid (serum, pus, blood) leaks out (either directly or into blisters that subsequently burst), then golden-brown or black crusts (scabs) form on the surface or at the edges of the damaged skin. *(See also Blisters, page 242)*

### PROBABLE

■ **Impetigo**

■ **Eczema**

■ **Injury**

■ **Herpes Simplex**
*(See page 243)*

### POSSIBLE

■ **Chicken Pox**
An infectious disease caused by the same virus that causes shingles *(see Herpes Zoster, page 102)*.
• Crops of spots at different stages.

- Spots are red, raised, and form vesicles, then pustules (vesicles filled with pus).
- Pustules burst and crust over.
- Fever.
- Malaise.

### ▨ Herpes Zoster
*(See page 102)*

## RARE

### ▨ Pemphigus Vulgaris
*(See page 244)*

### ▨ Psoriasis
A skin disorder of unknown cause.
- Multiple red lesions of varying size.
- The red areas are covered with thick silver scales.
- If the scales are scraped off, the underlying skin shows multiple, tiny bleeding points.
- May occur on any part of the body, but frequently on the back of the knees, elbows, and scalp.
- The nails are involved in about half the cases, though the changes can be quite subtle.
- Some individuals develop arthritis *(see page 286)* in association with the psoriasis.

Pustular psoriasis is an uncommon form of the condition in which pus-filled vesicles (pustules) arise from the affected skin. When these break down, some crusting may occur.

### ▨ Dermatitis Artefacta
Some people suffering from psychological disorders deliberately harm themselves, for example, by burning, scratching, or even applying caustic fluids. The resulting injuries may well include extensive scabs and crusts, for which there is no clear explanation. Sometimes, child abusers cause similar injuries to children.

## PEELING OR FLAKING SKIN

Occurs in association with many skin diseases, but typically blisters and rashes, whose other symptoms are just as, if not more, noticeable *(see under Blisters and Rashes)*. And, of course, peeling skin is the eventual and unfortunate outcome of sunburn.

Some skin diseases benefit from sunlight: psoriasis and acne are examples. However, it is now established beyond much doubt that sunbathing predisposes to skin cancer. No sunbathing can be considered entirely safe. You increase your risk considerably if you have fair skin and sunbathe (redheads with freckles should avoid the sun); you expose yourself to the sun around the middle of the day; or you develop any redness of the skin. This means you are burnt. Burnt skin means a higher risk of skin cancer.

It is wise to keep to the following rules when you are on holiday or during sunny spells:

- Increase your exposure to the sun very gradually.
- Wear T-shirts and hats.
- Use a high-factor sun protection cream, ensuring you use both a UVA and UVB filter.
- Cover children well.
- Reapply sun blocks after bathing.
- Avoid the midday sun.

Protective creams *are* effective and should be used.

## SKIN APPEARS PALE

*(See page 430)*

## SKIN APPEARS BLUISH

*(See page 250)*

## SKIN APPEARS BLACKENED

*(See Discoloration of the Skin, page 248)*

## YELLOW SKIN

*(See Yellowness—General, page 253)*

## LOCALIZED YELLOW AREAS IN THE SKIN

### ■ Xanthomata

Localized, well-defined deposits of fatty material just below the skin surface. May occasionally be a sign of excess lipids (fats) in the blood, which in turn may pre-dispose to arterial disease. Most commonly seen around the eyes, when the deposits are called xanthelasma.

### ■ Gouty Tophi

*(See Gout, page 284)*

## YELLOWISH SKIN—JAUNDICE

*(See page 253)*

# DISCOLORATION OF THE SKIN

Meaning any abnormal change in the color of your skin. This can happen because of a local problem or because of a general (systemic) disease of one or more of the body's organs or systems. There are several conditions where changed skin color is a major feature.

Well-known types of skin discoloration are listed here by the type of color change and by whether the change is local or general. Obviously, color changes will usually be more obvious in people with lighter skin than in those with darker skin.

Not listed here are spots and rashes, which are covered elsewhere *(see pages 263–265)*.

## BLACK—LOCAL

### ■ Mole

Common in adults, generally from a millimeter or two in diameter to a centimeter across. Typically brown/black in color, and some have hairs growing from them. They are harmless, but see malignant melanoma *(see below)*.

### ■ Malignant Melanoma

A form of skin cancer, manifesting usually as dark or black areas and most common in fair-skinned individuals who have had lengthy, frequent exposure to the sun. They are increasingly common, very probably because more people take vacations in the sun. The role of ozone depletion in the atmosphere is less certain, but may be an important factor. Some malignant melanomas are extremely aggressive.

Malignant melanomas start as small black areas and are often difficult to tell from moles. Even a vague suspicion that you may have one is reason enough to show it to a doctor without delay, as early diagnosis improves the chances of successful treatment. Once treated, you may need to be followed up for several years. The warning signs are:

- New appearance of a pigmented lesion.
- Bleeding within an existing mole (unless there is a clear history of trauma).
- Itching.
- Color change.
- Change in size or shape.
- Appearance of smaller lesions nearby.
- Ulceration.

Any one of these warning signs should prompt you to visit your doctor urgently.

## ■ Acanthosis Nigricans

Black pigmentation in the armpit, the groin, or on the face and neck, usually in the elderly. It can be associated with cancer elsewhere. A similar change commonly occurs on obese patients. Rare and untreatable.

## ■ Dry Gangrene

*(See also Itching or Numbness of the Fingers and Toes, page 329)* Gradual loss of blood supply to a toe or a foot, or any extremity, may cause this condition. The affected part becomes withered and black and may drop off—typically, a frostbitten toe.

## BLUE—LOCAL

## ■ Cyanosis

*(See Bluish-Purple Lips, page 74)*

## ■ Mongolian Blue Spot

A blue/black area typically seen on the buttocks and sacral region in West Indian and Asian children. May often be mistaken for a bruise; can be several centimeters across.

## ■ Blue Nevus

Occurs anywhere on the body; may be only a few millimeters in size. It is an innocent mole that happens to look blue.

## ■ Livedo Reticularis

An exaggeration of the body's normal response to heat and cold: white areas of skin surrounded by a "chicken wire" pattern of bluish blood vessels.

## BLUE—GENERAL

### ■ Cyanosis

*(See page 438)*

### ■ Drugs Side Effects

Amiodarone, a drug used for treating heart irregularities, may rarely cause a bluish-gray, slaty discoloration of the skin.

Similarly, prolonged courses of the antibiotic minocycline, formerly used frequently to treat acne, can produce a slate-gray skin color change that is permanent.

### ■ Methemoglobinemia

Can occur through exposure to certain drugs—for example, dapsone—for treating leprosy or dermatitis herpetiformis, or certain chemicals. Some people inherit the condition, which affects the oxygen-carrying capacity of the hemoglobin in red blood cells.

### ■ Ochronosis

Affects cartilage and other connective tissue, for example, the whites of the eyes. The cartilage underlying the skin looks bluish or blue-black, whereas normally the overlying skin color would predominate. Caused by an abnormality of amino acid metabolism called alkaptonuria.

## BROWN—LOCAL

### ■ Pregnancy

As pregnancy progresses, the nipples, the genitalia, and a line down the center of the abdomen become progressively darker, turning from pinkish to brownish. *(See also Chloasma, below)*

### ■ Chloasma

A brownish, patchy pigmentation of the face that occurs in some pregnant women and can occur with the combined contraceptive pill.

### ■ Venous Ulceration

Longstanding varicose veins in the legs *(see page 317)* cause brownish pigmentation of the lower legs and feet. Sometimes, there is ulceration as well, particularly on the inner side of the ankle.

### ■ Erythema Ab Igne

A reddish-brown, irregular discoloration that appears after long exposure of the skin to heat. May well be noticed on the shins of an elderly person who spends hours in an armchair close to an open fire.

## ■ Seborrheic Wart

A flat, brownish wart, slightly raised above the surrounding skin. Sometimes they occur in considerable numbers. Also known as senile warts because they appear during middle-age and later. Harmless.

## ■ Café-au-Lait Spots

Like large freckles; may be multiple. Occasionally associated with neurofibromatosis.

## ■ Addison's Disease

Caused by longstanding underactivity of the adrenal glands.

- Brownish/dark pigmentation of the skin, especially skin creases, nipples, genitalia, old scars, and gums (in the last, may appear gray).
- Weakness, fatigue.
- Weight loss, anorexia.
- Craving for salt.
- Nausea, vomiting, diarrhea.
- Low blood pressure.
- Occasionally, hair loss.
- Occasionally, vitiligo *(see page 253)*.

## BROWN—GENERAL

## ■ Freckles

May occur naturally or may appear in increased numbers after exposure to the sun. May grow darker than usual and may coalesce, if exposed to sun. Mostly found on the face, shoulders, and arms, but may cover the entire body. Most common on redheads.

Avoid the sun if you have freckles.
*(See Peeling or Flaking Skin, page 246)*

## ■ Hemochromatosis

Also called bronze diabetes. An abnormality of metabolism of iron from birth, it causes:

- Diabetes mellitus *(page 180)*.
- Bronze skin.
- Cirrhosis.
- Joint inflammation.
- Heart abnormalities.
- Shrunken testes, reduced libido.

## ORANGE—GENERAL

## ■ Carotenemia

Eating too much food containing carotene, typically carrots, causes an orange discoloration of skin. Carotene is the active ingredient of some sun-free self-tanning products.

## PINK—LOCAL

■ **Salmon Patch Nevus**

A salmon-pink birthmark. Can occur any-where but is often found on the neck.

Some persist, but most disappear after a few years.

## PURPLE—LOCAL

■ **Port-Wine Stain**

A permanent birthmark caused by an ab-normality of the capillary blood vessels, producing an often extensive discolored area on the face and neck. Permanent, but can be disguised with makeup.

■ **Kaposi's Sarcoma**

Bluish-red areas appear on the skin. This is a malignant tumor that used to be seen mainly in Africa, but is now encountered all over the world as one of the compli-cations of AIDS.

## PURPLE—GENERAL

Likely to be cyanosis *(see page 438).*

*(See also Blue—General, page 250)*

## REDNESS—LOCAL

Described as erythema.

■ **Flushing**

A response to heat or embarrassment; also, in association with menopause *(page 349).*

■ **Erythema Ab Igne**

*(See Brown—Local, page 250)*

■ **Palmar Erythema**

Redness of the palms of the hands. Seen in alcoholics and in others suffering from liver disease.

■ **Erythrasma**

Reddish-brown discoloration of the skin, particularly near skin folds (breasts, armpits, groin). The skin is dry and the areas are irregular and slightly scaly. Caused by bacterial infection.

■ **Paget's Disease of the Nipple**

Localized redness with scaling and inflammation, mimicking eczema. If you notice such changes on the nipple or areola (the pink area around the nipple), see your doctor urgently—the possibility of underlying breast cancer must be excluded. *(See also page 358)*

## REDNESS—GENERAL

### ■ Viral Infection

Many viruses will cause nonspecific reddening of the skin. Typically, the rash fades soon after the illness settles.

### ■ Drug Reaction

A diffuse reddening of the skin may be associated with medication. The reddening may be patchy or blotchy or widespread. Itching (pruritus) often accompanies these reactions. Penicillin and aspirin commonly cause this reaction.

## YELLOWNESS—GENERAL

This is never a local condition.

### ■ Jaundice

Yellowish whites of the eyes and yellow skin gradually progressing to a deeper, browner color. There may also be itching (with resulting scratch marks), pale stools, and dark urine.

### ■ Uremia

*(See page 266)*

### ■ Mepacrine

This anti-malarial drug can cause yellowing of the skin.

## WHITENESS OR PALENESS—LOCAL

### ■ Vitiligo

Destruction of pigment-producing cells (melanocytes) in the skin, leading to white patches. In those with darker skin, these can be quite disfiguring.

*(See also Addison's Disease, page 251)*

### ■ Halo Nevus

Some moles *(see Black—Local, page 248)* become pale and the area around them loses pigment. Moles and surrounding areas are known as halo nevi. Vitiligo *(see above)* may also develop.

### ■ Tinea Versicolor

A fungal infection of the skin.

• Initially, areas of irregular brown coloration.

• Predominantly found on upper body, arms, and neck.

• Later, these patches lose their pigment, leaving pale areas.

Treatable with antifungal creams.

### ■ Post-Inflammatory

Any inflamed or damaged skin—from a graze, burn, or herpes sore, for example—

may lose its usual color after healing. Normal pigmentation may return after a few months.

## ■ Leprosy

*(See page 327)*

## ■ Arterial Blockage

*(See Peripheral Vascular Disease, page 326)*

## ■ Phlegmasia Alba Dolens

This means blockage of the principal veins draining blood from the leg. Typically occurs after being bedridden.

- Initially, malaise.
- Pain in groin and thigh.
- Leg swelling follows.
- Leg is pale and feels cold.

## ■ Raynaud's Phenomenon and Disease

*(See page 304)*

# WHITENESS OR PALENESS—GENERAL

## ■ Anemia

*(See page 402)*

## ■ Leukemia

*(See page 497)*

## ■ Albinism

An inherited abnormality of metabolism that results in absence of pigment in body tissues.

- Fair skin.
- White hair.
- Pink irises of the eyes.
- Problems with vision.

## ■ Phenylketonuria

Caused by an error of metabolism resulting in an accumulation of chemicals that affect the brain. Children are screened at birth.

- Blond hair.
- Blue eyes.
- Mental deficiency and aggression, if untreated.

Treatment involves avoiding foods containing the amino acid phenylalanine.

## ■ Hypopituitarism

*(See page 271)*

## ■ Shock

*(See page 420)*

## PARASITES

Scabies and lice are the principal visible parasites of the human skin and body. *(See page 447)*

## LINEAR MARKS ON THE SKIN

These are the causes worth considering for clear, isolated, linear marks on the skin. There are others, but they are extremely rare.

■ **Lymphangitis**

Infection in a limb can track up the lymphatic pathways to the lymph glands. May be seen on the arm and forearm after a simple injury, even a cat scratch to the hand, for example.

• Site of wound may be apparent.

• A red line extends directly from the region of the wound continuing up toward the armpit.

• Tender lymph nodes may be felt in the armpit.

Antibiotic treatment is advised to stop the infection.

■ **Scabies**

Fine gray lines a few millimeters long. *(See page 265)*

■ **Acanthosis Nigricans**

*(See page 249)*

**PROBABLE**

■ Vitiligo

*(See page 253)*

**POSSIBLE**

■ Halo Nevus

*(See page 253)*

■ Tinea Versicolor

*(See page 253)*

■ Post-Inflammatory

*(See page 253)*

**RARE**

■ Lichen Sclerosus et Atrophicus

*(See page 265)*

■ Leprosy

*(See page 327)*

■ Morphea

*(See page 263)*

■ Raynaud's Phenomenon and Disease

*(See page 304)*

## MINIATURE RED SPOTS

■ **Campbell de Morgan Spots**

- Tiny and bright red, often raised above the surrounding skin surface.
- Present on the chest and abdomen.

Most common in elderly people. Of little significance.

■ **Spider Nevi**

These are essentially red spots with several tiny vessels emanating from the center. They can appear in children and in adults. Multiple nevi may be a feature of pregnancy and of liver disease; also of hereditary hemorrhagic telangiectasia.

## SORES OR ULCERS

These are described elsewhere in the book in relation to the part of the body on which they occur.

## VESICLES

Small blisters. *(See pages 242–244)*

## WHEALS

A term used to describe raised marks on the skin. *(See Urticaria, page 263)*

## WARTS

*(See Lumps in the Skin, below)*

## LUMPS IN THE SKIN

It is best to play safe and report any lump in the skin to a doctor: most are innocent, but some need expert evaluation to rule out the possibility of malignant disease. The earlier the diagnosis and treatment, the better the outlook. If a lump is pigmented, bleeding, irregular, ulcerated, or growing rapidly, all the more reason to see a doctor without delay.

Covered here are lumps that may

appear in skin anywhere on the body. Lumps specific to certain parts of the body are covered in the appropriate sections.

## PROBABLE

### ■ Sebaceous Cyst

Sometimes called a wen. A harmless lump caused by buildup of sebaceous material—solidified, waxy, body fluid—in a sweat gland near the surface of the skin. May well start as an unsqueezed pimple, which, if it does not become infected, can develop over many years into a sebaceous cyst. No relation to cancer.

• Smooth; not tender.

• Frequently, multiple cysts on scalp, neck, or scrotum.

• Size ranges from a few millimeters to several centimeters.

• A small black mark in the center, the punctum, marks the entrance to the gland.

### ■ Dermoid Cysts

These are congenital cysts that develop on the head and neck and are most common at the outside end of the eyebrow. They may also occur as benign tumors elsewhere on the body.

### ■ Papilloma

*(See page 355)*

### ■ Wart

Caused by a viral infection of the skin. Small, often multiple, pain-free thickening of skin, with rough skin on the surface growing out of the normal skin.

### ■ Verruca

A wart on the base of the foot. Because the foot is weight-bearing, the wart is pushed into the sole of the foot and can be painful.

## POSSIBLE

### ■ Lipoma

A benign, fatty tumor that may appear as a smooth, often soft, lump in or beneath the skin.

### ■ Pyogenic Granuloma

Possibly caused by minor injury. A soft, red, fleshy benign tumor that bleeds easily when knocked. Often found near a fingernail or toenail.

### ■ Ganglion

A local degeneration of fibrous tissue. Appears as a small, firm lump near tendons or joints. Commonly seen on the back of the wrist. Used to be treated by a blow from the family Bible to disperse the lump; now, a ganglion is either left alone, aspirated with a large needle, or removed surgically.

## ◼ Molluscum Contagiosum

Caused by a virus.
- Crops of small pink lumps.
- Often on trunk or face.
- Each lump has a depression in the middle.

They clear up of their own accord.

## ◼ Vascular Malformations

There are many different types: spider nevus, salmon patch (also known as strawberry nevus), port-wine stain, Campbell de Morgan spots, and hereditary hemorrhagic telangiectasia are examples. These are rarely seen as lumps, but a cavernous hemangioma may develop as a lump. It may be extensive, covering part of the face.

Rarely present at birth but appears during the first few months of life. Normally clears by about six years.

## ◼ Basal Cell Carcinoma

Commonly called a rodent ulcer. *(See page 97)*

## RARE

## ◼ Squamous Cell Carcinoma

A malignant tumor, most common in the elderly or those whose immunity is suppressed.
- Often on the head or neck.
- May be an irregular lump.
- May bleed.
- May ulcerate.
- Local lymph nodes may be enlarged.

## ◼ Malignant Melanoma

*(See page 248)*

## ◼ Secondary Tumor

Technical term, metastasis. This is cancer that has spread from a primary site to create tumors elsewhere in the body. Irregular, hard, fleshy nodules or plaques seen or felt in the skin of someone known to have a primary cancer raise the suspicion of metastases. It is rare for skin metastases to be the first symptom you notice of internal primary cancer, but it is possible.

## ◼ Lymphoma

One particular type of lymphoma starts in the skin. It is noted as an irregular thickening. Diagnosis can only be made by taking a sample and examining it under the microscope. *(See also page 496)*

# SKIN TENDS TO CRACK

This is a feature of inflammation or infection of the skin. The most common causes are fungal infection and eczema.

## ◼ Fungal Infection

Different fungal infections may affect all parts of the body, but commonly found on the hands, feet *(see Athlete's Foot, page 268)*, and groin.

- Discrete, dry, reddened, itchy, painful areas of skin.
- Skin macerates and rubs off.
- Sometimes, associated blisters.
- Some fissuring, cracking, and thickening of the skin.

Easily treated with antifungal creams and ointments.

### ■ Eczema

The term is often used interchangeably with dermatitis. May be confused with fungal infections and vice versa.

- Diffuse patchy redness.
- Red lumps.
- Weeping, crusting.
- Fissuring, scaling.

*(See page 269)*

## MOLES

*(See page 248)*

## BUBBLES FROM A SKIN WOUND

Bubbles and fluid oozing from a wound, or surrounding skin that feels "crackly" when pressure is applied, suggests a very severe infection known as "gas gangrene."

Pain, malaise, and discoloration will almost always be present.

Get medical help immediately.

## BLEEDING "UNDER" THE SKIN

Medical term, purpura. In fact, the skin has several layers and the term properly describes blood leaking into surrounding surface tissue. The cause is either an injury that did not pierce the skin surface or an abnormality of blood vessels or of blood.

When blood leaks into surrounding tissue, it is broken down and undergoes several changes of color, from red/purple/ black to brown, green, and yellow.

The significance of purpura ranges from the minimal to an indication of life-threatening disorders.

### PROBABLE

### ■ Bruise

Bruises can be divided (in order of size) into petechiae or ecchymosis. If there is also a visible or palpable swelling, the term hematoma is used. Bruising may be caused by direct injury, such as a blow, or by indirect pressure, such as strangulation.

### ■ Senile Purpura

- Blotchy, well-demarcated purple patches.
- Often seen on legs or arms.
- Part of the aging process.

## POSSIBLE

### ■ Drug-Related

May be associated with taking steroids.
- Well-demarcated red and purple blotches.

See your doctor if purpura develops.

### ■ Henoch-Schönlein Purpura

Cause unknown. In adults and children.
- Purpura.
- Urticarial rash.
- Painful joints.
- Abdominal pain.
- Bloody diarrhea.
- Blood in the urine.

Normally resolves of its own accord, although steroids may be advised. Complications may affect the kidney.

### ■ Meningococcal Septicemia

*(See also Meningitis, page 428)* A life-threatening condition occurring with or without meningitis. Affects preschool children and young adults most severely.

- Sudden onset of purpuric rash, which may be extensive or minimal.
- Malaise.
- Fever.
- Rapid deterioration and collapse.
- Death may occur within hours.

If suspected, and certainly if the child has had contact with another case of meningitis, see a doctor urgently.

## RARE

### ■ Blood Disorders

Blood disorders, such as leukemia or aplastic anemia, often show themselves with sudden onset of widespread bruising. *(See also page 429)*

### ■ Scurvy

*(See page 441)*

### ■ Ehlers-Danlos Syndrome

An inherited disease in which the body cannot make normal supporting tissue.
- Markedly "double-jointed" joints.
- Skin scars easily.
- Bruising is common.
- Skin is soft and velvety in texture.

### ■ Disseminated Intravascular Coagulation

A potentially fatal condition caused by failure of the blood clotting mechanism. Often associated with severe infection. Rarely seen outside of hospitals.

## BOILS AND CARBUNCLES

### ■ Boil

An abscess in a hair follicle. Also known as a furuncle.
- Prime sites are the neck, armpit, and buttocks.
- Local redness.
- Swelling.
- Pain.
- Develops a point and discharges yellow/green pus.

### ■ Carbuncle

A collection of boils that may interconnect under the skin. Recurrent boils or carbuncles suggest the possibility of underlying disease, particularly diabetes mellitus *(see page 180)*. Urine can be tested for sugar as a quick screening method.

Another cause of recurrent boils may be poor personal hygiene. Occasionally, the diagnosis of acne vulgaris *(see page 242)* may have been missed.

Boils and carbuncles will normally come to a head, discharge their fluid naturally and disappear. However, this may take so long or be so painful that it is tempting to lance the boil at an early stage—don't. It is important that this is done when the boil is "ripe." See your doctor to have a boil lanced—if it is done inexpertly, the result may be severe scarring.

Nowadays, antibiotics can often clear boils either before they become too painful or before they discharge.

## BULLAE

Medical term for a large blister. *(See page 242)*

## CORNS AND CALLUSES

Both words describe harmless thickening of the skin, which develops as a protective measure.

### ■ Corn

Typically appears on the upper surface of the little toe, where the toe rubs against shoes.

### ■ Callus

A thickening of the skin of the hands or feet. People who go habitually barefoot develop calluses on the pressure-bearing areas of the sole. Likewise, manual workers develop calluses on the palms of the hands, typically at the base of the fingers.

## FLAB

Apart from obvious folds of fatty tissue that go with obesity, flab is sometimes used to describe skin that has lost elasticity. You can pick it up in folds, and it fails to return immediately to its original contours. There are three main causes.

### ■ Aging

With age, skin loses its elasticity. Wrinkles, skin creases, and sagging jaw lines are part of the process, and provide limitless work for cosmetic surgeons.

### ■ Dehydration

The body needs a certain amount of water in order to function properly. Severe loss of fluid can arise because of reduced intake (for example, when someone is in a coma) or increased output (for example, with diarrhea or vomiting). The result is flabby, turgid skin, which will not unwrinkle when pinched. Naturally, this effect of fluid loss does not happen overnight.

### ■ Massive Weight Loss

If you are obese and manage, with a commendable spurt of willpower, to lose a large proportion of your weight very rapidly, you may be unjustly repaid with a new problem: the skin needs time to compensate for the loss of fat. Meanwhile, huge lax folds of skin develop, particularly on the abdomen, buttocks, thighs, and upper arms.

Cosmetic surgery may be helpful in some cases.

## HARD SKIN, LOCAL OR GENERAL

The obvious diagnosis is a corn or callus (see page 261). Here are the less self-evident causes.

### PROBABLE

### ■ Keloid

Describes excessive scarring after cuts or injury and is seen most commonly in African Americans. The site of the injury hardens, with an overgrowth of hard scar tissue above the level of the surrounding skin. Why some people develop keloid scarring and others don't is a mystery. It is harmless, but severe cases sometimes require treatment for the scar tissue, either by injection or by further surgery. There is no guarantee that this will lead to a more satisfactory appearance.

### POSSIBLE

### ■ Lymphedema

- **Post-Phlebitic Limb**

*(See Swollen Ankle, page 316)*

- **Myxedema**

Puffy swelling of the skin, particularly on the hands, feet, and ankles and around the eyes. May be seen with hypothyroidism *(page 351).*

## RARE

- **Vitamin A Deficiency**

- Night blindness.
- Abnormality of the cornea, leading to inflammation, scarring, and blindness.
- Rough, dry skin.

- **Morphea**

A localized variant of scleroderma *(see right).*
- Well-defined, pale areas.
- The skin in these areas is smooth and hard.
- Loss of hair at these sites may occur.
- Ulceration may occur.

- **Scleroderma**

An autoimmune disease.
- Hard, rigid skin develops.
- Tiny red spots (telangiectasia) are evident.
- Skin becomes shiny and smooth.
- Hands become stiff.
- Joints may become stiff.
- Skin of face is affected, making the mouth appear small.
- Face lacks expression.
- Raynaud's phenomenon *(see page 304)* develops.
- Swallowing is impaired and weight loss follows.

- **Cancer**

Secondary or metastatic cancer deposits (having spread from a primary site elsewhere) can arise in the skin, leading to small areas that are hard to the touch. They may be single or multiple. A somewhat specialized example is a secondary deposit in the navel called Sister Mary Joseph nodule, after the nun who first observed it at the Mayo Clinic.

## AN ITCHY RASH

## PROBABLE

- **Eczema**

*(See page 242)*

- **Urticaria**

Commonly called hives. A type of allergic reaction triggered by various agents. Typically, urticaria appears suddenly and dramatically. The wheal may come and go quite quickly, clearing in one area only to reappear in another.

• Red, blotchy areas with puffy, paler patches in the middle.

• Some swelling.

• Itchy, often intensely so.

There are several types, grouped according to cause or appearance. One form, dermatographia, is particularly severe: just stroking the skin firmly raises a wheal—you can even draw a picture on the skin.

The most common form is allergic urticaria. Common causes include plants, chemicals, food, and medicine colorants.

## ■ Scabies

## ■ Lichen Planus

Very itchy, flat-topped, purplish bumps on the skin, especially the wrists, and often associated with white patches in the mouth. The cause is usually unknown.

## ■ Lice

## ■ Insect Bites

Can occur as an itchy rash or with no obvious rash. *(See page 95)*

## ■ Fungal Infection

*(See page 258)*

## ■ Pityriasis Rosea

Most common in young people and may be associated with a viral infection.

• A single, itchy red lesion may appear anywhere on the trunk—the herald patch.

• After a few days, scattered patches of pinkish elevated areas develop. They characteristically lie along the line of the ribs.

• The rash persists for about six weeks.

Usually no treatment is required. Calamine lotion or, in severe cases, antihistamine drugs may help.

## ■ Lichen Simplex

You scratch an itchy place and the itchiness goes for a while, but as soon it comes back, you scratch again. A vicious cycle of scratching and itching develops, causing local inflammation. The inflammation causes thickening of the skin, with furrows or lines developing in chronic cases.

## ■ Pruritus Ani or Vulval Itch

These conditions are often characterized by itching plus rash. *(See page 348)*

## ■ Drug Reaction

If you are allergic to a drug, the classic reaction is:

• Widespread rash, but predominating on trunk.

• Patchy reddening.

• Some local swelling.

• Intense itching.

Reactions to drugs can occur even after long-term use.

## RARE

### ■ Nodular Prurigo

• Multiple warty areas.
• Intensely itchy.

Cause unknown, but possibly initiated by scratching.

### ■ Lichen Sclerosus et Atrophicus

• Involves skin around the vulva, anus, or penis.
• White, pale skin.
• Clearly delineated.
• Reddened areas within the affected skin.
• Itchy.

When seen on children, this may wrongly be attributed to abuse.

## ITCHING—WITHOUT A RASH

Covered here is persistent, severe itching that has become a nuisance. The medical term is pruritus. Close inspection with a magnifying glass may reveal either of the common causes—scabies and lice. Scratch marks are the obvious evidence of severe itching, and of course they also reveal to the doctor where the symptom is at its worst.

Excluded here are an itching scalp caused by a bad bout of dandruff *(see page 272)* and itching in the anal area *(see pages 159–160)*.

## PROBABLE

### ■ Scabies

Infestation with the scabies mite, which burrows under the skin.
• Severe itching is noted.
• Mite burrows may be seen as gray lines a couple of millimeters long.
• Burrows are often between fingers or front of wrists.
• Eventually, raised, reddened areas may appear all over the body.
• Scabs may develop because of scratching.

### ■ Lice

Commonly known as nits. There are three main types: head lice, body lice, and pubic lice.
• Persistent itching.
• Local lymph nodes may enlarge.
• Eggs may be seen on the bases of hairs or you may see lice themselves, although they are quite elusive.
• Spread by direct contact with other infected hairs or skin.
• The pubic louse may cause itching in the anal or vulval regions.

### ■ Insect Bites, Including Fleas

- Itching at the site of the bite.
- Reddened, hard nodules at the site of the bite appear later.

Fleas are commonly the culprits; most common in homes with cats.

### ■ Fiberglass

Glass fibers can become invisibly embedded in skin, causing itching. Protective clothing should be worn.

### ■ Senile Pruritus

The elderly sometimes complain of itching for which no cause can be found. It may be the result of the aging process.

### ■ Threadworm

*(See Worms, page 152)*

- Itching and irritation around the anus.

Most children have this common complaint at some time. Treatment is simple and available either directly from the pharmacy or from a doctor.

### ■ Strep Infection

Commonly in young children, a bacterial infection of the anal skin causes a chronic, itchy anal condition.

## POSSIBLE

### ■ Pregnancy

Many women complain of itching in the last months of pregnancy. Local causes such as thrush need to be excluded.

### ■ Liver Disease and Jaundice

Any condition that causes jaundice, usually liver disease, may also cause intense itching. The itching may arise before the yellow skin color is noticed.

### ■ Drugs

Some drugs—for instance, penicillin and aspirin—can cause severe allergic reactions, with itching. And some narcotic drugs, including cocaine and heroin, may cause itching, sometimes related to impurities.

### ■ Psychological

Itching without any cause found after full examination and investigation may be a sign of underlying psychological problems.

## RARE

### ■ Dermatitis Herpetiformis

*(See page 244)*

### ■ Uremia

High levels of urea in the blood are one of the end results of untreated renal (kidney) failure. A number of symptoms may be present:

- Dry, coated tongue.
- Breath smelling of urine.
- Hiccups.
- Nausea and vomiting.
- Dry, yellow-brown skin with a whitish "frost."
- Marked itching.
- Anemia.

## ■ Blood Disorders

A number of blood and related diseases may cause severe itching. They include polycythemia rubra vera, lymphoma, Hodgkin's disease, and leukemias.

## PRURITUS

The medical term for itching. *(See pages 19–20, 67, 159–160, 263–267, 348–349)*

## SKIN FEELS CLAMMY

If associated with coldness, see Itching or Numbness of the Fingers and Toes *(page 329)*.

## DRY SKIN

The two simple explanations are inflammation or failure of the sweat glands to work normally.

### PROBABLE

### ■ Eczema

*(See page 242)* When not in a phase of acute inflammation, patches of skin affected by eczema may feel dry and rough to the touch.

### ■ Fungal Infection

*(See page 258)*

### POSSIBLE

### ■ Heat (Sun) Stroke

Prolonged physical work in hot conditions or staying too long in the sun puts anyone, even the fit athlete, at risk of heat stroke. Most common in the very young and the elderly. Symptoms may develop rapidly.

- Dry skin, hot to the touch.
- High temperature.
- Weakness.
- Thirst.
- Headache.
- Confusion.

If untreated, it can be fatal. If you suspect this condition, seek medical help urgently.

It is important to protect yourself against the sun:

- Wear a hat and shirt, apply sun block, and maintain a high fluid intake (no alcohol).
- Keep cool by taking frequent showers or swimming; avoid exposure to the midday sun.

■ **Hypothyroidism**

*(See page 204)*

**RARE**

■ **Uremia**

*(See page 266)*

■ **Vitamin A Deficiency**

*(See page 263)*

■ **Ichthyosis**

A group of inherited disorders of the skin in which the skin is thickened, dry, and flaky. Often the inner aspect of skin overlying joints (typically, armpits and elbow creases) is spared.

Very occasionally, these changes, appearing in later life, may be associated with underlying malignant disease.

## BODY ODOR

This is possibly the most vague and most subjective symptom of all. Doctors and dentists see many people who believe that they smell, or that some part of them smells, even though no one else has commented. Some people seem to be abnormally sensitive to smells. And some people, notably small children, have a virtually nonexistent sense of smell.

Serious underlying disease is *very* rarely the reason for offensive body odor. If you put aside obvious cases of body odor caused by stale sweat, and if you also exclude psychological cases (where the smell is a belief rather than a physical fact), body odor usually comes down to three relatively common possibilities and one rare possibility.

■ **Athlete's Foot**

A fungal infection of the feet with reddened, itchy, painful areas between the toes, fissuring, and cracking. The feet and shoes give off a characteristic cheesy odor, which is sometimes strong enough for others to smell, even if the shoes are on.

Try self-help and commonsense use of over-the-counter medications.

■ **Bad Breath**

*(See page 82)* Self-help and over-the-counter medications usually work.

■ **Offensive Discharges**

For example, vaginal discharge.

Try self-help measures and over-the-counter medications.

**RARE**

■ **Fish Odor Syndrome**

Medical term, trimethylaminuria. One of several rare metabolic diseases.

Specialist treatment and advice on odor concealment is needed.

# THE HAIR

## LIFELESS HAIR

Loss of body or "life" in the hair is to some extent inevitable with advancing years. It is seen in association with medical conditions that cause baldness. Severe stress, such as that caused by major, prolonged illness, can affect the quality and thickness of hair. Vitamin deficiency and severe undernourishment will also affect hair quality.

## LOSS OF HAIR OR BALDNESS

Also known as alopecia. Hair loss, known as "male pattern balding," is part of the normal male aging process and is characterized by:

• Recession of the hairline at the forehead and temples.

• Thinning of the hair on the crown. It becomes a bit frizzy and loses body.

• A gradual meeting of the hairless areas so that hair remains only on the sides and back of the head.

Though women are not prone to baldness, thinning and hair loss also happen in most women as they get older.

Abnormal hair loss can of course be a sign (in women as well is in men) of scalp disease or more generalized disease. Most such cases, as this section shows, are fairly easy to distinguish from normal baldness.

### PROBABLE

■ **Eczema or Dermatitis**

Any inflammatory skin condition may cause loss of hair in the affected areas.
• Complete patches of hair loss.
• Skin is itchy, inflamed, weeping, and may have some crusting.
• There is often some dermatitis or

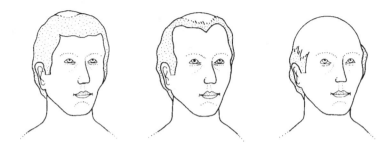

*Stages of Baldness*

eczema elsewhere on the body, though this can be a localized contact sensitivity on the scalp (for example, from a hair dye).

### ■ Alopecia Areata

The most common cause of patchy baldness.

• Local areas of total baldness, often only a few centimeters across and round.
• Normal "baby smooth" skin.
• Several patches may occur together.
• Regrowth normally occurs spontaneously after a few months, but if there has been damage to the pigment cells deep in the skin, the new hair may regrow white.

This is often seen at a time of stress, such as bereavement.

### ■ Childbirth

Many women notice changes in hair substance and texture before and after childbirth. Scalp hairs normally live for about three to seven years, and hairs are constantly reaching the end of their life cycle and entering the "falling-out phase," which only lasts a few weeks. During pregnancy, typically no hairs switch into this falling-out phase and so the hair density gradually increases, resulting in a lovely, thick head of hair by the end of the pregnancy. After childbirth, all those hairs that would have naturally fallen out over the previous nine months do so together, resulting in a rather dramatic hair shedding, which can be quite alarming. In rare cases, the original texture of the hair is never restored.

### Possible

### ■ Injury

Burns, skin loss, or even deep cuts can damage hair-bearing skin, so that hair may never regrow. Generally speaking, hair does not grow on scar tissue.

The only solution is to hide such areas by expert combing and styling.

### Trichotillomania

Nervous playing with the hair leaves it twisted, broken, or with bald patches.

### Psoriasis

• Hair loss in areas of psoriasis on the scalp.
• Silvery, scaly red patches seen in scalp.
• Other signs of psoriasis seen elsewhere on body *(see pages 240 and 348)*.

### Iron Deficiency

• Generalized hair loss or thinning.
• May improve after taking iron supplements.

*(See also Iron Deficiency Anemia, page 435)*

### Hypothyroidism

*(See page 351)*
• Hair is sparse.
• Hair may be dry and thin.

### Postmenopausal Change

Hair texture may change in and around the time of menopause due to alterations in hormone balance. The role of hormone replacement therapy in protecting against or reversing the effects of menopause is a subject of continuing research.

### Ringworm

Medical term, tinea capitis. A fungal infection of the skin of the scalp.
• Circular bald patches.
• Scaling of the skin.
• Brittle hair stumps remain.

Treatment is available with creams or tablets.

## RARE

### AIDS

Hair loss may be noted in the later stages of AIDS.

### Hypopituitarism

Underactivity of the pituitary gland may show itself in many ways, including:
• Absence of sexual function (loss of libido).

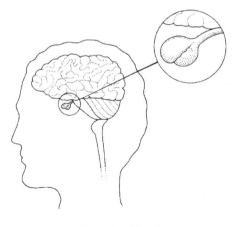

*Pituitary Gland*

- Absence of menstrual periods in females.
- Pale skin.
- Hair loss.
- Visual defects.
- Weight gain and fatigue.

*(See also page 431)*

■ **Anagen Alopecia**

Some drugs affect hair during their growth (anagen) phase, notably anti-cancer "cell poisons" given as courses of chemotherapy.

Vitamin A toxicity (for example, with the powerful acne drug isotretinoin) can rarely also cause diffuse hair loss. After stopping the drug, hair usually regrows.

Anticoagulant therapy is another, not uncommon, cause.

## DANDRUFF

The cause of this very common condition is a sensitivity to a *Malassezia* yeast. This yeast naturally lives on the scalp of about one in four persons; about 10 percent of people become sensitive to it and manifest this with dandruff. The only way to remain clear long-term is to use an anti-yeast shampoo, even if only once every two weeks.

The worst cases are accompanied by itching of the scalp, and sometimes a steroid-based scalp application may be necessary.

Rarely, other conditions are diagnosed, such as psoriasis.

## UNWANTED BODY HAIR

It is one of nature's many ironies that while baldness is almost universally an unwanted male symptom, unwanted body hair is almost exclusively a female symptom. Covered here is hirsutism in its specific sense of a male pattern of hair distribution on a woman.

**PROBABLE**

■ **Normal Pattern**

Patterns of hair growth on the face, limbs, and body vary according to country or region of origin. Individuals should compare themselves with others from a similar ethnic background before deciding that they have abnormally hairy bodies. For example, Japanese and Chinese women have very little body hair, whereas Mediterranean people typically may have much more.

## Possible

### ■ Polycystic Ovaries

Otherwise known as the Stein-Leventhal syndrome.
- Hairiness.
- Obesity.
- Acne.
- Absent or very infrequent menstrual periods.
- Ovaries have multiple cysts.

### ■ Menopause

Women going through menopause may note increased amounts of hair, typically fine hair that appears on the face.

## Rare

### ■ Drugs

A number of drugs may increase either fine hair on the face or body hair elsewhere. They include some steroid preparations, hormone treatments (including the pill), minoxidil (used to treat high blood pressure and as a hair restorer), and some anti-epileptic drugs.

### ■ Anorexia

Severe wasting conditions can cause an excess of hair growth. The most common situation is anorexia nervosa, where the excess growth of fine downy hair, known as lanugo hair, occurs (typically on the face).

### ■ Acromegaly

Caused by excessive production of growth hormone. In addition to other features of this disorder, women with acromegaly may have increased body hair.

### ■ Cushing's Syndrome

May be caused by a disorder of the adrenal gland or by taking steroids.
- Round, "moon" face.
- Fat deposited on back (buffalo hump).
- Fat deposited on body (not legs).
- Muscle fatigue.
- Easily bruised skin.

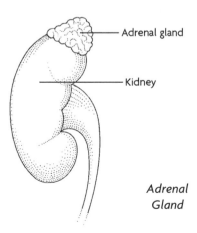

*Adrenal Gland*

- Stretch marks.
- Bone pain.

   Women also note:
- Increased body hair.
- Periods stop.
- Enlarged clitoris.

   Men may suffer from:
- Impotence.
- Acne.

## ■ Turner's Syndrome

A chromosomal abnormality. The individual has female characteristics and other changes including:
- Very short stature.
- No secondary sexual characteristics (with total absence of periods).

- Short web-necked appearance.
- Broad chest with widely separated nipples.
- Hirsutism.

## ■ Congenital Adrenal Hyperplasia

Excessive growth of the adrenal glands from birth.
- Mild hirsutism.
- Enlarged clitoris.
- Fused labia.

   May appear at a later age with:
- Acne.
- Early false puberty.
- Enlarged clitoris.
- Absent or scanty periods.

# THE BONES, JOINTS, AND MUSCLES

This section covers the body's "chassis"—the frame on which the tissues hang. Connected to the bones are the muscles, whose expansion and contraction, lengthening and shortening, provide movement. They have many common problems.

In this section, the usual order of symptoms has been varied in order to begin with some key general symptoms of muscles and bones occurring elsewhere in the body. We then move to specific bone, joint, and muscle symptoms as experienced in different parts of the body, working from the shoulders downward. Finally, under the heading Fingers and Toes are grouped symptoms affecting the outer reaches, or extremities, of the body, which are vulnerable in certain special ways.

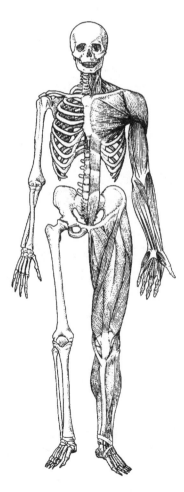

*Musculature and
Skeletal Structure*

275

## WASTING AND LOSS OF POWER IN THE MUSCLES

Muscular wasting, or atrophy, results from either damage to the nerve or blood supply to a muscle, to lack of use because of illness or injury, or to primary muscle disease.

### PROBABLE

■ Injury

The body's normal protective response to immobilization of the affected part. One of the best examples of this is a damaged knee. The knee is held slightly flexed, and you try to prevent movement for a few days. By the end of a week, you may well see some wasting of the quadriceps muscle at the front of the thigh. The weaker the muscle, the less safe the joint feels, and a vicious circle of disuse and further wasting then continues. This is why careful medical assessment and controlled exercises to maintain muscle bulk are important for all such injuries.

■ General Body Wasting

Bedbound patients can develop generalized disuse atrophy (wasting) of muscles. This can be aggravated by the underlying condition.

### POSSIBLE

■ Carpal Tunnel Syndrome

*(See page 300)*

■ Injury of a Nerve or Nerves

*(See page 327)*

■ Diabetes

*(See Diabetic Neuropathy, page 325)*

■ Alcoholic Neuropathy

*(See page 326)*

■ Rheumatoid Arthritis

*(See page 285)*

### RARE

■ Motor Neuron Disease

A disease of the nervous system. There are several forms, but the main features are:
• Progressive onset of muscular weakness, accompanied by muscle wasting.
• Small muscles of the hand are affected first.
• "Flickering" contractions of parts of muscles.

The disease progresses relentlessly, ultimately affecting speech, swallowing, and breathing muscles.

■ Duchenne's Dystrophy

This is a primary muscle disease affecting boys, which starts during the first few years of life.
• Wasting and weakness of back and pelvic muscles; affects both sides of the body.

- Failure of function affecting both sides of the body leads to a "waddling" gait while still mobile.
- Gradual degeneration leading to inability to walk and general immobility.

- Immobility leads to the muscles shortening, and deformity becomes inevitable. The outlook is poor.

■ **Subacute Combined Degeneration of the Spinal Cord**

*(See page 328)*

## CRAMPS, ACHES, AND PAINS IN THE MUSCLES

Most are of little significance. If they die away within a few days, they should not be taken seriously, unless they are recurrent.

### PROBABLE

■ **Simple Cramp**

- Sudden onset of muscle spasm, often while asleep.
- Muscle, often the calf, feels hard due to contraction.
- Relieved by massage.
- Often residual discomfort for a few hours.

■ **Viral or Bacterial Infection**

Fleeting muscular pains are a common accompaniment of any infection. Most resolve within a day or two. No specific treatment is required, apart from that for the underlying infection.

■ **Injury**

A direct blow to a muscle can cause painful local swelling and bruising. Indirect injury—for instance, straining to lift a heavy object—can make muscle fibers stretch and tear. Repetition of the movement reproduces the pain. Treatment for both is painkillers and resting the affected muscle.

### POSSIBLE

■ **Intermittent Claudication**

*(See Peripheral Vascular Disease, page 326)*

■ **Spinal Stenosis**

The spinal cord runs through a bony tunnel within each of the vertebra of the back; in later life, this tunnel often becomes narrowed, squeezing the spinal cord.

- Pain felt in the muscles of the buttock, thigh, or leg; worse when walking.
- Pain often improves when bending forward.

• Usually affects adults over the age of fifty.

• Associated with back pain and due to "wear and tear" degenerative changes in the back or associated with long-standing disc prolapse problems.

### ■ Biochemical Imbalance

Loss of salt, typically after strenuous exercise, can precipitate painful cramps.

### ■ Polymyalgia Rheumatica

A disease of the elderly.

• Painful, upper limb muscles.

• Extreme muscle stiffness, particularly in the morning (to the point where you have to roll out of bed).

• Malaise.

• Fever.

## RARE

### ■ Drugs

A number of drugs are known to cause muscle pains. The most widely used drugs associated with this are statins (used to lower cholesterol). Others include lithium, alcohol, amphetamines, and suxamethonium (used for general anesthesia).

### ■ Dermatomyositis

A disease associated with disordered immunity. May very rarely be associated with cancer.

• Inflammation and pains in multiple muscle groups.

• Muscular weakness.

• Rash often around the eyes and on the backs of the hands.

### ■ Polymyositis

Can be associated with many diseases, including collagen disorders and lung cancer. May remit and relapse.

• Progressive, painful inflammation of muscles; worse when used.

• Affects muscles in a variable manner, but those affected are weak.

• Fever.

• Malaise.

• Rapid heart rate.

### ■ Cushing's Syndrome

Caused by an excess of corticosteroids and often the result of doctors giving steroids to treat other diseases, such as rheumatoid arthritis.

• Weight gain, except for limbs.

• Moon face.

• Buffalo hump.

• Muscle weakness.

• Purple lines (striae) on abdomen, back, and upper thighs.

• Osteoporosis.

• Diabetes.

• High blood pressure.

• Hair grows on body.

• Occasional psychiatric disorders.

## ■ Primary Aldosteronism

A very rare disease, also known as Conn's syndrome, caused by excess secretion of the chemical aldosterone by the adrenal gland.

• Muscle weakness.
• Excessive thirst.
• Excessive urine output.
• High blood pressure.

## ■ Tetanus

Caused by the organism *Clostridium tetani* and acquired by contamination of open wounds. The damage is done by a powerful toxin that attacks the nervous system. Symptoms may take two weeks or more to develop.

• Local muscular weakness near site of infection.
• Facial muscles go into spasm; the individual appears to be forcing a grin.
• Muscles of the body go into spasm at the slightest stimulus.
• Fever.

Tetanus still claims victims, even when cared for in specialized units. Immunization is the essential precaution and needs to be repeated every ten years until you have had at least five tetanus vaccinations.

## POOR OR ABSENT MUSCLE CONTROL

*(See Brain and Nervous System, especially Convulsions, page 392, and Paralysis, page 415)*

## INVOLUNTARY TWITCHING OR TREMBLING MUSCLES

*(See page 451)*

## PAINFUL BONES

Pain in bones can be either localized (to part of one or more bones) or generalized.

### PROBABLE

## ■ Injury

Is it broken? Signs of a break (fracture) are:
• Pain at the site of injury.
• Possibly deformity—the limb looks bent.
• Loss of function—typically inability to bear weight.

Depending on the site and force of the injury, skin, nerves, and blood vessels may be involved.

Obviously, urgent medical attention is needed. Persistent pain following an injury, particularly when accompanied by swelling, should raise the suspicion of a fracture. Seek medical help.

Lesser injury may not cause a break, but can still cause pain and loss of function.

*(See also Subperiosteal Hematoma, below)*

### ■ Callus

New bone formed after a fracture.

• Previous, definite bone fracture.

• Forms within a few weeks.

• The larger the bone, the greater the amount of callus.

• Pain free when bone is fully healed.

### ■ Subperiosteal Hematoma

A direct injury to bone, typically the shin, but no fracture.

• Clear history of local injury.

• Swelling (bruising) noted almost immediately.

• Painful for several weeks after the injury.

• A hard lump still apparent for weeks or months afterward.

• Common in those who play "rough and tumble," or contact, sports.

### ■ Osteoarthritis

*(See page 307)*

### ■ Osteoporosis

*(See page 282)*

## POSSIBLE

### ■ Secondary Cancer

There is the possibility of localized bone pain being caused by a secondary (metastatic) deposit in someone with primary cancer. So, if an individual has a *known* cancer elsewhere in the body, this possibility needs to be considered. In an otherwise fit person, it becomes a Rare rather than Possible diagnosis.

### ■ Inflammatory Arthropathies

A term for joint inflammation, such as rheumatoid arthritis or ankylosing spondylitis *(see page 293)*.

### ■ Acute Osteomyelitis

A bone infection which, if suspected, requires immediate treatment. A primary site of infection elsewhere in the body may be apparent; the bone is affected by bacteria carried in the bloodstream.

• High, persistent fever.

• Sudden onset of pain in bone with swelling, which may not be obvious.

• Overlying redness and swelling of the soft tissues, not the bone.

• Extreme pain on movement.

• Rigors.

• Malaise.

## ■ Chronic Osteomyelitis

May occur after untreated or inadequately treated acute osteomyelitis, or after a compound fracture (a fracture and a cut down to the bone).

- Thickening of bone.
- Wound (sinus) discharging pus.
- Local pain.
- Inflammation around wound.

## ■ Malunion of Fracture

Failure of adequate reduction, meaning a poorly joined break. Sometimes this occurs despite careful realignment or setting of the broken bone. It may give the appearance of deformity or swelling.

## ■ Paget's Disease of Bone

*(See page 449)*

## RARE

## ■ Rickets and Osteomalacia

*(See page 294)*

## ■ Acromegaly

General enlargement of the skeleton caused by excessive growth hormone from the pituitary gland. Jaws and hands appear especially large.

## ■ Benign Tumor of Bone and Cartilage

Both bone and cartilage in any part of the body may give rise to benign tumors, which present as:

- Pain free hard lumps.
- Smooth surfaces.
- Slow-growing.

## ■ Cancer of the Bone or Cartilage

Individuals with known cancer of other organs of the body (for example, breast or lung) may develop secondary tumors (deposits) in the bones.

- Chronically and progressively painful.
- Pain may be very localized.
- A lump may *not* be present.

Other symptoms of advanced cancer may be present, but sometimes bone secondary tumors are the first indication of an as-yet undiagnosed cancer. This is why localized pain in a bone without a history of injury should be followed up with your doctor.

Primary malignant bone tumors are more rare than secondary tumors. They may form at any age, and there are several different types.

## ■ Tuberculosis

*(See page 472)*

## BONES BREAKING EASILY

Meaning fractures occurring without an obvious history of injury. They divide into two types: those that are the result of disease (pathological) and those in apparently normal bones (spontaneous or stress fractures).

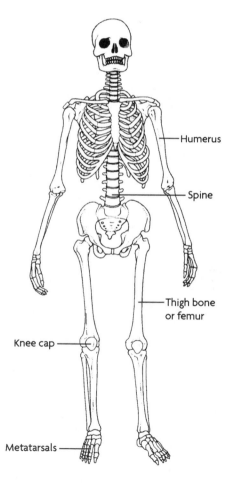

Humerus

Spine

Thigh bone or femur

Knee cap

Metatarsals

Spontaneous or stress fractures may occur because of repeated bending, as when athletes train, or after repeated compression (for instance, jumping and running) that acts on the spine.

- Local pain.
- Local swelling.
- Relieved by rest over a few days.
- Pain recurs when activity is repeated.
- May not be seen initially on an x-ray.

Typical sites include the small bones of the foot (metatarsals), upper arm bone (humerus), upper thigh bone (neck of femur), knee cap (patella), and spine.

In pathological fractures, the bone is abnormally weak because of either local abnormality (for example, malignant tumors, tuberculosis, osteomyelitis) or general abnormality (for example, osteoporosis, osteomalacia). These abnormalities can be congenital (brittle bone disease) or acquired (rheumatoid arthritis). Also, if a bone is unused, it becomes thinner and is prone to break.

### PROBABLE

#### ■ Osteoporosis

The idea of osteoporotic fractures as pathological fractures is a little controversial, but the simple fact remains that osteoporotic bone is not normal bone.

Gradual thinning of the bone, particularly in elderly females, may result in broken bones without significant injury. A fracture of the neck of the femur is very common. The symptoms are:

- Pain in the groin/hip (after or causing a fall).
- Apparent shortening of the leg.
- Inability to bear weight on the affected side.
- The foot on the affected side may be turned outwards.

Other common sites of osteoporotic fractures include the wrist (breaks easily after a mild fall) and the upper backbone (thoracic spine), which often breaks on its own, causing pain and the stoop often present particularly in elderly ladies.

Most commonly treated with an operation to realign and fix the broken bone.

## POSSIBLE

### ■ Osteomalacia

*(See Rickets and Osteomalacia, page 294)*

### ■ Disused Bone

Bone requires regular use to maintain its normal structure. If unused because of paralysis (for instance, by a stroke, multiple sclerosis, or spina bifida), the bones become weak and may even break when the individual is being carried or turned in bed.

So, bone pain in any bedridden or partially paralyzed individual may be caused by a fracture.

### ■ Bone Cancer

While uncommon in someone not known to have cancer, severe bone pain following a minor injury should be taken seriously in someone who has known cancer, and bone cancer in particular. *(See page 281)*

## RARE

### ■ Paget's Disease of Bone

*(See page 449)*

### ■ Osteomyelitis

### ■ Benign Bone Tumors

### ■ Brittle Bone Disease

Osteogenesis imperfecta. There are a number of types of this condition. In the most severe form, fractures develop in the womb and at birth. In the milder variant, fractures occur later in life. This is a hereditary disorder of connective tissue, often found in many family members, which prevents bones and other tissue from forming properly. The symptoms may include:

- Bones fracture with minimal injury.
- Whites of the eyes appear blue.
- Teeth may be deformed.

• General deformity because of repeated fractures.

• Other possible symptoms include hearing loss, teeth problems, and easy bruising.

■ **Marble Bones**

Also known as osteopetrosis. A very rare, inherited condition in which bones become even more solid and hard than usual. As well as an increased likelihood of fractures, growth may be affected.

## INFLAMED OR ACHING JOINTS

Virtually any generalized disease, such as influenza, gives symptoms of aching in the joints and muscles. These are often fleeting, moving from one joint or muscle to another. Many diseases have major or primary involvement with joints, the most significant of which are covered here.

### PROBABLE

■ **Viral Infection**

Any viral infection, such as the common cold or influenza, will give vague joint pains.

• General malaise.

• Fever.

• Cough, runny nose.

• Muscle pain.

• Joint pain.

Normally cures itself in a few days. Some viruses can lead to joint swelling for a longer period of time, such as German measles (rubella), slapped cheek disease (parvovirus), and glandular fever.

■ **Osteoarthritis**

*(See page 307)*

### POSSIBLE

■ **Gout**

Caused by excess uric acid in the blood. This may occur due to high alcohol use, medication (such as bendroflumethiazide used to treat high blood pressure), kidney problems, certain diets high in "purine foods" (such as Marmite, game meat), and other rare causes.

• One joint is affected at a time (monarticular); most commonly, first affects the big toe joint.

• Sudden onset.

• Joint is hot, shiny, red, and excruciatingly painful.

• There may be malaise and fever. Attacks recur and involve other joints. Each attack may last around one week.

• Gouty tophi, lumpy collections of uric acid crystals, form in the skin, particularly on the ears and adjacent to joints.

The high levels of uric acid, if untreated, can cause kidney stones and kidney failure. Blood tests or taking a sample of fluid from the swollen joint help to confirm the diagnosis. Lifestyle changes and medication can control the symptoms.

## ■ Rheumatoid Arthritis

The most common type of chronic, generalized inflammatory joint disease. It is actually a connective tissue disease and it may run in families. Symptoms are caused by persistent inflammation of the synovial membrane, which lines joint capsules. Most common in young women.

An immunoglobulin called rheumatoid factor is commonly present in the blood of affected individuals. Features include:
- Painful swelling of joints (often symmetrical).
- Early morning stiffness.
- Progressive joint deformity *(see also sections on specific joints).*
- Progressive loss of function.
- Lumps may appear in skin and around joints.
- Osteoporosis may develop.
- Anemia.
- Muscle wasting.
- Higher risk of heart disease later in life.

Treatment involves relief of pain and reduction of inflammation. Recent advances in medication have revolutionized the treatment of this condition. At later stages in severe cases, surgery may be necessary to improve function because of deformity.

## ■ Ankylosing Spondylitis
*(See page 293)*

## ■ Sickle-Cell Disease

An inherited disease found in African Americans. The red blood cells become sickle-shaped when low amounts of oxygen are available. These sickle cells are less pliable than normal cells and so block up capillaries (small blood vessels), causing damage to organs because of lack of oxygen and poor blood supply. Some individuals are less affected—they are described as having sickle-cell trait. Those with full-blown disease have recurrent attacks of severe pains in the limbs and abdomen (sickle crises).

Features of the disease include:
- Anemia.
- Increased predisposition to infection.
- Joint pains.
- Fever.
- Jaundice.
- Abdominal pains.

Treatment is mainly aimed at relieving the symptoms. Blood transfusions, administering oxygen, and strong painkillers are mainstays.

### RARE

### ■ Septic Arthritis

This is a very serious condition and should be seen by a doctor the first day it is noticed. A joint becomes infected with a bacteria. Most commonly this occurs after joint surgery (such as joint replacement) or in a joint otherwise damaged by arthritis. Symptoms include:

• Painful, swollen, hot, and possibly red joint. Usually only one joint is affected.

• Fever.

• Often feeling unwell.

Treatment involves antibiotics for many weeks, often in the hospital via an intravenous drip to start with.

### ■ Juvenile Idiopathic Arthritis

This is the juvenile form of rheumatoid arthritis and other similar conditions occurring in childhood.

### ■ Reiter's Syndrome

Occurs in adults, mainly in men. It occurs a few weeks after a bowel infection *(Salmonella)* or a sexual infection *(Chlamydia)*. There will be the following three symptoms:

• Urethritis (burning on passing water, often with a discharge).

• Conjunctivitis.

• Arthritis pain and swelling of two or three joints, such as a hip, knee, or ankle.

### ■ Psoriatic Arthritis

Occasionally, arthritis can be a complication of psoriasis, a skin disease.

• Various joints, in different parts of the body, are affected.

• The distal interphalangeal joints may be the only ones involved.

• Possibly nail pitting.

### ■ Gonococcal Arthritis

One of many complications of the sexually transmitted disease gonorrhea. In men, the main symptom is:

• Urethral discharge.

In women, up to 75 percent may have no symptoms. Those that do may have:

• Pain on passing urine.

• Vaginal discharge.

May develop in one joint with symptoms of infective arthritis *(see left)*.

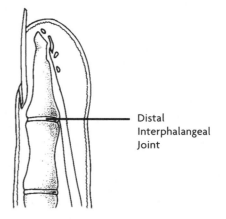

Distal
Interphalangeal
Joint

- Systemic Lupus Erythematosis (SLE)

*(See page 460)*

- Rheumatic Fever

*(See page 202)*

- Hemophilia

*(See page 441)*

- Syphilis

*(See page 379)*

## SWOLLEN JOINT WITH NODULES

### PROBABLE

- Bursa

Many joints have sacs, like empty balloons, overlying their surfaces. If damaged, these fill with fluid and enlarge. They feel like smooth, fluid-filled swellings and may be uncomfortable and irritating. In particular, the bursa in front of the knee may become swollen after kneeling, commonly known as housemaid's knee.

- Osteoarthritis

*(See page 307)*

### POSSIBLE

- Rheumatoid Arthritis

*(See page 285)*

- Gout

*(See page 284)*

### RARE

- Charcot Joints

Joints that have lost the sense of pain and position. If the joint is damaged, it can become progressively more deformed, as degeneration occurs rapidly. The joint looks as if it should be very painful, possibly with extreme swelling and deformity. Fluid, bony protuberances and loose pieces of bone may easily be felt in and around the joint. Dislocation is not uncommon. The more common causes include syphilis, spina bifida, or indeed anything that can damage the peripheral nerve system, including diabetes and excessive alcohol.

## PAINFUL JOINTS

*(See Inflamed or Aching Joints, page 284)*

## STIFF JOINTS

*(See Inflamed or Aching Joints, page 284)*

## PAINFUL SHOULDER

### PROBABLE

#### ■ Frozen Shoulder

Most common in later middle-age. Called "frozen shoulder" because someone with this condition tends to hold their shoulder very still, due to the pain.
• Slight injury to shoulder joint may or may not have occurred.
• Subsequently progressive pain and stiffness.
• Pain starts at shoulder tip and runs down outer arm toward the elbow.
• Can be very disabling, with reduced movement of the shoulder and pain on moving it or lying on it at night.

Tends to cure itself over a year or so, but may be treated with physiotherapy or a cortisone injection to encourage movement of the shoulder.

#### ■ Painful Arc Syndrome

Most common in a middle-aged or later middle-aged person.
• Pain at shoulder tip.
• Variable in intensity; worse at night.
• Limited shoulder movement.
• Local area of tenderness can be identified with one fingertip.
• Pain worse over part of the "arc" made by raising the arm from the side.

#### ■ Rotator Cuff Tear

Tendons lying at the upper part of the shoulder can tear or rupture without warning. Tends to occur with preexisting "wear and tear" changes, and thus typical of the elderly.
• May be associated with a fall or lifting.
• Sudden onset of pain.
• Arm cannot be moved outward.

#### ■ Dislocation of the Shoulder

A common injury in contact sports. The shoulder is a "ball and socket joint." Forceful injury makes the ball, which is found at the top of the humerus (upper arm bone), slip out of its socket.
• Pain on movement.
• Loss of shoulder contour.
• "Ball" (humeral head) may be felt below the outer end of the collarbone.
• Arm is held out from the body at elbow.

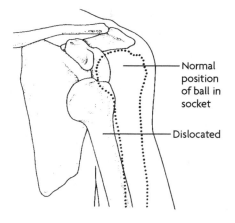

*Shoulder Dislocation*

### ■ Rheumatoid Arthritis

The shoulder joint can be affected in patients with rheumatoid arthritis. *(See page 285)*

### ■ Fractured Collarbone (Clavicle)

The clavicle may break as a result of direct or indirect injury.

- Pain at the point of the break.
- Pain on arm movement; often the individual holds the affected arm with the opposite hand to prevent movement.
- Deformity at fracture site.

### ■ Fractured Humerus

The upper end of the humerus can break in a number of ways, but the damage is almost always the result of a direct blow or a fall.

- Pain when attempting to move the shoulder or arm.
- Often, substantial tracks of bruising down the arm.
- Variable amount of deformity, dependent on the degree of displacement.

### ■ Polymyalgia Rheumatica

*(See page 278)*

### ■ Osteoarthritis

*(See page 307)*

### RARE

### ■ Ruptured Biceps Tendon

In the elderly. The top end of the biceps

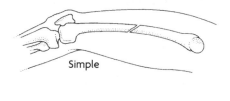

Simple

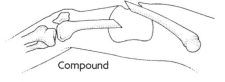

Compound

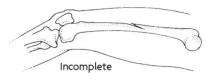

Incomplete

*Types of Fractures*

muscle runs over the top of the humeral head. Changes due to wear and tear can make it rupture.

- Sudden onset of pain at shoulder tip.
- Flexing arm against resistance allows upper end of biceps (now unattached) to bunch up and become visible in the upper arm.

### ■ Tuberculosis

(See page 472)

### ■ Internal Bleeding

Anyone who develops pain at a shoulder tip after abdominal injury, when lying flat, must be urgently investigated for internal abdominal bleeding. It is thought that blood from the bleeding point tracks up to the diaphragm, from where pain is referred to the shoulder, which shares the same nerve supply.

## CANNOT STRAIGHTEN BACK

(See Painful Back, below)

## ROUND OR HUNCHED SHOULDERS

(See Kyphosis and Scoliosis under A Lump on the Back, page 295)

## PAINFUL BACK

The back is taken here as the area from the neck down to the tailbone (coccyx). All of us will have at least one episode of back pain during our lives, caused by either injury or disease. Pain may prevent you from straightening up, but may also be felt when in a normal upright posture.

Back pain lasting more than two to three weeks and which does not respond to simple painkillers must be reported to a doctor.

### PROBABLE

### ■ Muscular

Tearing or bruising of muscles or ligaments.

- Distinct history of injury—typically a blow or from pulling or pushing.
- Dull ache initially, but the pain increases.
- Pain is local.
- Worse on movement, such as coughing or deep breathing.

Resolves after a few days. May need strong painkillers.

## ■ Acute Back Strain

- May develop after a sudden twisting or bending movement, or from lifting even a very small object.
- Often in the lower back.
- Often very painful at the beginning, then less so.
- Worse on movement—may be impossible to move initially.
- Difficult to say exactly where the pain is.
- Lifting the leg straight while lying flat may aggravate the pain.

Normally responds to gentle mobilization and painkillers, although it can take many weeks. A physiotherapist, osteopath, or chiropractor may be able to help.

## ■ Chronic Back Strain

Low back pain that recurs. The individual has had similar episodes over a number of years and will be aware of the types of activity that cause it and relieve it. Symptoms can be made worse by obesity.

- Similar symptoms to acute back strain, but may be less intense.

## ■ Osteoarthritis

The "wear and tear" disease. Particularly vulnerable are weight-bearing joints such as the hips and low lumbar spine, but any joint can be affected.

- Intermittent, nonspecific low back pain.
- Worse after standing and at the end of the day.
- Relieved by rest.
- However, it is possible that discomfort remains even while lying in bed.
- Gradually, as the joint becomes stiffer, pain decreases and some mobility is lost.

## ■ Sciatica

Really a symptom itself, rather than a diagnosis, and a common one for many who suffer from bad backs. Caused by pressure on the sciatic nerve, which has its origins in the lower back. Can rarely be caused by actual damage to lumbosacral nerves, lumbar spine, and the sciatic nerves. Persistent sciatica needs investigation as it can indicate serious underlying disease.

- Pain originates in low back or buttock.
- Pain radiates down the back or side of the thigh, calf, and sometimes into the foot.
- Tingling or numbness may also be noted in the leg.
- Symptoms can be made worse by raising and straightening the leg.

## ■ Cervical Spondylosis

*(See page 133)*

## POSSIBLE

### ■ Kidney Infection

Pain usually on one side of the loin (area on either side of the backbone, between the ribs and hip). This is often severely painful, associated with fever symptoms and urinary symptoms (pain on passing urine and passing small, frequent volumes).

This requires urgent antibiotics.

### ■ Prolapsed Intervertebral Disc

Often known as a "slipped disc" (as are acute and chronic back strains and sciatica). The fibrous disc that acts as a buffer between the vertebrae has a gelatinous center. Age or injury can cause this center to bulge out, applying pressure on the nerves that emerge between the vertebrae and supply sensation to the body.

• Minor episodes of backache are an early warning.

• Sudden onset of severe back pain when bending or stooping; you may be unable to stand.

• Sciatica *(see page 291)* may be present.

• Coughing and straining make the pain worse.

• Numbness or tingling may develop in a leg or foot.

• Very occasionally, a slipped disc may cause urinary retention. This is a medical emergency.

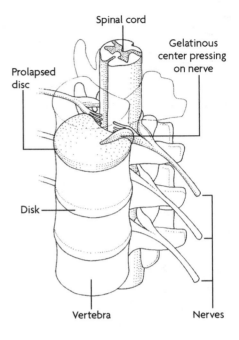

*Prolapsed Disc*

The symptoms may subside in a few days or weeks, although a few may persist. If you have numbness or tingling in the feet or legs or in the genital region, and/or your ability to pass urine seems to be affected, seek medical help urgently.

### ■ Shingles

Shingles is caused by the chicken pox virus. Those who have not had chicken pox can catch it from someone with shingles.

• Initially, skin irritation.

- Red spots develop in a band that is a few inches wide on one side of the body.
- The spots develop into fluid-filled vesicles, which burst and form crusts.
- Can become very painful.

If suspected, shingles can be treated with one of several antiviral drugs, but these are best given before the spots develop. Tends to cure itself.

### ■ Coccydynia

Pain associated with the coccyx or tail-bone.

- Persistent pain after a fall.
- Pain aggravated by local pressure.
- Pain aggravated by sitting.

### ■ Scoliosis

*(See page 295)*

### ■ Kyphosis

*(See page 295)*

### ■ Osteoporosis

Thinning of the bones often caused by aging. In women, this is especially a post-menopausal problem.

- Occurs in otherwise fit individuals.
- Increasing deformity as age increases.
- Shortening of the vertebral column; height loss.

### ■ Ankylosing Spondylitis

Essentially an inflammatory disorder affecting the spine and sacroiliac joints; most common in males during the late teenage years. It tends to occur in families.

- Intermittent backache or buttock pain at the early stage.
- Intermittent stiffness.
- Symptoms worst in the early morning, improving with movement and exercise.
- As the disease progresses, swelling and stiffness of other joints may develop.
- Occasionally, eyes, heart, and lungs may be affected.

## RARE

### ■ Cancer of the Spine (Primary or Secondary)

The spine is a well-recognized site of secondary cancer, meaning cancerous growth that has spread from another (primary) site. Anyone developing the following should see a doctor without delay (although most of these symptoms are *not* due to cancer):

- Severe continuous pain in the back that wakes you at night.
- Pain radiating from the back to the limbs.
- The development of pain, weakness, or altered sensation in the limbs.

Other symptoms of cancer, including weight loss, malaise, and loss of appetite may also be evident.

## ■ Benign Tumor of the Back

Although benign tumors rarely give rise to pain, large ones, or ones adjacent to pressure areas (for example, at the level of the waistband) may do so. Even if you think it is benign, report it to a doctor.

## ■ Discitis

An infection develops in the intervertebral disc. The pain often gradually gets worse over weeks. This can be difficult to diagnose. Sometimes it is associated with fever symptoms, weight loss, or feeling generally unwell.

Treatment is with antibiotics for many weeks, usually initially in the hospital.

## ■ Rickets and Osteomalacia

Both conditions represent similar disease processes in children (rickets) and in adults (osteomalacia) and are caused by lack of vitamin D.

The symptoms of rickets are:
- Skull deformity.
- Knee, ankle, and wrist thickening.
- Enlargement of the bony cartilages of the chest ("rickety rosary").
- Lower limb deformities.
- Rarely, spinal curvature and pain.

The symptoms of osteomalacia are:
- General bone pain.
- Backache.
- Muscle pain.
- Loss of height due to vertebral collapse.
- Stress fractures.

## ■ Gastrointestinal or Abdominal Disease

A number of unusual conditions may cause back symptoms, although very rarely in isolation. Inflammation of the pancreas and peptic ulcer may cause pain (often centrally in the small of the back). Inflammatory bowel disease, such as Crohn's disease or ulcerative colitis, can cause back pain, either by referred pain from the diseased bowel or because of the joint inflammation that, rarely, may be associated with them. An aneurysm (swelling) of the large aorta artery can cause back pain together with pulsation in the abdomen.

## ■ Tuberculosis

*(See page 472)*

## A LUMP ON THE BACK

### PROBABLE

#### ■ Benign Tumor of Skin Structures

Meaning a harmless lump, such as a lipoma or sebaceous cyst, which may occur in the skin anywhere on the body. Common features are:

• Pain free.

• Slow increase in size.

• Otherwise sound health.

#### ■ Infection

• Often sited on the upper back.

• Painful.

• Red.

• Localized swelling.

• Pus may ooze out.

Any infection may eventually become an abscess, a collection of pus. Often, it may discharge itself, but occasionally surgical drainage may be needed. Sometimes, cellulitis *(see page 317)* develops, which requires antibiotics. If recurrent infections occur, then a doctor should ensure that diabetes is not to blame.

#### ■ Normal Bony Prominences

Occasionally, a previously unnoticed lump may become apparent. This often occurs after a loss of weight. The spine itself is a rather knobby structure.

### POSSIBLE

#### ■ Kyphosis and Scoliosis

Deformities of the spine causing humps. Kyphosis:

• Spine is unusually curved.

• Curve of the upper spine is exaggerated when viewed from the side.

• Humpback appearance.

• Some pain.

There are various causes, including bad posture, osteoporosis, osteoarthritis, ankylosing spondylitis, or rare congenital disease.

Scoliosis is a sideways deformity of the spine:

• Sometimes there's a family history.

• Spine appears to curve more to one side when looked at from behind, particularly when the person bends forward.

• Some pain.

May be associated with any disease that affects the spine.

### RARE

#### ■ Spina Bifida

A congenital abnormality recognized at or soon after birth.

#### ■ Cancer

People with known malignant disease may develop secondary growths in either the skin or skeletal structures of the back. Pain, irregular contour, and rapid growth are ominous signs.

Usually the cancer will have already made itself known.

### ■ Tuberculosis

Unrecognized tuberculous infection of the spine or other bone(s) can cause sudden collapse of the affected part so that a bony lump can be felt. This may be known as a kyphus, a specific type of kyphosis *(see page 295)*.
- Develops rapidly.
- Often associated with general malaise and occasional fever.
- Pain is often slight in the early stages, but can then become severe and constant.

## BACK PAIN, WOMEN ONLY

### PROBABLE

### ■ Menstrual Period Pain

Also called dysmenorrhea.
- Low abdominal and back pain associated with periods.
- Occurs at each period and then resolves.
- Otherwise fit.

### ■ Mittelschmerz

- Low back and abdominal pain developing in the middle of the menstrual cycle.
- Believed to be associated with ovulation.

### POSSIBLE

### ■ Pelvic Inflammatory Disease

Infection of the female genital tract. If suspected, requires treatment to minimize the risk of infertility later.
- Fever.
- Low back and low abdominal pain, ranging from severe to very slight, or even nonexistent.
- Vaginal discharge—yellow/green/brown.
- Discharge is often smelly.
- Possibly malaise and fever.

### RARE

### ■ Cancer of the Cervix, Ovaries, and Womb

- There may be chronic, unremitting back or lower abdominal pain.
- Possibly offensive, bloody vaginal discharge (in cases involving the uterus and cervix).
- Abdominal swelling; fluid collects in the abdominal cavity.

Other symptoms associated with malignant disease may be present:

- Weight loss.
- Anorexia.
- Anemia.
- Malaise.

## PAINFUL ELBOW

A number of structures around the elbow can give pain. The elbow joint is made up of three bones: the humerus, the radius, and the ulna. A number of muscles and tendons attach near the joint and nerves pass close by.

A direct blow can, of course, break or bruise the bone; the olecranon is the most prominent part and is often damaged. The lower end of the humerus may be broken. The upper end of the radius may be broken indirectly if you fall on an outstretched hand, as force is transmitted up the arm to its top end. The symptoms of a fracture are:

- Local pain.
- Local swelling.
- Loss of function—flexing/extending and twisting the forearm.
- Deformity may not be particularly noticeable.

Bruising can give similar symptoms, but the pain disappears relatively quickly and function returns.

One other elbow problem lies outside our conventional analysis of probable, possible, and rare: knocking the "funny bone." The funny bone is not in fact a bone, but a nerve called the ulnar nerve, which runs round the back of the medial epicondyle. If you knock it:

- Exquisite pain on the medial epicondyle (and not knowing whether to laugh or cry).
- Pain and altered feeling (tingling)

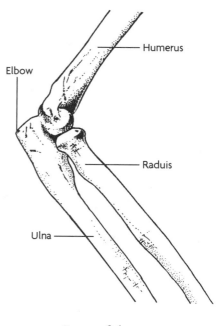

*Bones of the arm*

sensed down the forearm to the hand (mainly on the little and ring fingers), lasting a few seconds.

## Probable

### ■ Tennis Elbow and Golfer's Elbow

These are repetitive strain injuries typical of tennis players and golfers, but more commonly seen in anyone who uses their arms repetitively. Patients are often middle-aged.

• Local pain: in tennis elbow, the outer side of the elbow is involved; in golfer's elbow, the inner side.

• Pain worse on certain movements, such as turning a door handle, shaking hands, lifting, or serving at tennis.

May be treated with rest, physiotherapy, or (more rarely now) with a local injection of an anesthetic and steroid; occasionally, surgery may help. Acupuncture may also be of benefit.

## Rare

### ■ Loose Bodies

Pieces of bone may chip off and lie free in the joint as a result of injury, degeneration (perhaps from osteoarthritis), inflammation (perhaps from rheumatoid arthritis), or some unknown cause.

• Intermittent pain in joint.

• Joint locks.

• Cannot always fully extend or flex the elbow.

• Associated symptoms of other disease.

If symptoms persist or progress, surgical removal of the loose body may be necessary.

### ■ Infected Bursa

The bursa is a sac, like an empty balloon, that lies under the skin over the olecranon. Injury—a blow or friction—to the olecranon makes the bursa fill with fluid, which can then be seen as a lump on the point of the elbow. This is often pain free. Occasionally, enlargement is associated with other diseases such as gout or rheumatoid arthritis. If the overlying skin is damaged (cut or grazed), then the fluid may become infected.

## PAINFUL WRIST

## Probable

### ■ Sprain

Usually the result of a twisting or bending injury.

• Uncomfortable on movement, but no real limitation.

• No specific local tenderness.

Will resolve within a few days.

### ■ Colles' Fracture

Common in postmenopausal females who fall onto an outstretched hand. The ends of the radius and ulna are broken.

- A "dinner fork deformity."
- Pain in wrist.
- Lump on back of wrist.
- Pain on movement.
- Swelling can be extensive.

Requires realigning and immobilization in a plaster cast.

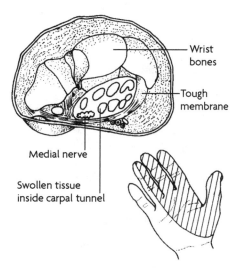

*Carpal Tunnel*

### ■ Scaphoid Fracture

After falling onto an outstretched hand.

- Pain in the wrist.
- Swelling.
- Pain on movement.
- Local pain at base of the back of the thumb.

If this fracture is untreated, the scaphoid, a small bone in the wrist, will degenerate, causing early osteoarthritis. Suspected scaphoid fractures must be immobilized initially, and x-rays reviewed after a week or so.

### POSSIBLE

### ■ Osteoarthritis

(See page 307)

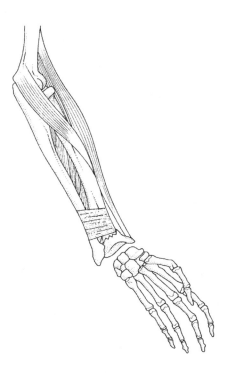

*Colles' Fracture*
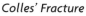

■ **Rheumatoid Arthritis**

*(See page 285)*

■ **Carpal Tunnel Syndrome**

Although mainly causing symptoms in the hands and fingers, carpal tunnel syndrome may cause pain in the wrist and forearm as well.

• Pressure on nerves passing to the hand through the wrist gives rise to tingling and numbness.

• Common in pregnancy and premenstrually or when fluid retention is a symptom.

*(See also Swollen Hands, page 301)*

**RARE**

■ **Tuberculosis**

*(See page 472)*

## SWOLLEN WRIST

*(See Painful Wrist, page 298)*

## A SWELLING AT THE WRIST

**PROBABLE**

■ **Ganglion**

A small, usually pea-sized or larger, fluid-filled swelling adjacent to the wrist joint, capsule, or tendon sheath.

• Localized smooth lump, normally on the back of the wrist.

• Cystic.

• Can shine a light through it.

• Mild discomfort; worse if knocked.

Usually no treatment is required; occasionally removed by surgery. Used to be treated by a firm blow from the family Bible, but this is best avoided.

**POSSIBLE**

■ **Osteoarthritis**

*(See page 307)*

■ **Rheumatoid Arthritis**

*(See page 285)*

**RARE**

■ **Pseudogout**

This is caused by the deposition of calcium crystals in the joint. The joint becomes red, hot, painful, and swollen over hours.

It is treated with strong painkillers and usually resolves in a few days.

■ **Septic Arthritis**

*(See page 310)*

## UNUSUALLY LARGE HANDS

If these have increased in size in adulthood, this may be a feature of acromegaly *(see page 281).*

## SWOLLEN HANDS

### PROBABLE

#### ■ Normal Variation

Intermittent swelling of one hand, or both, is a common, noticeable symptom. You may find it difficult to remove rings or a wrist strap may make an indentation on the wrist. May be worse in hot weather or, for women, premenstrually.

#### ■ Pregnancy

Particularly in the later stages of pregnancy, the body's normal response is to retain fluid and this tends to make the hands look puffy. It is important to have your blood pressure and urine checked by your midwife/general practitioner to ensure that your blood pressure has not risen during pregnancy.

#### ■ Injury

Swelling would be a normal response to direct physical insult, such as bruising, a fracture, or tendonitis.

### POSSIBLE

#### ■ Hypothyroidism

Carpal tunnel syndrome *(see page 300)* can be a feature of this condition, which is caused by an underactive thyroid gland. (Do not confuse this with *hyperthyroidism,* an overactive gland.) Other symptoms are:

- Skin becomes dry and rough.
- You "feel the cold."
- Voice becomes gruff, features coarsen.
- Weight gain, constipation, slow speech, slow thought.

The disorder is easily treated. For further details, see hypothyroidism *(page 426).*

### RARE

#### ■ Axillary Vein Thrombosis

Blockage of the main vein in the armpit or upper arm. May have no apparent cause or occurs after vigorous exercise.
- Swelling of entire arm.
- No pain, but there may be a dull ache.
- Superficial veins of arm may appear more prominent because the deep veins are blocked.

#### ■ Lymphedema

Primary or secondary. *(See page 318)*

## TREMBLING HANDS

*(See Trembling or Shaking, page 450)*

## CLUBBED OR CURVED FINGERS OR NAILS

This means that:

• The end part of the finger becomes rounded.

• The nails appear larger and more curved lengthways and side to side.

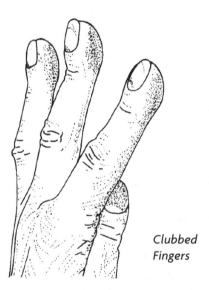

Clubbed Fingers

• The angle between the nail bed and the skin on the back of the finger is lost.

If the fingers have been clubbed since birth, and there are similar finger shapes in the family, then the symptom is not significant. But if clubbing develops during life, it may well be associated with other diseases, some of which are listed below. It is rare for clubbing alone to be the first indicator of these diseases. Medical science has not yet explained this phenomenon. Diseases in which clubbed fingers is a symptom include lung diseases such as bronchiectasis, lung fibrosis (fibrosing alveolitis), cystic fibrosis, or lung cancer; heart disease (congenital heart disease, endocarditis); gastrointestinal disease (Crohn's disease, cystic fibrosis, liver cirrhosis, ulcerative colitis); and malignant disease. See relevant sections for further details.

## PROBLEMS WITH FINGERNAILS

It is said that over sixty diagnoses can be made from examining the nails alone. The appearance of the nail may be a clear sign of certain diseases, and the most common variations are listed here, along with the disease with which they are associated.

- Bitten fingernails: may, of course, be no more than a habit, or may point to an underlying tension, even anxiety or depression, particularly if of recent onset.

- Paronychia (sometimes known as "a whitlow"): an abscess of the fingertip, which becomes red, tender, tense, and throbbing; pus may accumulate. Often needs to be released by a surgical incision. Antibiotics may be required.

- Transverse fissures (lines): quite common after any illness and may be present for many months.

- Transverse ridges: often in association with eczema.

- Subungual hematoma: discoloration after injury. The classic injury to a nail is a hammer blow or an object dropped on the toes. Within a few minutes, a blue, then a purplish, then a dark brown or black area may appear. The toe feels painful and throbs, because blood, which causes the discoloration, builds up pressure under the nail. The symptoms are easily relieved by piercing the nail over the hematoma with a heated sterile needle, allowing the blood to escape. This should be done by a health professional, as it would be unsafe to do this in the presence of a finger fracture.

- Pale nails or leukonychia: in association with pale mucosa and conjunctiva in the eye, this symptom suggests anemia.

- Bluish nails: suggests cyanosis. Often accompanies lung or heart disease. Examine also the lips and the ears; breathlessness may be a feature.

- Koilonychia or spoon-shaped nails: iron deficiency, anemia.

- Glomus tumor: an exquisitely tender, red- or violet-colored area a few millimeters across under the nail.

- Pitting of the nails: often occurs in association with psoriasis.

- Onycholysis (the nails separate from the nail bed): another feature of psoriasis, particularly at the end of the nail.

- Fungal infections of the nails: these give a markedly thickened, irregular, and discolored nail. The nail loses its usual color, becoming uniformly cream-colored and opaque. Other fungal infections may be present elsewhere.

- Onychogryphosis: enormous overgrowth and thickening of (mainly) the big toenail, most commonly seen in the elderly. Advanced cases end up looking like a ram's horn.

- Brittle nails: may be due to excess manicuring and application of polish and polish remover.

- Splinter hemorrhages (longitudinal

areas of redness that look like small splinters at the tips of the fingernails): may be associated with infection of the heart lining. Heart murmurs, malaise, shortness of breath, fever, and anemia are other signs.

• White lines (short, white lines are frequently seen across nails): the exact cause is unclear. They may be a sign of a blow to the nail or may appear after an illness. They are of little significance.

Other diseases associated with nail deformities are:

• Lichen planus: a rare, itchy skin disease that also affects the nails. The whole skin may be affected. The nails in about 10 percent of cases become flaky, striated (lined), spoon-shaped, or may be destroyed.

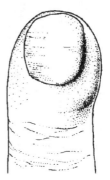

*Paronychia*

• Alopecia areata: hair loss from the scalp, in patches. The nails may be pitted.

• Nail-patella syndrome: a rare hereditary disease. Rudimentary or absent nails and small or absent patella (kneecap).

• Paronychia congenita: nails are thickened, as is the surrounding skin.

## EXTREMELY COLD OR FROZEN FINGERS

This symptom occurs with chilblains and frostbite *(see under Itching or Numbness of the Fingers and Toes, page 329).*

■ **Raynaud's Phenomenon**

This is where the hands go cold and painful. The fingers change color, initially white, then blue, then when they recover, red. This condition can occur on its own (Raynaud's disease) or due to other causes, such as drugs (beta-blockers), connective tissue disorders such as lupus (SLE) *(see page 460)* and scleroderma *(see page 263),* use of vibrating tools, or sometimes due to the presence of an extra rib in the neck.

## SWOLLEN OR MISSHAPEN FINGERS

**PROBABLE**

### ■ Pulp Space Infection

Infection, typically after a prick from a plant or needle in the soft tissue at the finger tip.

- Swelling.
- Pain.
- Redness.
- Throbbing.

May require drainage or antibiotics.

### ■ Trigger Finger

Thickening or inflammation of part of a flexor tendon in a finger or thumb, which causes:

- The digit to "stick" when bending or straightening.
- May "unstick" with a snap, spontaneously, or may need to be forced to straighten.

> If a finger or thumb is severed, place it in a clean, sealed plastic bag or wrap it in clean material or plastic wrap, surround it with ice, and rush to the nearest hospital. (Do not put the ice directly next to the finger as this can damage it). With new microsurgical techniques, it is sometimes possible to save the digit.

- A small tender nodule may be felt at the base of the digit on the palm.
- This nodule can be felt clicking as the digit is flexed.

Recovery may be spontaneous, but per-

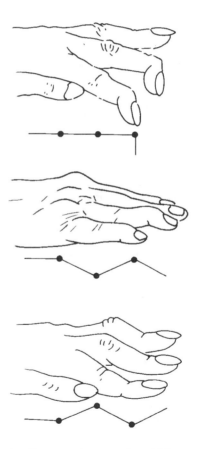

*Mallet, top; Swan neck, middle; Boutonniere, bottom.*

sistent symptoms can often be treated with a cortisone injection or sometimes surgery.

### ■ Heberden's Nodes

Caused by osteoarthritis.
• Distal interphalangeal joints are painful.
• Bony overgrowth makes the joints appear enlarged and knobby.

## POSSIBLE

### ■ Mallet Finger and Thumb

Damage to the tendon (extensor) that attaches to the dorsal surface of the end bone of each digit. The damage may be caused by injury to the end of the digit or, indirectly, after a wrist fracture. Occasionally, it happens in association with other disease, such as rheumatoid arthritis.
• Terminal phalanx of digit appears bent but cannot be straightened.

Splinting for six weeks may help cure cases caused by direct trauma. In other situations, surgery may be needed.

### ■ Rheumatoid Arthritis

This disease affects the fingers and hands in a number of ways, including:
• Ulnar deviation of the fingers: the fingers appear to drift toward the side of the little finger, and the knuckle joints appear pronounced.

• Swan neck deformities.
• Boutonniere's deformities.
• Drop finger (the finger cannot be extended at the knuckle joint).
• Mallet thumb *(see left)*.

### ■ Dupuytren's Contracture

• A fibrous contracture of (commonly) the little and ring fingers, which cannot be completely straightened.
• Sometimes, the fingers are so bent that washing the hand is a problem.
• Thickening can be felt on the palm side of affected fingers and on the palm.

Usually of unknown cause, but has been linked with excessive drinking and with certain drugs. It may also be hereditary.

### ■ Gout

A generalized disease that may affect joints and skin. In the fingers and hands, the following may be seen:
• Tophi: lumps in the skin containing waxy, yellow material.
• Deformed joints of the fingers and hand.

## RARE

### ■ Flexor Sheath Infection

Infection in the sheath surrounding the tendons that bend the fingers (flexor tendons).
• Entire finger is red and swollen.
• Pain.

- Loss of function.
- Pain worse on movement; finger is held crooked, the most comfortable position.
- Infection (untreated) may spread back into the palm of the hand.

This is an orthopedic emergency, needing immediate treatment to prevent long-term loss of function and deformity.

### ■ Ischemic Contracture

Also known as Volkmann's contracture. Direct or indirect injury to the blood supply of the forearm damages muscle, making it atrophy and shrink.

- Pale or bluish-looking skin on hand.
- Thin forearm.
- Hand is clawed: fingers flexed at both finger joints.
- Sensation diminished.
- Fingers can only be straightened when the hand is flexed at the wrist.
- Only able to grip when hand is flexed.

### ■ Congenital Deformities

Present at birth.

- Failure of development: part or all of the fingers and hand may be deformed or absent.
- Syndactyly or webbing: fusion of adjacent fingers.
- "Extra" digits, ranging from small lumps of flesh to entire digits (usually on the outer part of the limb).

### ■ Congenital Contracture

Present from birth.

- Fingers may be bent.
- Thickened tissue may be felt on the surface of the palm.
- May only affect one digit.

### ■ Malignant Tumors

*(See Lumps in the Skin, page 256)*

### ■ Benign Tumors

*(See Lumps in the Skin, page 256)*

## PAINFUL HIP

Likely to have different causes at different ages. Pain is often felt in the groin or the front of the hip and may radiate down the thigh and to the knee. In children (who may not complain of pain), a limp may be the only evidence of pain. Accidental dislocation is excluded from this section because the cause—severe injury—is obvious.

### PROBABLE

### ■ Osteoarthritis

From about fifty years of age. Osteoarthritis is a problem of growing old—

of degeneration. All of us are affected to some degree by this form of arthritis, sometimes described as "wear and tear" arthritis. Some preexisting conditions predispose to an early appearance of osteoarthritis, including congenital dislocation of the hip, infective arthritis, Perthes' disease *(see right),* and slipped epiphysis *(see page 309).* The risk is increased if the diagnosis is missed or treatment delayed.

• Pain radiating from the groin to the knee.

• Initially after exercise, progressing to pain at rest or disturbing sleep.

• Progressive stiffness of leg.

• Difficulty in putting on shoes and socks.

• Progressive limp.

• Apparent shortening of leg.

Treatment is first aimed at relieving the pain (painkillers), then at improving function (exercises and physiotherapy); eventually, severe cases may require joint replacement.

### ■ Fractured Neck of Femur

*(See information on pathological fractures under Bones Breaking Easily, page 282)*

## POSSIBLE

### ■ Irritable Hip

Typically in children.

• Pain in the groin or front of thigh, often to the knee.

• Limp.

• All movement of hip limited by pain.

This diagnosis tends to be made if investigations for other causes lead to nothing. The hip resolves with bed rest and, occasionally, traction. A child with a new limp should be taken to see a doctor the same day to exclude other more serious problems, such as infection.

## RARE

### ■ Perthes' Disease

The blood supply to the femoral head is compromised and it dies. The course of the disease is up to four years. Surprisingly, the symptoms can be quite slight.

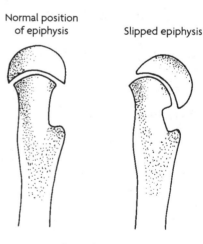

Normal position of epiphysis

Slipped epiphysis

*Slipped epiphysis*

- Patient aged five to ten years, occasionally older or younger.
- Intermittent ache in hip.
- Intermittent limp.
- Painful movements.

It is important to distinguish between this serious disease and irritable hip.

### ■ Slipped Epiphysis

- Hip pain and limp.

Diagnosis is by x-ray.

### ■ Congenital Dislocation of the Hip

*(See Dislocated Hip, below)*

## DISLOCATED HIP

May be congenital (hereditary) or acquired, caused by accident or infection.

### ■ Congenital Dislocation of the Hip (CDH)

CDH tends to run in families and arises because of an abnormally shaped hip socket, combined with lax joint ligaments. Breech birth (when the baby's feet, rather than the head, emerge from the birth canal first) increases the likelihood. Babies who have family histories of CDH or who have been breech during pregnancy are often screened a few weeks after birth with an ultrasound scan to ensure that this condition is not present.

Symptoms before walking:
- Asymmetry of hip, seen at skin creases.
- Legs will not part fully.
- The baby may be late to start walking.

Symptoms after walking:
- Asymmetry of legs.

- Limp.

If both hips are dislocated, the waddling gait could pass as normal, in which case the dislocation will go undetected, causing damage. So, the problem needs to be recognized at an early stage. Treatment is with different forms of splint. If untreated, the limp remains and the hip joint is progressively distorted and damaged. Ultimately, severe osteoarthritis develops and hip replacement may be needed as an adult.

### ■ Acquired Dislocation

Acquired dislocation of the hip is caused either by injury or infection. Typically, a car or motorcycle accident, in which the individual is sitting with the knee bent, results in the femoral head being pushed backward out of the acetabulum. Extreme force is needed.

- Extreme pain.
- Deformity in extreme cases.

- Leg is shortened and twisted inward.
- The knee is slightly bent.
- The leg cannot be moved.

The femoral head can be replaced in the acetabulum, but recovery can be a lengthy process, often because there are other injuries.

Much less commonly, the hip may also dislocate forward; also centrally, when the femoral head pushes through the acetabulum into the pelvis.

### ■ Septic Arthritis

Infection of the hip. This most commonly arises after hip surgery, but can arise on its own in adults and children. Untreated infection in any joint requires urgent orthopedic attention to remove pus and clear the infection, as the joint surface and surrounding structures can be rapidly destroyed.

Features include:
- Pain (of variable intensity).
- A limp.
- Eventually, loss of function.
- Malaise.
- Fever.

Neglected, or mistreated, episodes of infective dislocation may mean surgery at a later date to correct deformity.

## BOW-LEGGEDNESS

In most cases, this is an innocent variation of normal, occurring in childhood. Most children grow out of it.
- Feet together.
- Knees splayed.

May also, but much more rarely, be seen in rickets *(page 294)*, osteoarthritis *(page 307)*, and Paget's disease *(page 449)*.

## LIMPING

Limping can be a symptom of many disorders and is caused by pain, deformity, or both. Look for a specific site of pain or deformity and then refer to that section.

## PAIN WHEN WALKING

*(Consider explanations in the following pages covering the leg and knee; also, see the preceding pages covering the hip)*

## WALKING WITH A WADDLING GAIT

*(See Congenital Dislocation of the Hip, page 309, and Duchenne's Dystrophy, page 276)*

## PAINFUL LEG OR THIGH

*(See the general bone and muscle symptoms, page 277; also, see back symptoms, page 290)*

## PARALYZED LEG

*(See pages 415–416)*

## VEIN OR VEINS STANDING OUT IN LEG

*(See Varicose Veins, page 317)*

## SWOLLEN LEG

*(See Swollen Ankle, page 316)*

## WEAK LEG

*(See Wasting and Loss of Power in the Muscles, page 276)*

## LEG UNUSUALLY WHITE

This may indicate sudden blockage of an artery—a medical emergency—as a result of peripheral vascular disease *(see page 326)*.

## KNEE PAIN AFTER INJURY

The precise cause of the pain will be governed by the force of the injury, and its site—so the categories of Probable, Possible, and Rare are not relevant here.

The knee is made up of bones (lower femur, upper tibia, patella), ligaments (medial and lateral collateral, anterior and posterior cruciate), the joint capsule, the medial and lateral menisci, and the surrounding soft tissues. All can be damaged.

The most significant injuries are listed below, plus their symptoms and an indication of the type of injury that may cause them. All require immediate treatment. Delaying treatment, especially if the injury is severe, will increase the risk of complications. All injuries to a joint increase the risk of early onset of osteoarthritis.

### ■ Dislocation of the Knee

Enormous force is needed to disrupt the knee joint, including its capsule and ligaments.
• Severe pain.
• Marked deformity.
• Marked bruising.

Nerves and arteries to the leg may be damaged.

### ■ Dislocation of the Patella (Kneecap)

*(See Locked or Locking Knee, page 314)*

### ■ Femoral Condyle Fractures

• May be sustained after a fall from a height.
• Severe pain in the knee, which cannot be moved.
• Immediate swelling and deformity.

### ■ Ligamentous Tear

Can be complete or partial, and is often missed—the symptoms of swelling, pain, and reduced function being put down to sprain. Often, the worse the damage (for example, a complete rather than a partial tear), the less the pain felt. If

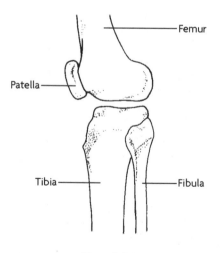

*Knee Joint*

someone has a severe injury to the knee that still allows some movement, the knee should be assessed for stability by an expert when symptoms have settled and before any sporting activities are started again.

### ■ Fractured Patella (Kneecap)

Probably caused by falling onto knee or by a direct blow.
- Immediate swelling.
- The knee is bent.
- May be unable to straighten leg, either because of pain or due to disruption of the straightening mechanism.

### ■ Supracondylar Fracture of the Femur

Caused by severe, direct injury.
- Severe pain—knee cannot be moved.
- Immediate swelling and deformity.

### ■ Fractured Tibial Plateau

Caused by a direct blow or a fall from a height.
- Severe pain—knee cannot be moved.
- Immediate swelling and deformity.

### ■ Upper Tibial Epiphysis and Apophysis

Injury to the upper part of the lower leg, below the kneecap (the shin just below the knee), can damage the point of attachment of the quadriceps tendon to the tibia.

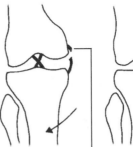
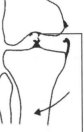

Medial ligament     Cruciate ligament

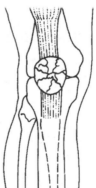
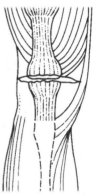

Star-shaped fracture     Transverse fracture

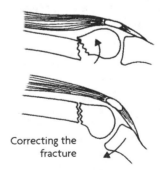

Correcting the fracture

*Knee Injuries (top to bottom): Ligamentous tear, Fractured patella, Supracondylar*

- Knee swollen, particularly below the kneecap.
- Local tenderness at the upper tibia.
- Raising the leg when it is straightened is painful or impossible.

A similar condition in young adults, which develops spontaneously, is known as Osgood-Schlatter disease.

## KNEE, SWOLLEN

*(See Knee Pain After Injury, (page 312); Locked or Locking Knee, below; and Inflamed or Aching Joints, page 284)*

## LOCKED OR LOCKING KNEE

The knee joint gets fixed at a particular angle. If it is completely locked, it is not possible to straighten it. Some knees lock intermittently; that is, they may appear to "catch" and then to straighten. These symptoms invariably suggest a problem within the knee itself, either a damaged cartilage (meniscus) or a loose body, which might be bone or cartilage. If injury to the knee predates the symptoms, it is important to remember exactly how it happened.

### PROBABLE

#### ■ Ligament Damage

The most common reason for the knee to lock, collapse, or give way is damage to one of the internal ligaments. Symptoms are often similar to those of damage to the cartilage *(see Torn Medial Meniscus, right)*.

#### ■ Torn Medial Meniscus

Typically, the meniscus is crushed and twisted between femur and tibia. Common in football and rugby players.
- Often immediate pain at the inner aspect of knee.
- Knee may lock (cannot be fully straightened).
- Swelling of the joint within a few hours.

After the first incident, symptoms may subside, only to recur with increasing frequency.

### POSSIBLE

#### ■ Loose Body

Trapped between femur and tibia.
- Intermittent sudden pain on climbing or descending stairs.
- Inability to straighten leg.

- Swelling due to fluid may accompany each attack.
- Each attack resolves as the loose body moves from between the joints.
- The loose body may be felt in the joint, often above or at the side of the patella.

### ■ Osteoarthritis

Degenerative or osteoarthritic changes in the joint can cause formation of loose bodies *(see above)*. Common in later middle-age and onwards.

## RARE

### ■ Recurrent Dislocation of the Patella (Kneecap)

Anatomical peculiarities (often, in fact, normal variants of the ligaments, muscles, tendons, or bones around the knee) may allow the kneecap to slide sideways. Most common in young females.

- Kneecap may appear very mobile from side to side.
- Knee gets stuck in a bent position (maybe only briefly), causing the individual to fall (collapsing knee).
- Kneecap can be felt to one side, and then moves.
- May occur in both knees.

### ■ Torn Lateral Meniscus

Less common than a torn medial meniscus *(see page 314)*. Symptoms are the same, except pain is on the outer side of the knee.

### ■ Discoid Lateral Meniscus

An abnormally shaped lateral meniscus slips between the femur and tibia and the knee gives way. A "clunking" sensation is experienced. Eventually, surgery will be needed.

### ■ Chondromalacia Patella

Degeneration of the cartilage at the back of the kneecap. Young females are often affected.

- May have had recurrent patella dislocation *(see left)* or a knee injury.
- Intermittent pain at the front of the knee, with swelling.
- Occasional locking of the knee.
- Knee occasionally gives way.

### ■ Osteochondritis Dissecans (OCD)

The lower part of the articular surface of the femur (the condyle) may be damaged after injury. Part of the articular cartilage flakes off, creating a loose body. The individual is often in his or her late teens.

- Intermittent ache.
- Intermittent swelling.
- Intermittent locking.
- Knee feels unstable, as though it will collapse.

## "KNOCK-KNEES" AND BOWLEGS

In the great majority of cases, knock-knees (genu valgum) are a normal feature of childhood. As the child grows, the knees gradually begin to look normal, usually by the time the child is seven.

- Feet appear splayed.
- Knees press against each other. Doctors often watch the leg shape over a period of six months to see how the appearance changes.

May also, but rarely, be seen in rickets *(page 294)*, osteomalacia *(page 294)*, Paget's disease *(page 449)*, and Charcot joints *(page 287)*.

## BOWLEGS

Bowlegs are common in infants. If the child is lying flat, with feet together, and there is a gap of more than 2 inches (5 cm) between the bottom of the femurs at the knee, an x-ray may be a useful precaution to exclude rare causes, such as rickets and problems of bone development.

Bowing on one side only should always be investigated by a doctor.

## PAINFUL KNEE

*(See Inflamed or Aching Joints, page 284; Locked or Locking Knee, page 314; and Painful Hip, page 307)*

## SWOLLEN ANKLE

Can be one or both sides.

### PROBABLE

■ **Acute or Chronic Injury**

*(See Weak and Painful Ankle, page 319)*

■ **Isolated Dependent Edema**

The calf muscles play an important role in helping to prevent ankles from swelling. When these are not used regularly, the feet and lower legs tend to swell with fluid (edema). This commonly occurs when sitting for long periods on an airplane and is common in the elderly who sit for long periods of the day. This can be improved by keeping mobile and keeping the legs elevated on a stool if this is a problem. Support stockings can reduce this problem. It is important to consider other causes of ankle swelling, such as heart failure or the causes listed below.

## POSSIBLE

### ■ Varicose Veins

Enlarged leg veins caused by damage to valves in the veins. Blood fails to return to the heart at the proper rate and stays in the leg. This, in turn, can cause a swollen ankle and lower leg, often only on one side.

• Varicose veins visible.
• Increases during the day or after exercise.
• Discomfort rather than pain.
• Disappears when leg is elevated and at night.
• May be associated with ulcers, particularly inner ankle swelling.
• Long-standing varicose veins cause brownish discoloration of the lower legs and feet. Sometimes described as varicose eczema.

### ■ Deep Venous Thrombosis

Blockage of the veins by a thrombosis or blood clot deep inside the leg. May occur for no reason or after an operation or prolonged bed rest. More likely in the elderly, the obese, smokers, and those on the contraceptive pill or with known

cancer. If suspected, requires urgent medical attention.

• Sudden onset.
• Initially no pain, then mild/moderate discomfort.
• Calf and sometimes the thigh also swell.
• Pain may be aroused by pressure on the back of the calf.
• Swelling is persistent and does not decrease.

If a piece of the clot moves from the legs to the chest, there will be chest pain and shortness of breath *(see Pulmonary Embolus, page 227)*. If the clot in the lung is large enough, death can follow in rare cases.

### ■ Post-Phlebitic Limb

For months or years after a deep venous thrombosis *(see left),* the limb may remain swollen and tender. Ulcers may develop at the ankle, plus discoloration of the skin. It is best treated with support bandages.

### ■ Cellulitis

A bacterial infection of the soft tissues. It may be localized in part of the foot, ankle, or leg, or it may spread. Caused by a simple puncture wound or by bacteria gaining access through broken skin on the foot or ankle (for example, via an ulcer or athlete's foot).

- Redness, swelling.
- Can be very painful.
- Skin may be shiny, due to stretching.
- Malaise.
- Fever.

Rest and antibiotics will be needed to treat this condition.

## ■ Heart Failure

If the heart fails to pump as well as it should, the body retains fluid. At worst, this can cause congestion of the lungs, which makes breathing difficult. A mild case may cause ankle swelling.
- Swelling on both sides.
- Legs feel cool.
- May be intermittent.
- May be associated with shortness of breath.
- In bad (and untreated) heart failure, swelling may progress all the way up the leg.
- Associated symptoms can include distended neck veins and cyanosis.

The symptoms can be treated with diuretics and other heart medications.

## RARE

## ■ Anemia

Ankle swelling may be the first symptoms noted by an anemic individual. This is because anemia may precipitate mild heart failure *(see above)*.

## ■ Lymphedema

Obstruction to drainage of fluid via the lymphatic system. It may be primary (no underlying cause), the result of a congenital abnormality, or it can arise from absence of the lymphatic system in that limb. A congenital form known as Milroy's disease also exists. Secondary lymphedema can be caused by surgery on the lymph glands in the groin (for example, to control malignant disease), by obstruction to the lymph glands (by cancer, for example), or by parasite infection (filariasis).
- Firm swelling.
- Does not vary in size.
- Infection or inflammation may develop *(see Cellulitis, page 317)*.
- Skin becomes thickened.
- In severe cases, the skin may acquire the texture of elephant hide (elephantiasis).

## ■ Missed Fracture

Occasionally, a small fracture of an ankle bone may go unrecognized at the time of injury, resulting in long-term swelling, pain, and instability.

## ■ Nephritis

Damage (acute or chronic) to the kidneys caused by disease, not injury, may also cause swelling of the ankles. Other symptoms may include:

- Puffy face (particularly around the eyes).
- Protein and/or blood in urine.
- Malaise.
- Shortness of breath.
- Nausea and vomiting.

### ■ Hypoproteinemia

Low levels of a protein called albumin can cause ankle swelling. This can occur with kidney disease, liver disease, or due to conditions causing less protein to be absorbed from the gut.

## WEAK AND PAINFUL ANKLE

Almost always the result of injury, such as a twist (often caused by slipping on a step) or jumping from a height. The ankle joint is made up of three main bones: the tibia, the fibula, and the calcaneum. Each may be damaged. The injury also damages the soft tissues (ligaments, tendons, and muscles) surrounding the ankle. Pain originates from these structures. The ankle feels "weak" and likely to give way. The symptoms only relate to the affected ankle.

Ankle injuries should be regarded seriously, since even untreated sprains can cause long-term disability. Painkillers, rest, and physiotherapy are often appropriate treatments if there is no fracture.

### PROBABLE

#### ■ Acute Trauma (Sprain)

- Clear history of injury.
- Painful to stand or bear weight.
- Swelling, local or general.
- Swelling appears after a few hours or the following day.

- Ankle feels as though it will give way.

### ■ Achilles Tendonitis

The Achilles is the tendon that joins the calf muscle to the back of the foot. It often gets inflamed in those who walk a lot, particular in sedentary older athletes recently taking up sport again or after

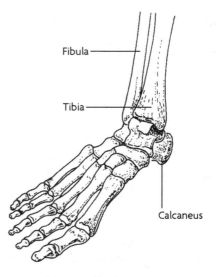

*Foot and Ankle Bones*

recent calf injuries. Overpronation *(see page 321)* predisposes to this. The tendon is often painful, worse on walking/ running, and can become swollen.

Treatment is with rest, stretching, painkillers, physiotherapy, and treatment of the overpronation, if present.

The Achilles tendon can rupture. Usually, this happens while walking or exercising, and no cause is found. It is more common in those who have had Achilles tendonitis and in those taking long-term steroid medication. Presents with sudden onset of severe pain on the back of calf/heel, associated with a snapping noise as if they have been shot. Often immediate difficulty with walking occurs and the area will swell.

## POSSIBLE

### ■ Chronic Injury

• Injury at some time in the past (weeks, months, or even years).

• Symptoms have persisted for some time.
• Feeling of weakness or "about to give way" predominates.
• Pain not so intense as with acute trauma.
• Swelling after exercise.

### ■ Fracture

In general, the symptoms are very obvious and confined to the affected bone.
• Pain severe.
• Unable to bear weight.
• Immediate swelling.
• Bruising within a few hours.

A break to the lower end of the tibia will cause symptoms on the inner aspect of the ankle; a break to the lower fibula on the outer aspect; and a break to the calcaneus (heel bone) on both sides and at the back over the heel.

## UNUSUALLY LARGE FEET

### PROBABLE

### ■ Normal Variant

Most individuals worried about their foot size have no physical abnormality or underlying disease. The size of their feet merely reflects the variation in size

that would be expected in any population. And many people worry that their feet are too small.

### RARE

### ■ Acromegaly

*(See page 281)*

## FLAT FEET

The term really means flattening of the arches. It can be a postural problem, in association with knock-knees and a short Achilles tendon. It may occasionally be congenital, in association with spina bifida, but this is rare. It may also develop as a result of general lack of fitness, say, after being bedridden. The muscles and tendons that support the arches become wasted and flat feet develop.

- Feet look flat—no arch on instep.
- Shoe soles wear badly.

- Pain is rare but may develop later in the foot and leg muscles.

Treatment is rarely needed, although instep supports may be of some help. Most commonly, no cause for flat feet is found and, unfortunately, specialists can offer little in the way of help.

The French believe in encouraging very young children to walk barefoot on different surfaces (sand on a beach is a favored one) to help develop the arches. Flat feet often run in families.

## PAINFUL ARCHES OF FEET

*(See Flat Feet, above)*

## OVERPRONATION

This condition is increasingly being recognized and is more common in those with flat feet. Pronation refers to the slight inward rolling motion the foot makes during normal walking or running. The foot and ankle rolls slightly inward to accommodate movement. Some people, however, overpronate and roll more than normal. With overpronation, the arch of the foot flattens and causes excessive stress and pressure on the soft tissues of the foot. Overpronation can cause problems with foot pain, plantar fasciitis, Achilles tendonitis, shin splints, as well as aggravating knee, hip, and back problems.

Overpronation can often be treated effectively by wearing appropriate insoles in your shoes (orthotics).

## PAINFUL FEET

### PROBABLE

#### ■ Verruca

Also called a plantar wart. Caused by a viral infection, hence outbreaks in schools and swimming pools.

• Local tenderness on sole of foot, where the verruca is pushed into the surface.

• The plantar wart is visible and there may be several, normally on the weight-bearing areas.

• May vanish spontaneously.

Most schools no longer undertake verruca checks. There is no need to prevent a child from swimming because he or she has a verruca. As this is a viral infection, the body will eventually overcome it, and the verruca will go.

Only painful or unusually troublesome verrucas need to be treated. An old, hard verruca is not very infectious. Over-the-counter treatments are best, but may take many weeks to work.

### POSSIBLE

#### ■ Plantar Fasciitis

Also called policeman's heel. An inflammation of the layers of membrane called fascia, which lie in the sole of the foot.

• Common after the age of forty.

• Local tenderness underneath the heel.

• Worse on walking/running.

• Often associated with overpronation *(see page 321).*

• Most common in occupations requiring individuals to be on their feet for long periods—a penalty for being a policeman or nurse.

Treatments may include a heel raise, foot stretches, physiotherapy, orthotics, and occasionally a steroid injection.

#### ■ Hallux Valgus

The big toe becomes deformed; most common in women beyond middle-age.

• Tip of big toe points to outer side of foot.

• Base of big toe is prominent.

• The end of the metatarsal bone points to the inner side of the foot.

• A lump of bone is therefore felt under the skin.

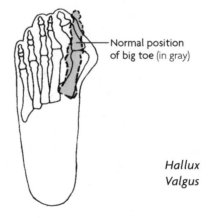

Normal position of big toe (in gray)

*Hallux Valgus*

- The overlying skin becomes thickened and painful (bunion) as does the bone on the sole of the foot.

May eventually need surgery.

### ■ Hallux Rigidus

Caused by osteoarthritis of the first metatarsophalangeal joint.
- Pain on movement.
- Bony outgrowths may develop, appearing as lumps around the joint.
- Thickened skin may develop on the upper surface of the joint.
- Range of movement of the joint is eventually limited by stiffness and pain.

### RARE

### ■ Claw Toes

*(See Pes Cavus, right)*

### ■ Morton's Metatarsalgia

Affects the middle-aged.
- Enlargement of the nerve (neuroma) between the heads of metatarsal bones.
- Local pain between two toes, worse if the foot is squeezed from side to side.
- Tingling of the two toes affected.

May require a cortisone injection or surgery.

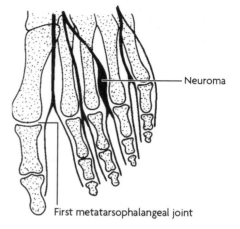

First metatarsophalangeal joint

*Morton's Metatarsalgia*

### ■ Pes Cavus

The opposite of a flat foot—the arch of the foot is raised. Often associated with curling of the toes (claw toes). Thought to be caused by imbalance of the muscles that support the arches, and most likely to be seen in those with neurological disease of the lower limb, such as poliomyelitis, spina bifida, or cerebral palsy.
- Curled or clawed toes.
- High arch on instep.
- Callosities eventually develop on pressure points.

## SWOLLEN FEET

*(See Swollen Ankle, page 316)*

## ULCERATED OR INFECTED FEET

### PROBABLE

■ **Ingrown Toenail**

The big toe is the one almost always affected. The side of the nail cuts into the toe tissue causing local infection (paronychia). Caused by ill-fitting shoes, cutting the nail too short, or picking at the nail.

• Outer side of nail most commonly affected.

• Often on both feet.

• Recurrent pain.

• Recurrent infection, with redness, swelling, and pus.

May ultimately need surgery to nail bed.

■ **Athlete's Foot**

*(See Itching or Numbness of the Fingers and Toes, page 329)*

■ **Verruca**

*(See page 322)*

### POSSIBLE

*(See Diabetic Neuropathy, page 325, and Peripheral Vascular Disease, page 326)*

### RARE

*(See Alcoholic Neuropathy, page 326; Multiple Sclerosis, page 326; Raynaud's Disease, page 304; Frostbite, page 329; Syphilis, page 379)*

■ **Buerger's disease**

Buerger's disease is a painful ulceration caused by obliteration of blood vessels in the limbs; particularly in young male smokers of Eastern European origin.

## CORNS ON THE FEET

*(See page 261)*

## FINGERS AND TOES

Collected here is a group of symptoms that can particularly affect the fingers and toes (but also the arms and legs), parts of the body at the outer reaches of the blood's circulation. The nose and ears are similarly placed, and certain symptoms such as numbness, itching, or discoloration (for example, chilblains) can affect them just as they do the fingers and toes.

## NUMB FINGERS AND TOES

The onset of numbness in any part of the body should be taken seriously. It is not a common symptom in isolation and may be an accompaniment to underlying disease. Its main danger is that the "warning sign" of pain is not present, therefore skin damage, skin breakdown, and ulcers may develop because the individual cannot feel the discomfort. This is particularly common over pressure points (heel, medial and lateral malleolus, sole of the foot).

Numbness of fingers and toes accompanied by back pain is a serious symptom and should be reported to your doctor immediately. It can be a sign of direct pressure applied to a nerve by a disc or from a bone injury.

### POSSIBLE

■ **Cervical Spondylosis**

*(See page 133)*

■ **Diabetic Neuropathy**

A long-standing complication of diabetes, neuropathy means disease of the nerves. If you have diabetes, you may notice:

• Some tingling and pain (lower limbs).
• Stocking anesthesia (numbness over a leg up to the knee—the area covered by a stocking).

• Some muscle wasting and weakness.
• Painless ulceration over pressure points on feet.
• Cellulitis *(see page 317)* associated with ulcers.

Occasionally, only one nerve may be affected, causing numbness, muscle wasting, and weakness in one limb.

Other neurological symptoms of diabetes may be:
• Radiculitis—localized scalding and painful sensory changes.
• Irregular shape to pupils.
• Impotence.
• Failure of orgasm.
• Nocturnal diarrhea.
• Feeling of dizziness on standing or changing position (postural hypotension).
• Loss of sweating in lower limbs.

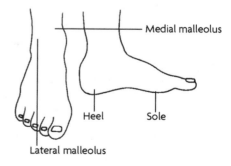

*Pressure Points of the Feet*

## Multiple Sclerosis

Formerly known as disseminated sclerosis. Nervous tissue in the central nervous system is affected. Features may include:
• Numbness and tingling in hands or feet (allowing ulcers to develop if pressure points are not treated carefully).
• Visual disturbances (poor vision, double vision).
• Weakness in limbs.
• Loss of postural sense.
• Vertigo.
• Bladder disturbance.
• Tremor.
• Speech disturbance.
• Swallowing difficulties.

May take several years to be diagnosed as it remits and relapses. The outlook is mixed: some unfortunate cases suffer, eventually, from paralysis and disability; in many, symptoms remain mild and many can be helped with medication.

## Peripheral Vascular Disease

As individuals age, the arteries begin to "fur up" with fatty and calcified deposits; a normal part of the aging process known as atherosclerosis. In certain individuals, particularly smokers and those with a genetic disposition, the arteries fur up more extensively and at a younger age. Progressive atherosclerosis will result particularly in reduction of blood supply to the legs, with:

• Cold limbs (predominantly the legs).
• Legs may appear pale if lifted in the air.
• Cramp-like pain, particularly in the calf muscles, on walking any distance (intermittent claudication).
• Pain settles when walking stops.
• Occasionally, sensory changes, including numbness.
• Pulse may not be felt in the usual places.

## Alcoholic Neuropathy

Most chronic alcoholics have damaged nerves, leading to:
• Numbness in the lower limbs; ulcers may develop.
• Tingling in the lower limbs.
• Burning in the lower limbs (especially in the feet).
• Weakness of the lower limbs.
• Wasting of the muscles of the lower limbs.

Walking will be affected. The problems can be reversed by giving up alcohol, eating a proper diet, and taking B vitamin supplements.

## RARE

## Guillain-Barré Syndrome

Also known as acute inflammatory polyneuropathy. An illness affecting the peripheral nervous system. It can occur at any age, often one to three weeks after an acute viral or bacterial (such as food poisoning) infection.

- Initially, tingling in the hands and feet.
- Weakness develops in the arms and legs and, ultimately, in severe cases, the muscles controlling the lungs. Sometimes, the individual needs artificial ventilation.
- Loss of sensation may be severe or minimal.
- Facial weakness is a possibility.

Gradual improvement takes place over weeks or months. Most people make a full recovery.

■ **Frostbite**

*(See page 329)*

■ **Leprosy**

Essentially a disease of underdeveloped countries, leprosy is acquired by close contact with an infected individual over a prolonged period. Under these circumstances, the diagnosis will probably be obvious. One of the early signs is numbness and tingling in the ends of the arms and legs. There are many other symptoms.

## COLD FINGERS AND TOES

*(See Feeling the Cold, page 495)*

## ALTERED SENSATION IN THE FINGERS AND TOES

Any disease or injury of a nerve can cause altered sensation in the area of the skin supplied by that nerve. It can take many forms, from tingling, through pins and needles and burning, to complete absence of sensation if the nerve is destroyed.

### PROBABLE

■ **Disease or Injury of a Nerve or Nerves**

Perhaps the most common form is pres-sure neuropathy or nerve palsy. This can occur if you fall asleep in an awkward position. Nerves usually affected are the ulnar (at the elbow), the radial (at the upper arm), and the peroneal nerve (by the knee). Common to all these palsies are:

- On waking, initial numbness in the area served by the nerve.
- Initial loss of function of the affected part.
- Within a few minutes, sensation returns.

• At first, this is a mild tingling, but it progresses to painful pins and needles.

• After several more minutes, or longer, the sensations settle and full function returns.

Occasionally, if the local pressure on the nerve has been unduly prolonged, full function may take weeks to return.

■ **Cervical Spondylosis**

*(See page 133)*

■ **Carpal Tunnel Syndrome**

*(See page 328)*

**POSSIBLE**

■ **Diabetic Neuropathy**

*(See page 325)*

■ **Multiple Sclerosis**

*(See page 326)*

■ **Peripheral Vascular Disease**

*(See page 326)*

■ **Alcoholic Neuropathy**

*(See page 326)*

**RARE**

■ **Subacute Combined Degeneration of the Spinal Cord (SACD)**

SACD is a result of vitamin $B_{12}$ deficiency caused by a number of factors, the most significant being pernicious anemia. Other causes include poor diet, extreme vegetarianism, and malabsorption. Damage is done to parts of the white matter in the spinal cord, leading to:

• Pins and needles (paresthesia) in the feet (hands and arms are rarely affected).

• Inability to feel vibration and to sense position, affecting legs and body.

• Weakness in the legs; muscle wasting.

• Unsteady gait.

Other symptoms of the disorder causing SACD may also be present.

■ **Guillain-Barré Syndrome**

*(See page 326)*

■ **Frostbite**

*(See page 329)*

■ **Leprosy**

*(See page 327)*

## TINGLING FINGERS AND TOES

*(See Altered Sensation in the Fingers and Toes, page 327)*

# ITCHING OR NUMBNESS OF THE FINGERS AND TOES

In an otherwise normal individual.

## ■ Athlete's Foot

A fungal infection of the feet.
- Irritation between the toes.
- Burning and itching between the toes.
- Some redness, as a result of inflammation.
- Crusting and further infection can take place.
- Smelly feet.
- Cracking of skin, particularly between the toes.

## ■ Chilblains

Damage to blood vessels in the skin caused by exposure to cold.
- Local pain in fingers or toes.
- Itching and burning at first.

    Followed by:
- Swelling.
- Local discoloration (reddish/purple) at the site of pain.
- Blister formation.

Treated best by slow rewarming.

## POSSIBLE

## ■ Dermatitis

Acute dermatitis (inflammation of the skin) may be caused by an allergy to chemicals (for instance, deodorant or laundry detergent). So, dermatitis can be caused by socks washed in a detergent to which an individual is allergic.
- Irritation.
- Burning.
- Inflammation, including weeping and crusting skin.
- Symptoms confined to areas that come in contact with the source of the allergy.

## RARE

## ■ Frostbite

In prolonged exposure to below-freezing temperatures, all extremities are at risk, including ears, nose, toes, and fingers. People with poor circulation, typically the elderly, or those who lose heat fastest (for instance, children), are most at risk.
- Initial pain and tingling in affected part.
- May become numb (pain free)—a bad sign.
- Discoloration: may at first be reddish purple, but when the affected part becomes white, then the frostbite is serious.
- If untreated, the frostbitten areas will develop gangrene—death of tissue—because blood is no longer supplied. Ulcers develop and rapidly become infected.

Urgent medical help is needed to supervise the rewarming of the affected part and to minimize the final damage.

# THE REPRODUCTIVE
# AND SEXUAL ORGANS

This chapter is divided into symptoms in women, symptoms in men, symptoms common to both and related to sexual relations, and miscellaneous problems.

*Female and Male Reproductive Organs*

# SYMPTOMS IN WOMEN

## MENSTRUATION

During the monthly cycle, the lining of the womb thickens and prepares to accept a fertilized egg. If conception does not take place, the lining breaks down and is shed—this is the menstrual discharge. This complex process involves hormones from the brain, the ovaries, and the egg, all directed toward a common goal: a successful pregnancy. It is aptly said that menstruation is the womb crying for want of a pregnancy.

Problem-free menstruation depends on a healthy balance between mind and body—it is more likely to be upset by psychological factors than most other bodily functions. The length, frequency, and heaviness of menstruation vary from person to person and from month to month, and this is not necessarily a symptom of abnormality. Sudden changes are a different matter and should be heeded.

## PREMENSTRUAL TENSION

Feelings of tension and stress are just two from an array of physical and mental changes that appear up to two weeks before menstruation and go on after bleeding begins. Among the many possible symptoms, the most common are:
- Feeling bloated.
- Irritability and tension.
- Tiredness.
- Headache.
- Tender breasts.
- Depression.

No one reason satisfactorily explains the symptom, nor is there any agreed to or predictably useful treatment. Possibilities include vitamin $B_6$, evening primrose oil, herbal treatments, and alternative or complementary therapies. Hormonal preparations, such as the contraceptive pill, are also used. Other drugs, such as diuretics, antidepressants (selective serotonin-reuptake inhibitors or SSRIs), or tranquilizers, have also been tried with varying degrees of benefit. The use of symptom diaries, where women record their feelings, can identify other gynecological symptoms or psychiatric symptoms, which may in turn lead to specific treatments or cures. Some women find that simply knowing that they have a real condition, albeit one that medicine is relatively ignorant about, enables them and their families to adjust to their symptoms.

## PAINFUL PERIODS

Lucky is the woman who has no pain with her periods. Otherwise, levels of pain vary widely, as does the amount of pain that different women can tolerate. Pain can certainly be regarded as abnormal when time is regularly lost from work or when periods are accompanied by debilitating cramps, faintness, and vomiting. In older women, these symptoms should be investigated, particularly if previously acceptable periods become intolerable and are accompanied by pain on intercourse or heavy bleeding.

### PROBABLE

#### ■ Unknown Origin

• Painful periods are common in young women for the first few years of menstruation, possibly related to release of prostaglandin hormones and muscle contraction in the wall of the womb.
• Typically, the pain begins twelve to twenty-four hours before bleeding and continues for the first one or two days.
• Pain is usually felt in the lower abdomen, tops of legs, and lower back.

Anti-inflammatory drugs that counteract the effects of prostaglandins (ibuprofen, aspirin, mefenamic acid) may help. The contraceptive pill is also useful and usually lightens and shortens the periods.

### POSSIBLE

#### ■ Endometriosis

A condition where tissue identical to the lining of the womb is found outside its normal location—commonly in the ovaries, fallopian tubes, and pelvis—and "bleeds" in synchrony with menstruation.
• Most common in women in their twenties and thirties.
• Pain often lasts throughout the period, but can occur before or after.
• Often, pain deep in the pelvis on intercourse.
• Sometimes causes difficulties with fertility.

Treated with hormones (contraceptive pill) or other drugs that stop the periods. Surgery is sometimes required to destroy or remove endometrial tissue.

#### ■ Pelvic Inflammatory Disease

Usually sexually acquired, for example, *Chlamydia* infection. Can follow intrauterine coil use, termination of pregnancy, or childbirth.
• Accompanied by pain deep in the pelvis on intercourse.
• Sometimes with vaginal discharge or other symptoms of sexually transmitted diseases (STDs).
• Periods may be irregular.

• Risk of infertility and ectopic pregnancy.

Treatment is with antibiotics; it is essential to treat sexual partner and contacts to prevent reinfection.

## ■ Fibroids

A condition where benign growth of the muscle wall of the womb occurs. Most commonest in ages thirty-five to fifty, especially in non-Caucasian ethnic groups.

• Associated with heavy periods and sometimes fertility problems.
• Sometimes swelling or a lump is felt in the lower abdomen.
• Can become suddenly painful due to twisting or interruption of blood supply.

Many women need no treatment as fibroids regress after menopause. Alternatively, they can be treated with hormones that induce a menopausal state. Occasionally, treated by surgery.

## HEAVY PERIODS

The amount of blood lost during a period is very variable, but as a rule of thumb heavy periods are defined by blood loss that interferes with life. Loss of blood clots or flooding is a common feature, as are periods lasting longer than a week or accompanied by anemia (felt as tiredness or observed as pallor in the complexion).

### PROBABLE

## ■ Dysfunctional Bleeding

This refers to an abnormal pattern of bleeding in the absence of any structural abnormality in the reproductive organs. It is common at the beginning and end of reproductive life and may be associated with failure to ovulate.

May respond to hormone treatment or may resolve with time as a teenager or with menopause later.

### POSSIBLE

## ■ Fibroids

*(See above)*

## ■ Pregnancy and Miscarriage

Sudden or severe bleeding in any woman of childbearing age can relate to pregnancy or its complications. Twenty to forty percent of all pregnancies miscarry, mostly in the first twelve weeks. Heavy bleeding or a "late" period may be a miscarriage.

• Pregnancy may or may not be accompanied by other symptoms, such as nausea, vomiting, missed periods, and breast tenderness.

• Consider the possibility of contraceptive failure.

• Do a pregnancy test—urine, ultrasound scan, or (rarely) a blood test. A negative test may become positive if it is repeated after an interval.

### ■ Endometriosis

*(See page 333)*

### ■ Pelvic Inflammatory Disease

*(See page 333)*

## RARE

### ■ Thyroid Disease

Underactive glands are associated with heavy periods.

### ■ Abnormal Blood Clotting

Heavy menstrual flow may result from any condition that makes the blood clot less well than it should. Also, look for:

• Easy bruising.

• Gums that bleed easily.

• Pallor.

• Enlarged lymph glands.

• Blood in urine, vomit, or from bowels.

### ■ Tumors of the Cervix and Womb

Though heavy periods are a possible symptom, these diseases are more likely to cause:

• Irregular bleeding or post-coital bleeding.

• Unusual discharge.

• Postmenopausal bleeding.

Routine investigation of heavy periods will discover these tumors.

## IRREGULAR PERIODS

Irregular periods are common at the beginning and end of a woman's reproductive life. Other causes of irregular periods need to be distinguished from bleeding between periods (inter-menstrual bleeding), bleeding after intercourse (post-coital bleeding), and bleeding after menopause (postmenopausal bleeding), which are all potentially serious symptoms. It is best to report irregular bleeding to a doctor to help distinguish whether the cause is important. If tests are suggested, these might include an ultrasound scan, hysteroscopy (looking into the womb with an endoscope), colposcopy (examining the cervix with a microscope), or endometrial biopsy (sampling the lining of the womb).

Irregular periods may also be infrequent or become absent, so check the section on Absent or Infrequent Periods *(see page 336).*

## PROBABLE

■ **Dysfunctional Bleeding**

*(See page 334)*

■ **Breakthrough Bleeding on the Contraceptive Pill**

*(See page 340)*

■ **Hormone Replacement Therapy**

May need investigation to exclude other gynecological causes. May be used as treatment for irregular periods before menopause.

## POSSIBLE

■ **Pelvic Inflammatory Disease**

*(See page 333)*

■ **Polyps of the Cervix or Womb**

*(See page 340)*

■ **Cervical Erosion**

*(See page 340)*

■ **Atrophic Vaginitis**

*(See page 342)*

## RARE

■ **Cancer Occurring Anywhere in the Female Sexual Organs**

While cancer is rare, it is serious. Early diagnosis improves outlook and can offer a complete cure. Routine investigation of irregular bleeding should discover this.

## ABSENT OR INFREQUENT PERIODS

This section concerns women who have had previously normal periods. In the case of periods that have never started, see Delay in Beginning Menstruation *(page 339)*. In young women, stress is so often the reason for absent or infrequent periods that further investigation is usually unnecessary, except for reassurance or to exclude pregnancy. Irregularities in women in their late thirties or early forties are likely to have a physical or hormonal cause. In particular, women with infrequent periods should be examined to make quite sure that normal but infrequent periods are just that and are not in fact occasional, abnormal episodes of bleeding from the womb or cervix. Bleeding out of the blue, without your usual premenstrual symptoms, should definitely be investigated. Absent or infrequent periods may first be noticed as irregular periods so it is advisable to cross-check with that section *(see Irregular Periods, page 335)*.

## PROBABLE

### ■ Pregnancy

It is a useful and proven medical rule of thumb that, if in doubt, any woman of child-bearing age with absent periods should have a pregnancy test if intercourse has taken place. After any missed period, you should be on the lookout for other symptoms of pregnancy, such as:

• Morning sickness.
• Tender breasts.
• Lethargy.
• Weight gain.
• Passing urine more frequently than usual.
• Appetite changes.

Have a pregnancy test if you are uncertain.

### ■ Stress

An extremely common reason, especially in young women. Stress is caused not just by obvious emotional turmoil but by major changes in lifestyle, such as changes of job, travel, or illness. Even what appears to be "everyday stress," such as preparing for school exams, can be sufficient to stop periods. In conditions of obvious tension, the absence of periods for two or three months should not be a worry, as long as pregnancy is excluded.

Investigations are rarely needed, unless symptoms persist for more than six months.

### ■ Exercise

Commonly seen in athletes or fitness fanatics. Associated with osteoporosis in the long term.

### ■ Major Weight Change

Both excessive weight gain and dieting leading to weight loss will disrupt periods, because they affect some brain centers. The most extreme form is anorexia nervosa: typically, there is a distorted body image, self-induced vomiting, laxative abuse, and excessive exercising, all resulting in significant weight loss.

### ■ Breastfeeding

Periods can stop or become scanty during breastfeeding, since breastfeeding hormones delay the normal return of the menstrual cycle. It is, however, possible to become pregnant while breastfeeding, for ovulation may still occur.

## POSSIBLE

### ■ Menopause

The most common age of menopause is fifty-one. Premature menopause due to ovarian failure can happen from the age of thirty.

• Often preceded by irregular periods.
• Sometimes, there is a family history of early menopause.

### ■ Raised Prolactin

Prolactin is a hormone that normally

contributes to the production of breast milk.

- Absent periods, plus a milky discharge from the breasts, suggest an excess of prolactin. Can be caused by a tumor in the pituitary gland at the base of the brain.
- Some drugs can cause it: major tranquilizers used to treat mental illness or anti-emetics.

Blood tests and magnetic resonance imaging (MRI) of the pituitary gland help with diagnosis. Can be treated by medication or sometimes surgery.

## ■ Polycystic Ovary Syndrome

- Infrequent or absent periods.
- Excessive body hair.
- Acne.
- Weight is critical; more common and severe in the overweight, but can affect women of normal weight.
- Associated with infertility, diabetes, and increased risk of heart disease.

Diagnosed with blood tests and ultrasound scanning. Treated with weight reduction, drugs that modify hormone levels, and antidiabetic drugs. Rarely, surgery may be used.

## ■ Post-Pill Absent Periods

- Most common in women whose periods were irregular before they began to take oral contraception.

- Otherwise sound health.
- Periods return after three to six months.

If you have not had a period for more than six months after you stop taking the pill, seek professional advice.

## ■ Serious General Disease

The strain of another serious physical illness, such as cancer, or a major psychiatric illness or drug addiction may well cause absent or infrequent periods. Other symptoms of serious illness might include:

- Weight loss.
- Tiredness.
- Chronic cough.
- Fever, diarrhea.

Periods should return after recovery.

## RARE

## ■ Thyroid Disease

Overexcitability or lethargy, combined with disturbed periods, may suggest an overactive or underactive thyroid gland.

## ■ Adrenal Disease

A possibility if absent periods are accompanied by:

- Hairiness.
- Weight gain.
- Weakness.

## DELAY IN BEGINNING MENSTRUATION

By the age of sixteen, most Western girls are menstruating, and it is reasonable to be concerned about those who are not.

### PROBABLE

#### ■ Normal but Delayed

This is likely if there is:

- Normal development of breasts and pubic hair (including in armpits).
- Normal growth.
- Family history of menstruation starting late.

In addition, hormone tests would be normal. In these circumstances, it is a matter of "wait and see," sometimes using hormones to kick-start the system.

### POSSIBLE

#### ■ Hormone Disorders

Suggested if the girl has the following symptoms:

- Short stature.
- Poor development of breasts.
- Either an absence or an excess of body hair.
- Obesity.
- Very severe acne.

Investigation of the girl's hormones and treatment with hormones may be needed.

#### ■ Anorexia Nervosa

*(See page 437)*

### RARE

#### ■ Obstruction to Menstrual Flow

A membrane across the vagina can block the discharge of normal menstrual blood. There is normal sexual development and recurrent lower abdominal pain at period time.

- A bulge may protrude from the vagina, containing menstrual blood.

Treatment is simply the removal of the membrane.

#### ■ Genetic Disorders or Congenital Malformation

There are a wide range of disorders that can lead to malformation of the womb, ovaries, and vagina, or even a complete absence of these organs. There are no characteristic symptoms; it is a matter of specialist assessment, after all other causes have been excluded.

## BLEEDING BETWEEN PERIODS OR AFTER INTERCOURSE

The older the woman, the greater is the significance of this symptom. Causes are frequently obvious to the trained eye—you should always get your doctor's advice with this pattern of abnormal bleeding. Check that the cause is not blood in your partner's semen.

### PROBABLE

#### ■ Breakthrough Bleeding on the Pill

• Often when commencing the pill or for the first few cycles.

• Remainder of the cycle is normal.

• Scanty, painless show of blood for a day or two.

• Often occurs about the same time each month, usually toward the end of the pill packet.

If this appears for more than a few months, a change of pill may be advised. This bleeding does not, however, mean that the pill is not working. Don't stop taking the pill because of the bleeding; finish the packet normally.

#### ■ Erosion of the Cervix

A harmless and treatable alteration of the surface of the cervix sometimes associated with pregnancy or contraceptive pill use.

• Heavy, clear vaginal discharge.

• Bleeding after intercourse.

• Brief, irregular blood spotting between periods. Blood appears on underclothing and toilet paper unexpectedly.

Treatment involves cauterizing that part of the cervix, an outpatient procedure.

#### ■ Hormone Imbalance

Caused by changes in natural hormone levels during the cycle. A possibility in young women.

• Regular, scanty, intermenstrual bleeding.

• Periods are otherwise normal.

The diagnosis is made only after the other possibilities have been ruled out.

#### ■ Ovulation Bleeding (Mittelschmerz)

Occurs at the time of ovulation, midway between periods when an egg is released from the ovary.

• Sometimes accompanied by lower abdominal pain.

• Sometimes followed by a change in the nature of vaginal discharge.

• Doesn't occur when on the combined contraceptive pill.

### POSSIBLE

#### ■ Polyp of the Cervix

A small fleshy outgrowth from the cervix, which causes no other symptoms, and which may be visible to a doctor during a gynecological examination. Unusual in young women.

Polyps usually need to be removed, though they are rarely cancerous.

## ■ Inflammation of the Vagina

May be due to infection. In postmenopausal women, when vaginal skin becomes thin and raw, and is often accompanied by:

- Dryness of the vagina.
- Itch.
- Sometimes, a thin, watery, blood-tinged discharge.

Treatment aims to eradicate the infection and put female hormones back into the walls of the vagina, using estrogen cream or hormone replacement therapy (HRT).

## ■ Cancer of the Cervix

Cervical cancer is one form of cancer that should be largely preventable by having regular cervical cytology (Pap smear) tests. There is also an effective vaccine, which can be given to girls before they become sexually active.

It is associated with infection by the human papilloma virus types 16, 18, and 33. More common in women with many sexual partners; those who have sex at a young age; those who have many children; or those with HIV or other sexually transmitted diseases (STDs).

There is a precancerous stage (cervical intraepithelial neoplasia or CIN), which has no symptoms but can be detected by having regular cervical cytology tests—at least every three years. If tests are abnormal, women are advised to have a more detailed examination of the cervix with a microscope (coloscopy). If needed, simple outpatient treatment may be given during colposcopy to destroy the abnormal cells. Sometimes, the precancerous stage reverts to normal without treatment.

Cervical cancer in its early stages may have no symptoms, but later may present with:

- Bleeding after intercourse or bleeding between periods.
- Unusual vaginal discharge.
- In advanced cases, there may be pain in the pelvis or pain from secondary spread to adjacent structures or other parts of the body.

Early treatment is simpler and can be curative, while more advanced disease carries a worse outlook and requires more extensive intervention.

## ■ Cancer of the Womb

*(See page 342)*

## Rare

## ■ Urethral Caruncle

*(See page 342)*

## BLEEDING AFTER MENOPAUSE

Bleeding that occurs more than a year after periods have apparently finished is a very important symptom that should not be ignored, even if it happens only once or if the blood looks pink rather than the usual full red. Always seek medical advice if this occurs. There can be confusion with bleeding in urine or from the anus or bowel, so be prepared for your doctor to examine those regions, too.

### PROBABLE

■ **Atrophic Vaginitis**

Thinning of the vaginal lining associated with menopause.

• Associated with dryness of the vagina, soreness, and pain with intercourse.

• Pinkish discharge is more common than outright bleeding.

Responds to estrogen creams or hormone replacement therapy (HRT).

■ **Polyp of the Cervix**

*(See page 340)*

### POSSIBLE

■ **Cancer of the Womb**

About 10 to 20 percent of women with bleeding after menopause will have cancer of the lining of the womb (endometrium).

• Pain is a sign of advanced disease and so the usual first symptom is painless bleeding.

Diagnosis is confirmed by sampling the endometrium—dilation and curettage (D&C)—usually as an outpatient or sometimes under anesthetic. Treatment is usually by hysterectomy and radiotherapy. If it is caught early, the outlook is positive, but in advanced disease the prognosis is poor, underlining the need to report postmenopausal bleeding as soon as possible.

■ **Cancer of the Cervix**

*(See page 341)*

### RARE

■ **Urethral Caruncle**

This occurs when the outlet from the bladder, the urethra, lying just in front of the vagina, becomes swollen and inflamed.

• The swollen area is painful to the touch.

• Pain when passing urine.

• Pain on intercourse.

The treatment is usually surgical.

## BLEEDING FROM THE VAGINA

This topic refers to bleeding that is un-expected. Menstrual problems are dealt with under specific headings.

### PROBABLE

■ **Miscarriage**

Pregnancy is a possibility for any woman of childbearing years who experiences unusual vaginal bleeding. There is often great difficulty in deciding between a miscarriage and an ectopic pregnancy *(see below)*. Miscarriages up to the twelfth week after conception are common, occurring in up to 20 to 40 percent of pregnancies. They are emotionally traumatic. The chances are increased in the presence of:

- A missed period.
- Tender breasts, morning sickness.
- Lower abdominal pain.

■ **Ectopic Pregnancy**

Occurs if a fertilized egg implants not within the womb but somewhere else, usually inside the fallopian tube. Risk factors include a history of pelvic inflammatory disease, endometriosis, or use of the contraceptive coil (intrauterine device) or progesterone-only contraceptive pill. Typical symptoms include:

- Usually one or two missed periods.
- Abdominal pain, which may be severe.

- Vaginal bleeding; sometimes the bleeding is internal and, if heavy, may cause may cause faintness or shoulder tip pain.

This is a life-threatening emergency. Treatment is usually surgical, with removal of the pregnancy and sometimes the tube. Occasionally, an early ectopic pregnancy is treated with a drug called methotrexate or by observation without the need for an operation. Later, fertility can be affected.

### POSSIBLE

■ **Complications Late in Pregnancy**

In an established pregnancy, bleeding suggests a possible abnormality of the placenta. Painless bleeding happens if the placenta is lying too low in the womb (placenta previa). Painful bleeding, especially after twenty-six weeks, may mean that part of the placenta has detached from the womb (abruption). In either case, a full and urgent obstetric assessment is essential.

■ **Disease of the Cervix**

A possibility if the symptoms include any of the following, each of which is dealt with under specific headings:

- Heavy vaginal discharge.
- Irregular bleeding.
- Bleeding after intercourse.

## ■ Disease of the Womb

This is the likeliest cause of vaginal bleeding after menopause, an extremely important symptom.

## ■ Atrophic Vaginitis

*(See page 342)*

## RARE

## ■ Abnormal Blood Clotting

*(See page 335)*

## DISCHARGE FROM THE VAGINA

Normal discharge from the vagina is clear or slightly yellow. It varies in volume and consistency during the monthly cycle, reaching a peak at the time of ovulation, which is roughly mid-cycle. Vaginal discharge is also increased by sexual activity and ejaculation of semen into the vagina during intercourse. If you have a contraceptive coil (intrauterine device) fitted, the amount of discharge may increase. Any change in the amount, consistency, or smell of the discharge from what you would normally expect can be considered abnormal.

## PROBABLE

## ■ Thrush

Caused by a yeast infection, usually *Candida albicans,* which commonly live in small numbers around the genital area. Symptoms occur when the yeasts multiply and inflame the skin. Usually not sexually transmitted and a male partner does not need treatment unless sympto-

matic himself. Risk factors include recent antibiotic use and diabetes. Typical symptoms include:

- Vaginal itching.
- White discharge (sometimes "curd-like").
- Redness or soreness in the vulva and vagina.

Can be self-treated with pessaries, creams, or tablets that kill the yeasts. Consider the possibility of other sexually transmitted infections, especially if the symptoms do not resolve with treatment.

## ■ Bacterial Vaginosis

Caused by an imbalance of the normal bacteria in the vagina, with an overgrowth of anaerobic types, typically *Gardnerella vaginalis.* Not thought to be sexually transmitted, so partners do not need to be treated routinely.

- Produces a smell sometimes described as fishy or cheese-like.

Treated with oral antibiotics—metronidazole or clindamycin cream in the vagina. Consider the possibility other sexually transmitted infections, especially if the symptoms do not resolve with treatment.

## POSSIBLE

### ■ Atrophic Vaginitis

*(See page 342)*

### ■ Erosion of the Cervix

*(See page 340)*

### ■ Polyp of Cervix or Womb

*(See page 340)*

### ■ Vaginal Infections and Other Sexually Transmitted Infections (STIs)

*Chlamydia* and rarely *Trichomonas* or gonorrhea.

You need specialist assessment and contact tracing and treatment. Always seek medical advice if you suspect STIs.

### ■ Pelvic Inflammatory Disease

*(See page 333)*

### ■ Foreign Body

Probably the most common is a tampon lodged deep inside the vagina. Young children sometimes push small things inside themselves. Occasionally, condoms slip off and are retained in the vagina.

• Yellow or green discharge, increasingly heavy.
• Very smelly.
• Possible fever.

Tampons and the like are easily removed; children may need a specialist's help.

## RARE

### ■ Tumor

Growths in and around the vagina may be a rare cause of a persistent discharge, but should be visible on gynecological inspection. Occasionally, tumors of the womb, cervix, and ovaries can present with a discharge.

### ■ Sexual Abuse

This upsetting possibility needs to be considered for girls who have recurrent or unusual vaginal discharges. Signs of sexual interference might include:

• Tears, bruising around the vagina or back passage.
• Disturbed behavior.

This highly charged topic needs the utmost care, both to avoid false conclusions and yet to uncover hidden misery. If suspected, the case should be placed in professional hands.

## VAGINAL PROTRUSION AND SWELLING OF THE VULVA

### PROBABLE

#### ■ Prolapse of the Womb

Occurs typically in women who have had children or after menopause and is due to weakening of the muscles in the pelvis and around the vagina.

- The cervix is felt as a firm lump, coming down into the vagina.
- Worse on coughing, straining.
- Lessens on lying flat or relaxing.

Surgical repair is possible.

### POSSIBLE

#### ■ Prolapse of the Bladder or Rectum

Bladder prolapse is felt in the front of the vagina.

- Usually causes leakage of urine on coughing, laughing.

Rectal prolapse is felt at the back of the vagina.

- Surgical repair is possible.

#### ■ Vulval Varicosities

Seen in pregnancy, where the veins and tissues in the vulva become engorged with blood. Usually resolves after childbirth.

#### ■ Labial Cysts, Bartholin's Cyst

- Presents as a swelling on the vaginal lips, usually on one side only.
- Commonly gets infected and may be painful or discharge pus.

May need antibiotic or surgical treatment.

#### ■ Genital Warts

*(See Warts, page 378)*

### RARE

#### ■ Tumor

The growth could arise from the womb or the walls of the vagina or adjacent organs. Examination will pinpoint this.

## VAGINAL ODOR

### PROBABLE

#### ■ Normal

Some vaginal odor is unavoidable and is probably a sexual cue.

### POSSIBLE

#### ■ Infection

- Suggested by odors which are very smelly, or fishy.
- Accompanied by itch and discharge.

*(See Discharge from the Vagina, page 344, for causes)*

■ **Foreign Body**

*(See page 345)*

■ **Psychological**

• An odor is apparent to you but your partner or doctor smell nothing unusual.

• A worry that the odor is obvious to others or feeling the need to wash or clean the genital area too frequently.

A sympathetic ear may allow worries to be expressed, typically about the fear of sexually transmitted infections or cancer.

**RARE**

■ **Cancer**

Cancer of the cervix, womb, or even the bowel may cause:

• A persistent, foul-smelling vaginal discharge, bleeding, and pain.

Things should not reach this stage unless warning symptoms have been neglected, such as unusual vaginal bleeding, discharges, and changes of bowel habit.

## VAGINAL PAIN

The causes overlap with those symptoms described under Adverse Sexual Experiences *(see page 373)*.

**PROBABLE**

■ **Infections**

*(See Discharge from the Vagina, page 344, for causes)*

■ **Atrophic Vaginitis**

*(See page 342)*

**POSSIBLE**

■ **Vaginismus**

Spasm of the muscles around the vagina, which contract so tightly that intercourse is difficult or impossible.

Treatment involves psychological techniques to improve relaxation and sexual confidence.

**RARE**

■ **Cancer**

Cancer growing within the vagina can cause pain, but it is highly unlikely to be an early or sole symptom. Previously, there is likely to have been:

• Bleeding after intercourse, between periods, or after menopause.

• Usually, there will be discharge, which may be bloodstained.

## VULVAL ITCH

### PROBABLE

#### ■ Infection

- Rapid onset of intense itch.
- White or colored discharge.

Most commonly due to thrush *(see page 344).*

### POSSIBLE

#### ■ Allergy

The sensitive skin in and around the vagina may itch due to allergy to over-vigorous washing, bubble baths, vaginal deodorants, or condoms. Diagnosis is arrived at by cutting out all possible irritants and then testing each one individually. Special low-allergy condoms are available.

#### ■ Threadworms/Crab Lice

Threadworms are extremely common, particularly in childhood. Itching is intense, especially at night, and usually felt in and around the anus.

Crab lice are sexually transmitted and may be visible on close inspection in the pubic area. Consider the possibility of other sexually transmitted infections if you find them.

Treatment of both is straightforward.

#### ■ Eczema/Psoriasis

Common skin disorders, causing:

- Dry, flaking areas.

- Psoriasis spreads around back passage.
- Usually skin elsewhere is affected.

### RARE

#### ■ Lichen Sclerosus (LS) or Leukoplakia

LS is typically whitish or shiny thin-looking skin, sometimes with cracking and soreness. Leukoplakia is whitish skin with thickening. Most common in the elderly, but LS can also occur in children.

Specialist assessment and followup is essential as complications can include cancer.

#### ■ Cancer

Skin cancer may present the following symptoms:

- An itchy sore.
- Grows slowly.
- Bleeds.

Treatment is usually curative, but the earlier the diagnosis, the better.

#### ■ General Disease

Several disorders may cause generalized itch. Specific features might include:

- Swollen lymph nodes suggest infection or lymphoma.
- Jaundice suggests liver disease.
- Changes in volume of urine produced suggests diabetes.

- Widespread skin involvement may be due to other skin diseases.
- Joint pains suggest rheumatological diseases.

*(See also Itching—Without a Rash, page 265)*

## PAIN IN THE PELVIS

Pains in the lower abdomen are common in women and are frequently difficult to diagnose. Apart from gynecological causes (problems in the womb, tubes, ovaries, and vagina), there are other pelvic organs to consider: the intestines and the bladder. In addition, pain from other abdominal organs, such as the kidney, can be referred to the pelvis, as can pain from irritation of nerves in the back and diseases of the major arteries that run through the lower abdomen. The abdomen is also a sensitive index of emotional turmoil, at all ages and in both sexes.

Pain associated with the following symptoms suggest a gynecological cause:
- Painful periods.
- Unusual vaginal discharge.
- Abnormal vaginal bleeding.
- Pain on intercourse.
- Infertility.

*(See the sections referring to these symptoms for further details)*

Symptoms pointing to a non-gynecological cause are:
- Diarrhea, constipation, or bleeding from the bowel.
- Frequent or painful urination or the presence of blood in the urine.
- Pain varies depending on your posture—suggests a muscular or back-related cause.
- Pulsation in your abdomen, pain in your legs on walking.
- Depression, anxiety, or relationship problems.

Your overall condition may point to one of the many non-gynecological diseases that can cause recurrent abdominal pains. Your doctor will rely on the pattern of symptoms, and the results of tests, before making a diagnosis.

## HOT FLASHES

### PROBABLE

#### ■ Menopause

Known also as "the change" or "the change of life" and linked to the drop in levels of estrogens present in the blood. It marks the end of fertility. Average

age of menopause is fifty-one years, although this varies. In addition to hot flashes, symptoms include the following:

• Periods become irregular with variable flow before stopping.

• The skin of the vagina becomes drier and thinner—atrophic vaginitis *(see page 342)*.

• There is atrophy of other estrogen-dependent tissues in the genital area and breasts, leading to urinary leakage—stress incontinence and prolapse *(see page 346)*.

• There is weakening of the bones, leading to osteoporosis and risk of fractures.

Some features are more controversial, perhaps a reflection of personal adjustments to this major event in a woman's life:

• Loss of sexual desire.

• Depression.

• Irritability.

Hot flashes usually continue for about two years; a few unlucky individuals continue to have them for longer. This is not a symptom of disease. For some women, it is a relief for periods to end; for others, it is a matter of deep emotion, a signal of the beginning of old age. The reaction of the majority of women lies somewhere between the two, and it is intimately connected with support from their partners and families and their own self-esteem.

Overall, about 80 percent of women manage without any medical intervention. For others, hormone replacement therapy (HRT) is an effective treatment for the symptoms of menopause, relieving hot flashes and vaginal dryness and slowing the development of osteoporosis. Whether it relieves the psychological symptoms is more controversial. A decision about HRT needs detailed discussion with your doctor about the likely benefit versus the adverse risks, such as increased breast cancer risk in long-term users. Women wanting mainly to reduce the risk of osteoporosis have the option of other non-HRT treatments. Alternative or complementary therapies are widely used to good effect.

## POSSIBLE

### ■ Overactive Thyroid Gland

Symptoms include:

• Sweating, increased appetite, weight loss.

• Intolerance to heat.

• Tremor of hands.

• Consistently rapid pulse, possibly palpitations.

• Protruding eyes (in some cases).

Treatment aims to reduce the output of thyroid hormone from the thyroid gland.

## RARE

### ■ Persistent Fever or Sweats

It is worth considering whether any of the many causes of fevers or sweats might be responsible. The subject is covered in detail elsewhere, but your suspicions might be aroused by:

• Hot flashes occurring in the presence of a measurable fever.

• Hot flashes beginning abruptly while periods are still normal and regular.

• Drenching sweats at night.

• Malaise, weight loss.

• Symptoms starting after foreign travel to areas of endemic disease, such as malaria areas.

• Occupational risks, such as in health workers exposed to ill patients.

• The presence of enlarged lymph glands.

## MASCULINE CHANGES IN WOMEN

The development of male features in a woman may reflect upsets in the balance between male and female hormones in the body, unless this is clearly a feature of your family or race. If periods are normal, then a serious underlying hormonal problem is unlikely. However, the expectations and acceptability of certain features such as body hair vary enormously between different women and depend to some extent on external factors such as fashion and also age. Typical masculine changes are:

• Growth of hair on the face, chest, abdomen.

• Balding.

• Deepening voice.

• Disruption of periods.

## PROBABLE

### ■ Hereditary and Racial Differences

Racial and family differences in hairiness are well known; for example, both men and women from Mediterranean races tend to be hairier than Nordic peoples. There is no effect on fertility.

## POSSIBLE

### ■ Polycystic Ovary Syndrome

*(See page 338)*

### ■ Menopause

Some women approaching or going through menopause notice an increase in facial hair or loss of feminine features.

### ■ Hypothyroidism

An underactive thyroid gland may often

be the reason for masculinization, as it causes:

- Gruff voice, coarse dry skin.
- Periods become heavy or irregular.

Additional features of an underactive thyroid gland are:

- Weight gain.
- Slow thought.
- Slow pulse.
- Weakness.
- Constipation.

The diagnosis is made on the basis of blood tests.

### ■ Drugs

Hairiness is a side effect of several widely used drugs; for instance, steroids used to treat certain arthritic diseases can cause it.

### RARE

### ■ Ovarian Tumor

Suspected in a previously healthy woman who develops signs of masculinization. There are no other symptoms of an early tumor, which must be detected by examination and ultrasound investigation.

### ■ Cushing's Syndrome

There are many causes of this syndrome, which is due to the effects of excessive amounts of steroid hormones, either produced in the body or more commonly as a side effect of steroids given to treat other diseases. Among its symptoms are:

- Obese body, but thin limbs.
- Masculine features.
- Easy bruising.
- Excessive production of urine.
- Purple stripes or stretch marks across the hip and other fat-bearing areas.

## BREAST DISORDERS

It is wise for women to check their breasts from time to time, aiming to familiarize themselves with how they feel normally so that changes can be spotted early. Remember that the breast is sensitive to hormones present in the body and that these vary with the different phases of the menstrual cycle, thus the breasts feel slightly different at different times of the month. Any change from the "normal" feel of the breast tissue should prompt a visit to the doctor. Remember also that the tissues of the breast extend into the armpit, so checks should include that area.

Mammography (x-ray examination of the breast) is used to detect changes before *you* notice a problem. Such screening programs are not 100 percent reliable and may turn up abnormalities which, on further investigation, prove harmless. However, these false alarms are a price worth paying in order to detect more serious disease, such as cancer, at an earlier stage, when treatment is more likely to produce a cure. Further tests include fine needle aspiration cytology (FNAC), in which a syringe needle is used to sample cells from the breast, and breast ultrasound may help to clarify or confirm the exact diagnosis.

Breast cancer is undoubtedly the most feared and serious cause of symptoms in the breast, but it is not necessarily the most likely cause. Overall, the best advice is to seek medical help if you develop any breast symptoms that differ from what you know as your norm.

## LUMP IN THE BREAST

At some time in their life, most women will feel a lump in one of their breasts. Breasts are frequently lumpy, and some of these lumps are easily felt. In eight out of ten cases, it will be entirely harmless. Where cancer is diagnosed, you should remember that the outlook is much more likely to be good than bad and that most women can look forward to successful treatment with the real possibility of a cure. Breast cancer is one of the most closely studied forms of cancer, but doctors will admit that there is still an enormous amount they do not know about it. Fundamental questions remain unanswered, such as why the cancer starts, how quickly it grows, and how best to treat it. Expert opinion about therapy is constantly changing and improving, following the results of treatment trials, which are being carried out worldwide.

### PROBABLE

■ **Fibroadenoma**

Most common in women between twenty-nine and forty years old.
• Firm, painless lump.
• Freely mobile, which is why this lump has been described as a "breast mouse."

Some women have several of these over many years, but each one should be checked by a doctor and is usually removed. They are not thought to lead to cancer.

■ **Fibrocystic Disease**

This is a misleading technical term for something that is not really a disease at all. The breasts are generally lumpy, and within that lumpiness there may be more definite, large lumps that are usually fluid-filled cysts. Most common in women thirty to fifty years old.

- Lumpiness varies during the menstrual cycle.
- Often pain before a period.
- Often areas of the breast are tender.

Mammography is useful in differentiating these lumps from cancer. Many surgeons will drain obvious cysts, using a needle and syringe, then send the contents for detailed analysis. No other treatment is necessarily needed.

### ■ Breast Abscess
- A painful lump that enlarges over several days.
- Overlying skin is hot and red.
- Fever or flu-like symptoms.
- Sometimes a bloody discharge mixed with milk from the nipple.
- Most commonly occurs when breast-feeding, usually following an episode of "mastitis."

## POSSIBLE

### ■ Cancer
You feel a lump; it may be tiny but you are sure it has appeared recently. Some of the features that would suggest that a lump is likely to be cancerous are:
- A firm, irregular lump.
- Skin over it is dimpled and puckered.
- A newly indrawn nipple or any nipple changes occurring at the same time.
- Swollen glands felt in the armpit.

- Pain in the region of the lump, though the majority of early cancers are painless.
- Bleeding from the nipple.

Risk factors for developing breast cancer include family history of the disease and increasing age—80 percent of cases occur in women over fifty.

Tests to confirm the diagnosis include biopsy using fine needle aspiration cytology (FNAC), where a syringe and needle are used to sample cells from the lump, mammography, breast ultrasound, and sometimes other scans and blood tests.

Treatment depends on the type of cancer, its size and location (including whether it has spread to other areas), and other important factors, such as the age, general health, and, most importantly, the preference of the patient. Possible surgical treatments include lumpectomy (removal of the lump), mastectomy (removal of the breast), and exploration and sampling of the lymph glands in the armpit. Surgical reconstruction of the breast may also help with cosmetic and psychological well-being. Surgical treatment may be combined with radiotherapy or chemotherapy and may be followed by a course of medication (such as tamoxifen) to modify hormone levels. Every case is different and the treatment needs to be matched to the needs and preferences of the woman concerned.

### ■ Duct Papilloma

A lump felt just below the nipple and associated with a bloody discharge from the nipple. This should always be reported to your doctor.

## RARE

### ■ Fat Necrosis

A hard knock to the breast can damage fat cells, leading to a lump that feels indistinguishable from a cancer.

• First sign is often bruising visible on the skin.
• A firm lump.
• Does not move freely.
• Skin over it may be dimpled.

The only safe way to deal with this is a biopsy.

### ■ Other Tumors

It is possible for cancers elsewhere to spread into the breast. The diagnosis will probably only be made on biopsy.

## PAIN IN THE BREASTS

If pain is widespread and felt in both breasts, it is usually caused by a variation in hormone levels. If it is confined to one area, then you should feel for a localized abnormality, such as a lump or dimpled skin. Breast pain may be no more that a nuisance, but for some women it can be a great problem. Persistent pain should always be discussed with a doctor to establish its cause and whether further tests are needed. Once serious causes have been excluded, there will often be a simple solution such as a change in contraceptive pill or the recommendation to take evening primrose oil.

## PROBABLE

### ■ Hormonal Variation

• Commonly seen when starting the oral contraceptive pill or hormone replacement therapy (HRT).
• Cyclical variation, typically with premenstrual tenderness.
• Can be an early symptom of pregnancy.
• Common in late pregnancy or after childbirth as milk production occurs.

### ■ Fibrocystic Disease

*(See page 353)*

## POSSIBLE

### ■ Breast Cancer

*(See page 354)* Most early breast cancers present as painless lumps.

### ■ Breast Abscess

*(See page 354)*

### ■ Pain from the Ribs or Muscles

Inflammation of the muscles between ribs or where the rib and the breastbone meet. An injury or strain may be the cause.

- One breast affected.
- Pain is sharp and highly localized.
- Pain reproduced by pressing between the ribs or by pressing on the breastbone.

A harmless symptom that resolves over a few weeks.

---

# BREAST SIZE

As with any part of the body, there is considerable biological variability in breast size. Furthermore, the perception or appreciation of breast size is influenced by cultural and popular expectations. Breast size does not affect the ability to breastfeed a child, nor is it related to fertility. It is normal for the two breasts to be slightly different in size and shape.

## PROBABLE

### ■ Hereditary

Breast size is mainly determined by in-built factors, in other words, genetic control and expression. Race also plays a part, with Asian women generally having smaller breasts.

Reasons for breast surgery to increase or decrease breast size or modify breast shape might include: psychological distress, neck and back pains from very heavy breasts, or for cosmetic enhancement.

## POSSIBLE

### ■ Hormonal

The contraceptive pill and hormone replacement therapy (HRT) often cause a slight increase in breast size. Pregnancy, of course, makes the breasts enlarge, also under the influence of hormones. Many women notice a slight variation in size during their menstrual cycle.

## RARE

### ■ Lymphatic Obstruction

Interference with normal drainage of tissue fluid from the breast via the armpit will lead to one swollen breast. Often after radiotherapy to the chest wall, when the arm on that side is very swollen.

- You may feel glands in the armpit; if so, report it immediately.

- Breasts become generally firm.

Unfortunately, little can usually be done to cure this problem.

## DISCHARGE FROM THE NIPPLE

During pregnancy, it is normal for a milky fluid to ooze from the breasts. Mothers who breastfeed will find not only that suckling causes a discharge of milk, but that even the sound of the baby crying will trigger this response, and again this is entirely normal. Abnormal discharges may be of milk in the absence of pregnancy, clear fluid, blood, or yellow/green pus. Discharges are commonly due to disease of the duct system, that is, one of the twenty or so channels through which milk flows to the nipple from the milk-producing glands deeper within the breast. Abnormal discharge from the nipple should always prompt a visit to the doctor.

### PROBABLE

#### ■ Hormone Disturbance

Milk production is controlled by the hormone prolactin, secreted by the pituitary gland within the brain. An excess of prolactin causes:

- Discharge of milk from both breasts for months on end.

- Periods become scanty or stop altogether.

Blood tests will show abnormal levels of prolactin. The usual reason is a tiny growth in the pituitary gland; this can be controlled with appropriate drugs or surgery. A few medically prescribed drugs can cause this problem, particularly neuroleptic medication used to treat mental illness.

#### ■ Breast Abscess

*(See page 354)*

### POSSIBLE

The three following possibilities cause similar symptoms, and in all cases will require further investigation, since examination alone is not enough to decide definitely between them.

#### ■ Duct Ectasia

In this condition, enlarged ducts allow the buildup of normal secretions, which then appear as:

- A brown or green discharge.
- Discharge is firm and cheese-like.

■ **Duct Papilloma**

A benign, wart-like growth within one of the ducts leading to the nipple.

• A bloody discharge, perhaps just a spot of blood on the bra.
• Sometimes just a clear, yellowish discharge.
• A lump may be felt near the nipple.

■ **Cancer of Ducts**

• Bloody discharge.
• Possibly a pricking sensation behind the nipple.

## RARE

■ **Breast Cancer**

Occasionally, a breast cancer some distance from the nipple causes bleeding.

• A breast lump is likely.
• Some discomfort is possible.

■ **Paget's Disease of the Nipple**

A distinctive condition, most common in older women.

• Cracked, dry, red skin around one nipple.
• Oozes blood.
• The nipple becomes distorted.

This disease is nearly always due to breast cancer.

---

## RETRACTION OR INVERSION OF THE NIPPLE

Both nipples normally project a little, becoming flatter when warm or relaxed, and more protuberant if cold or in response to touch or sexual stimulation. Retracted or inverted nipples appear sunken into the breast.

## PROBABLE

■ **Congenital**

Commonly seen in baby girls who grow up with one or both nipples retracted or inverted; this persists into adulthood and tends to be lifelong. It is not a sign of disease, but might affect the ability to breastfeed.

There are many "cures" for retracted nipples, but there is little evidence that they work.

## POSSIBLE

■ **Breast Cancer**

The retraction or inversion of a previously normal nipple must be taken as a symptom of breast cancer until proven otherwise. You should search for:

• Lump in the breast.
• Discharge from the nipples.

Always inform your doctor of any such changes to your nipples.

# SYMPTOMS IN MEN

## LUMPS IN THE TESTICLE OR SCROTUM

In the same way that women should be encouraged to be aware of and familiar with the normal feel of their breasts, men are advised to familiarize themselves with the normal feel of the contents of the scrotum. This is best done when the muscle contained in the scrotal wall is relaxed, such as in a warm bath. Both testicles should be approximately the same size, with the left one commonly lying slightly lower than the right. It is possible to feel the epididymis, which is a somewhat firm, slightly irregular structure wrapped around the back of the testicles and attaching to the spermatic cord above. It is common to find small lumps in the skin of the scrotum; these are usually harmless cysts in the skin or sebaceous glands at the roots of pubic hairs.

Any variation in the contents of the scrotum from normal should be reported to a doctor, who will examine you and may recommend an ultrasound scan for confirmation of the diagnosis.

### PROBABLE

#### ■ Epididymal Cyst

A harmless swelling, arising from the epididymis.

- The swelling feels separate from the testicle.
- May be multiple and present on both sides of the scrotum.

Once confirmed, nothing needs to be done about a cyst unless it is causing discomfort.

#### ■ Varicocele

A harmless swelling caused by enlarged varicose veins; feels like "a bag of worms" above and behind the testicle. Rarely associated with fertility problems. Sometimes treated surgically.

### POSSIBLE

#### ■ Cancer of the Testicle

Overall, this is a rare tumor, but among cancer victims it is the most common malignancy affecting men between fifteen and forty years of age. Elderly men are also at risk. A lump in the testicle is cancer until proven otherwise and always requires medical assessment. Typically, cancer of the testicle presents as:

- A firm, painless enlargement of one testicle.
- Depending on the size of the cancer, the scrotum may appear swollen or there may be a sensation of heaviness.

The treatment depends on the precise type of tumor but carries a very positive outlook, particularly if any changes are spotted early.

## RARE

■ Tuberculosis

Uncommon, though increasing among the poor and homeless.

- A painless, enlarged testicle.
- May discharge like an abscess but without throbbing pain.
- Other features of tuberculosis, such as cough, malaise, sweats, and weight loss.

## SWOLLEN TESTICLES OR SCROTUM

This means swelling without any obvious lump *(for lumps in the testicle or scrotum, see page 359)*. Swellings may be due to an underlying cancer and should always be medically examined. Don't delay in reporting to your doctor any changes you notice in your testicles—early treatment has a very significant effect on the likelihood of a complete cure.

## PROBABLE

■ Hydrocele

An accumulation of fluid around the testicle.

- Tense, swollen testicle.
- Pain may or may not be present.
- If chronic, can be very large.
- In children, often accompanies a hernia.
- Not uncommon at, or soon after, birth.

Specialist opinion should be sought, since there may be an underlying cause, such as infection or cancer of the testicle.

■ Orchitis

A general term for swollen or inflamed testicle. Underlying causes include injury, infection, and mumps.

- Pain builds up over a few hours.
- Scrotum also usually swells with fluid.
- An acutely painful testicle may be twisted *(see Torsion, page 361)*, with a risk of future sterility.

Urgent medical attention is essential, especially for children.

## POSSIBLE

■ Hernia

When the bowel bulges through a weakness in the wall of the abdomen, usually in the groin.

- Commonly just a lump in the groin but may extend into the scrotum.
- In children, commonly extends to the scrotum, which appears to be swollen.
- Swelling may disappear after lying flat.

May require surgical repair, especially in children.

## RARE

### ■ Filariasis

A parasite that blocks the drainage of tissue fluids, leading to swelling of the affected region. Originates in tropical areas only.

- Repeated inflation of the testicles and epididymis.
- After several infections, the scrotum remains permanently swollen.

Advanced disease needs surgical treatment.

## PAIN IN THE TESTICLES

In boys and young men, pain, especially if it is one-sided, equals torsion *(see below)* until proven otherwise. In older adults, there is a wider range of possible diagnoses. If torsion is suspected, medical advice should be sought immediately as an emergency.

## PROBABLE

### ■ Epididymitis

The epididymis is a structure involved in the transport of sperm from the testicles, and it can normally be felt at the back of the testicle. Inflammation or infection usually occurs for no obvious reason, but if there is also discharge from the penis, a doctor must test for sexually transmitted infections (STIs). Epididymitis is an unsafe diagnosis to make for a boy before puberty, in whom torsion is far more likely.

- Pain, initially behind testicle, builds up over a few hours.
- There is swelling of the testicle and scrotum, which become exquisitely tender.
- The scrotum feels hot and there may be fever and nausea.
- Sometimes the testicle becomes infected or inflamed (epididymo-orchitis).

Antibiotic treatment is needed, plus rest, for a couple of weeks.

### ■ Torsion

The testicles hang on a cord, which can twist. Other structures near the testicles can also twist, giving a similar condition. Deciding which has happened can often only be done during an operation. Sometimes Doppler ultrasound is used first to check the blood flow to the testicle, which becomes compromised with a torsion. Typical features are:

- Sudden, severe pain in one testicle.
- Nausea, vomiting.
- Affected testicle swells and is tender.

An urgent operation is nearly always needed to untwist the testicle and to anchor it into place to prevent recurrence. It is usual to operate on the other testicle at the same time; if one has twisted, the other is likely to do so in the future. Neglected torsion will inevitably lead to death of the affected testicle, with future effects on fertility.

## Possible

### ■ Injury

- A definite history of injury to the scrotum, such as a kick in the crotch.
- Pain, tenderness, and visible bruising.
- Normal urinary stream and no blood.

Support and time to heal are the only remedies.

### ■ Varicocele

*(See page 359)*

### ■ Stone

A stone in the urinary system gives rise to:
- Pain of rapid onset and often of great severity, lasting an hour or so.
- Pains recur over days and weeks.
- Appears to radiate from the low back (kidney region) to the testicles or to the tip of the penis.
- Nausea, vomiting.
- Blood in urine.

Small stones will pass spontaneously, whereas larger ones may need surgical removal.

## Rare

### ■ Mumps Orchitis

Mumps is an increasingly rare disease because of immunization programs. A few cases give rise to inflammation of the testicles (orchitis).
- Mumps causes swellings, like hamster cheeks, just in front of the jaw joint.
- After three to four days, one or both testicles may swell.
- Fever, pain.

The risk of orchitis is much less than once thought. Although sterility may follow, it appears that this too is much less of a risk than was once feared.

### ■ Pancreatitis

*(See page 478)*

## PAIN BETWEEN THE LEGS

### PROBABLE

■ Injury

Injury between the legs may irritate the prostate gland, giving rise to:

• A dull ache between the legs.

• Slight discomfort or difficulty passing urine.

• Blood in the urine if there has been a severe injury, such as falling astride something.

### POSSIBLE

■ Prostatitis

Prostatitis is an infection or inflammation of the prostate gland. Symptoms include:

• Pain in the saddle area between the anus and scrotum.

• Burning sensation or difficulty when passing urine.

• Urine may appear cloudy and laboratory tests may show infection.

• Sometimes fever, muscle or joint pains.

• May be a recurrent or chronic problem.

This can be an awkward problem to eradicate, often needing extended courses of antibiotics.

### RARE

■ Cancer of the Prostate

An advanced cancer may produce the following:

• Ache or pain between the legs.

• Pain in the back or pelvis because of spread to the bones.

More usually, cancer of the prostate is painless and is found on investigation after difficulty passing urine caused by enlargement of the prostate, which obstructs the passage of urine.

## ABSENT TESTICLE

Absence should be discovered at routine child health checks from birth onwards. A testicle that is not brought down into the scrotum is at risk of decreased fertility and also at greater risk of a malignant change in later life.

### PROBABLE

■ Undescended Testicle

• Normal general development.

• Testicle often felt as a lump in the groin.

Three to four percent of male babies have undescended testicles at birth;

some of these descend spontaneously by the age of one. Medical advice should be sought early to establish the diagnosis and to get advice on the need for an operation. Surgical treatment reduces the risk of damaged fertility and subsequent testicular cancer.

## POSSIBLE

### ■ Retractile Testicle

An exaggeration of a normal reflex, which pulls the testicles up into the groin.

- Testicle is present at certain times.
- Cold and strong emotion can cause retraction.

Usually no treatment is needed for this condition.

## RARE

### ■ Ectopic Testicle

The testicle may lodge itself somewhere in the lower abdomen. It may be felt in the groin, at the base of the penis, or even the upper thigh. Surgical correction is recommended to preserve fertility.

## SMALL TESTICLE

Testicles vary in size and the left testicle usually hangs lower than the right one. Fertility may be normal unless both testicles are very small or defective in their function. Alcoholism and drugs used in treating cancer of the prostate may cause previously normal testicles to decrease in size.

## PROBABLE

### ■ Previous Injury or Infection

Likely if:

- Only one testicle is small.
- Previous pain.
- Previous swelling.
- Sometimes occurs in undescended

testicles that are surgically brought down into the scrotum, especially if this is done late.

Possible causes include twisted testicles and orchitis *(see Pain in the Testicles, page 361).*

## POSSIBLE

### ■ Hormone Disorders

- Both testicles are small.
- Individual is often very tall.
- Absent or decreased body hair.
- Breast development.
- Infertility.

Hormone testing is needed to pinpoint the root cause.

## ■ Genetic Disorders

A fascinating, highly complex area, touching on intersexuality and ambiguous sexual development.

- Testicles and penis may be abnormally formed.
- Male is likely to be abnormally tall or short.
- Infertility.

## DISCHARGE FROM PENIS

Whether clear or colored, discharge from the penis is highly suggestive of sexually transmitted infection (STI), with nonspecific genital infection and gonorrhea being the most likely causes. Must be seen at a specialist clinic; partner is also likely to be infected.

## DISEASED FORESKIN

The foreskin is subject to infection, resulting in cracking and scar tissue formation. It may cause pain, interfere with passing urine, and make sexual intercourse difficult.

### PROBABLE

### ■ Balanitis

An infection of the foreskin and adjacent penis. Diabetes may underlie recurrent balanitis.

- Mild pain, itching, and redness.
- Discharge around the foreskin, not from the opening of the penis itself.
- Sometimes associated with skin disease—seborrheic dermatitis or psoriasis.

Antibiotics, plus salt baths, are the treatment.

### ■ Phimosis

Phimosis is an inability to retract the foreskin over the tip of the penis. A non-retractile foreskin is normal in boys up to five years old and it is wrong to attempt to do so. It may be abnormal if there is:

- Recurrent balanitis.
- Ballooning of the foreskin on passing urine.

Circumcision or stretching of the foreskin is then advisable.

## POSSIBLE

■ **Paraphimosis**

The foreskin becomes stuck, rolled behind the tip of the penis.

• Pain.

• Swelling of tip of the penis prevents unrolling the foreskin back over the tip.

This calls for rapid treatment to replace the foreskin in its correct position; local anesthetic gels help a doctor to do this; sometimes surgery is necessary.

## RARE

■ **Cancer of the Penis**

A rarity in the West, but common in some Far Eastern countries. It is unusual among circumcised men, with the exact reason being unclear.

• Begins as a red area on the tip of the penis or hidden within the foreskin.

• Grows, ulcerates.

• Discharge, pain, bleeding.

Treatment is radiotherapy and surgery.

## BLOOD IN SEMEN

A fairly common symptom, which looks alarming but hardly ever has a serious underlying cause. In fact, the reason remains unknown for the vast majority of cases. It is most common in elderly men. It may be mistaken for bleeding from the vagina after intercourse.

It is sensible to have your genitalia examined, plus a urine test, to ensure that the blood does not come from the bladder. Otherwise, nothing else needs to be done unless the symptom recurs, when an internal check of the bladder and prostate gland may be advisable.

## PAINFUL PENIS

### PROBABLE

■ **Infection**

• Pain, burning on passing urine.

• Need to urinate frequently.

• Possibly blood in the urine.

• Urine cloudy or smelly.

These symptoms suggest a urinary tract infection. Such infections, whether in a boy or adult, should always be investigated, usually by ultrasound scan or x-ray examination, since underlying physical causes are common. A discharge suggests a sexually transmitted infection (STI).

■ **Diseased Foreskin**

*(See page 365)*

**POSSIBLE**

■ Stone

*(See Kidney Stones, page 184)*

**RARE**

■ Peyronie's Disease

*(See below)*

## CURVED PENIS

Known medically as chordee. Minor degrees are very common and may cause embarrassment, especially in teenagers. The curvature may be more apparent when the penis is erect. Extreme curvature may make sexual intercourse difficult.

**PROBABLE**

■ Congenital

• Noticed at birth.

• The opening for urine (external meatus) may be underneath the penis not at the end (hypospadias).

Delicate surgery to correct these abnormalities makes use of the foreskin, which should therefore not be circumcised.

**POSSIBLE**

■ Peyronie's Disease

A band of firm tissue forms on part of the shaft of the penis. In the middle-aged or older.

• Pain and curvature on erection.

• A firm or nodular area felt on the shaft.

Treatment is difficult. Occasionally, it disappears spontaneously.

**RARE**

■ Injury

Vigorous sexual intercourse or other injury may fracture the erect penis.

• Sudden pain, bruising, and deformity.

Needs early treatment to prevent permanent deformity.

## SMALL PENIS

An objective assessment of penis size is difficult because of variations at different temperatures and degrees of erection. Nevertheless, there is some biological and racial variation in size, though this rarely correlates with fertility or sexual performance. Adolescent boys and men beginning sexual activity often present to the doctor worrying that their penis is abnormally small, though examination almost always shows the penis to be within the normal size range. There is less variation in the size of the erect penis among men compared to variation in the non-erect state—in other words, most penises end up a similar size when they become erect. Worry about a small penis may be justified in the presence of some of the following features:

- Absent or small testicles.
- Absence of body hair.
- Excessive height.

- Breast development.
- Obesity.
- Previous injury, torsion of testicles.
- In boys, a small penis may appear very small if it is sunk in fat in the groin.

Investigations such as chromosome analysis, hormone profiles, and brain scans may be needed. As treatment is possible for boys, cases of true micropenis are worth reporting to a doctor, sooner rather than later.

## PROLONGED ERECTION

Also known as priapism. A very painful, prolonged erection in the absence of sexual desire. The tip of the penis may remain soft. Whatever the cause, it needs urgent treatment to avoid long-term damage to the penis.

### PROBABLE

#### ■ Cause Unknown

Accounting for about three out of five cases.

- It may follow prolonged sexual activity.
- Otherwise sound health.

### POSSIBLE

#### ■ Blood Disorders

Blood tests will seek leukemia or sickle-cell disease.

- Easy bruising, malaise, and large glands suggest leukemia.
- Recurrent joint or abdominal pains suggest sickle-cell disease (occurs almost exclusively in African American men).

### RARE

#### ■ All Other Causes

A routine search is always made for growths in the pelvis, drugs affecting erection, or damage to the spinal cord.

## FEMINIZATION IN MEN

Adult men who start to develop female features need a full hormonal assessment. Female features include loss of body hair, development of breasts, loss of sexual drive, and shrinking testicles and penis.

### PROBABLE

#### ■ Drug Effects

Some drugs have estrogenic (female hormone type) or anti-androgenic (anti–male hormone type) side effects. Common culprits are spironolactone, digoxin, and beta-blockers used in heart disease, estrogens and anti-androgens for treating cancer of the prostate, and chlorpromazine used to treat mental illness.

### POSSIBLE

#### ■ Alcoholism

A history of heavy, prolonged alcohol consumption or alcohol dependency.
- Impotence.
- Breast development.

- Decreased fertility due to diminished sperm count.

Tests may show cirrhosis of the liver. May reverse or partially reverse with alcohol avoidance.

#### ■ Genetic Problems

Men with genetic problems may be:
- Unusually tall individuals.
- Infertile.

Problems may be apparent from birth. Specialist investigation will identify the diagnosis.

### RARE

#### ■ Tumors

If the above causes are excluded, it is essential to search for cancers in the testicles, lungs, or elsewhere, which may be secreting female hormones. Possible symptoms include:
- Lump in or on a testicle.
- Coughing blood, chest pains, weight loss.

## PRECOCIOUS PUBERTY

Sexual development before the age of nine years is likely to be abnormal; that includes the appearance of body hair, enlarged penis, and deepening voice. Cases are rare but all require specialist investigation.

### POSSIBLE

#### ■ Hypothalamic Disease

The hypothalamus gland in the brain controls many hormones. A disorder is likeliest if:

- The boy was normal at birth and in early childhood.
- Later shows abnormal growth, either too short or too tall.
- Sometimes tumors in this part of the brain cause visual disturbances.

## RARE

### ■ Testicular Tumors

- A lump may be felt.
- There may be a change or swelling in one testicle.

Blood tests may detect abnormally high levels of hormones in the blood.

### ■ Adrenal Disease

Disease of the adrenal glands, which lie over the kidneys, usually makes a baby very ill within days of birth.

Hormone treatment prevents masculine changes appearing during very early childhood.

# SYMPTOMS COMMON TO BOTH MEN AND WOMEN AND RELATED TO SEXUAL RELATIONS

## FERTILITY PROBLEMS

Low fertility or infertility can be a cause of much heartache to both men and women and can put a relationship under tremendous strain. Furthermore, its investigation can be traumatic and difficult and needs to be handled with the utmost sensitivity and skill. A young healthy couple having regular sexual intercourse can expect about an 85 percent chance of achieving a pregnancy within a year, a figure that increases to 92 percent after two years. The remainder may need investigation and assistance.

It is important to remember that fertility in women decreases with age and this also applies to the success rates of assisted fertilization techniques. In this respect, men are luckier as the potency of their sperm shows only a marginal decline with age.

Overall, low fertility in a couple falls under the following causes (with approximate percentage of occurrence):

- Ovulation problems in women (20 percent).
- Tubal problems in women (14 percent).
- Hostile mucus in women (6 percent).
- Endometriosis in women (6 percent).

- Sexual difficulties (6 percent).
- Male factors (24 percent).
- Unexplained (24 percent).

Paradoxically, if a couple falls into the unexplained category, then statistically they have a 60 to 70 percent chance of a pregnancy within three years of investigation, a figure that is higher than where a cause is found.

When considering asking for medical help with fertility, it is always worth checking on general health and lifestyle matters: couples should try not to smoke, keep alcohol intake to a minimum, and optimize diet exercise and weight. Women should take folic acid supplements to help prevent neural tube defects when a pregnancy occurs.

## FEMALE FERTILITY DIFFICULTIES

### PROBABLE

#### ▪ Ovulation Problems

This involves a hormone imbalance and would be suspected if there are:
- Absent periods.
- Irregular periods.
- Infrequent periods.
- Very light or very heavy periods.

Ovulation can be monitored by a blood test looking for a rise in progesterone on day twenty-two of the cycle, or by using ovulation predictor tests mid-cycle, or by means of temperature charts. Ovulation problems may be treated with clomifene or gonadotropin medications.

#### ▪ Blocked Fallopian Tubes

These are the tubes through which the eggs travel to the womb. Blocked tubes usually follow repeated pelvic infection causing pelvic inflammatory disease *(see page 333)*, suspected from:
- Recurrent pelvic pain.
- Recurrent, infected vaginal discharges.
- Deep pain on intercourse.

Blocked tubes can be investigated by laparoscopy or x-ray (hysterosalpingogram). Tubal surgery or in vitro fertilization (IVF) techniques may provide a solution.

#### ▪ Cause Unknown

Despite thorough investigation, many cases remain unexplained.

### POSSIBLE

#### ▪ Endometriosis

*(See page 333)*

■ **General Disease**

Any serious, general disease can reduce fertility, but it should already be obvious.

■ **Womb Abnormalities**

Investigations sometimes show a range of unsuspected abnormalities, such as a malformation of the womb, which prevents implantation of the egg.

## MALE FERTILITY DIFFICULTIES

An early semen analysis is always advisable, looking for low numbers of sperm, increased numbers of abnormal sperm, or sperm motility problems. Temporary infertility can follow a severe illness, after which it takes a few months for sperm production to recover.

The main treatment for male infertility is intracytoplasmic sperm injection, where a sperm is recovered from the epididymis or testicle and introduced directly into an egg.

### PROBABLE

■ **Unknown Cause**

The majority of cases of male infertility have no identifiable cause.

■ **Damage to Testicles**

Suggested by:
• Small size, abnormally soft feel.
• History of undescended testicle or testicular surgery.
• History of mumps orchitis.

• History of sexually transmitted infection (STI).
• History of drug use (chemotherapy or illicit drugs).

Cigarette smoking, alcohol, cannabis, and high temperatures in the area of the scrotum can also decrease sperm production.

### POSSIBLE

■ **Varicocele**

*(See page 359)*

■ **Hormone Disorders**

A possibility if there is:
• Absent body hair.
• Development of breasts.

### RARE

■ **Chromosome Disorders**

• Unusual height.
• Enlarged breasts.
• Small or absent testicles.
• Absent body hair.
• Abnormally formed penis.

## LACK OF INTEREST IN SEX AND REDUCED LIBIDO

Most enduring relationships eventually balance the partners' sexual desires so that neither partner is left feeling frustrated or guilty. The road to that adjustment can be a difficult one. Blame does not enter into this, nor is it ever the fault of one party alone; recognizing that there is a problem is the first step to resolving it. Natural variations in a woman's sexual desire occur during the monthly cycle, reaching a peak in mid-cycle (before ovulation) for some women. Major illness and childbirth will usually decrease sexual desire. Sexual desire and libido also tend to reduce with advancing age.

### PROBABLE

■ **Psychological Factors**

Psychological factors are most likely if you feel:
• Sex is dirty.
• An aversion to being touched sexually by your partner.
• That things should be better than they are.
• Guilty about your lack of enjoyment of sex.

Psychosexual therapy can help this problem. Other counselors, including individual and relationship counselors, can also contribute.

### POSSIBLE

■ **Adverse Sexual Experiences**

Meaning traumatic events such as painful intercourse, misunderstanding about sexual anatomy and sexual response, or fear of becoming pregnant. Most important is the memory of early sexual experiences, particularly if either partner was abused. The techniques for dealing with such problems involve explanation, honesty, and patience. Gradually exploring your anatomy and sexual response, without initially indulging in sexual intercourse, may be helpful.

### RARE

■ **Depression**

A decreasing interest in sex in either a man or woman may signal depression. Some other features of depression are:
• Feelings of sadness and low mood.
• Loss of ability to enjoy things.
• Loss of sense of self-worth.
• Disturbed sleep.
• Easy crying.
• Thoughts of suicide.
• Slowing of thought.

Depression may respond to psychological treatments (talking therapy) or antidepressants. Unfortunately, some antidepressants (such as SSRIs) also adversely affect sexual performance.

## ORGASMIC FAILURE

Achievement of orgasm is only one part of a successful sexual relationship. Orgasm is a complex physiological process: in men it coincides with ejaculation of sperm, while in women the changes are more subtle. Men may be unable to achieve orgasm for many of the same reasons as women.

Some facts about female orgasm:
• It is a real physical and psychological event.
• Stimulation of the clitoris is usually important.
• It is not necessary for enjoyable sex each time.
• It may take longer to achieve for a woman than for a man.
• Women are capable of multiple orgasms; they do not need a resting period like most men.

Failure to achieve orgasm may be due to difficulty with the partnership or because of the techniques used during intercourse. Some people are unable to experience orgasm without masturbation. It is helpful to share and explore with your partner what forms of stimulation lead to orgasm so that they can be enjoyed together.

### PROBABLE

■ **Psychological**

This refers to an array of experiences that make a relationship, such as affection, trust, and previous positive experiences. It is common knowledge that uncertainty in these and other aspects will lead to problems with sex and orgasm.

■ **Poor Technique**

It is necessary to take anatomy into account. Orgasm usually requires:
• Adequate foreplay.
• Clitoral or penile stimulation.
• Avoidance of pain.
• Proper lubrication.

### POSSIBLE

■ **Partner's Problem**

Failure to achieve orgasm in a woman can be a result of a man's:
• Premature ejaculation.
• Impotence *(see page 375)*.

■ **Drugs**

SSRI antidepressants, such as fluoxetine, have a blocking or delaying effect on orgasm. Other drugs, such as those used to treat major psychiatric illness, may also adversely affect it.

## IMPOTENCE

Impotence means difficulty in achieving or maintaining a firm erection. It is a common disorder, admitted to far less often than it is experienced. Brief episodes of impotence accompany tiredness and any serious, general ill-health. After ejaculation, there is loss of erection, which takes longer and longer to recover with age, perhaps several days by old age. This may cause confusion if the true disorder is premature ejaculation. Psychological factors are still the most likely reasons for impotence, but it is increasingly clear that physical disorders, especially with advancing age, are more common than once thought, especially problems with blood flow to the penis. This probably reflects an openness to discuss and investigate sexual activity in the elderly.

There are a range of treatments now available, including drugs such as Viagra and preparations injected into the penile urethra or penis itself. Pump devices may also help.

(See also Premature Ejaculation, page 376)

### PROBABLE

#### ■ Psychological

Factors here include depression, problems between partners, and especially the vicious circle of past impotence causing impotence again. Symptoms strongly suggestive of a psychological cause are:

- Normal erections during sleep or on awakening.
- Ejaculation during sleep.
- Impotence with one particular partner.
- Sudden onset of impotence.
- Young age.

Therapy will include explanation, exploration of psychological problems, and gradual return to sexual intercourse.

### POSSIBLE

#### ■ Diabetes Mellitus

Diabetes affects the nerves and blood supply involved in an erection. Undiagnosed diabetes may cause:

- Excessive passage of urine at night and during the day.
- Thirst.

#### ■ Blood Flow Problems

An erection is caused by engorgement of the penis's spongy tissues with blood. If the veins carrying this blood supply are leaking, inadequate erection may follow. Arterial disease can also affect the blood supply, both to the penis and to the nerves controlling erection. Sophisticated tests of blood flow are available.

## ■ Drugs

Many drugs used to treat high blood pressure may cause impotence, as do tranquilizers and heroin. Numerous other drugs may be implicated and are worth looking into.

## ■ Alcoholism

Shakespeare sums it up in *Macbeth:* "It provokes the desire, but takes away the performance." Chronic alcoholism actually leads to hormonal and neurological changes that make permanent impotence a risk.

## ■ Postoperative

Surgery to the bowel or the prostate gland runs the risk of damaging the nerves involved in an erection.

## RARE

## ■ Neurological Disease

Of these, the most common is multiple sclerosis, giving rise to:

- Numbness in various parts of the body.
- Unsteady gait.
- Visual disturbances, transient blindness in one eye.
- Difficulty in controlling passage of urine.

Anything else damaging the lower spine may cause impotence.

## ■ Hormone Disorders

There are a wide range of possibilities. A possible cause if the person has:
- Absent or small testicles.
- Lack of body hair.
- Breast development.
- Unusually short or tall stature.
- Extreme obesity.

Hormone treatment may help such cases.

## PREMATURE EJACULATION

This means ejaculation before the penis enters the vagina or very soon after entry. While this is not a disease, it can be very troublesome for many men. Considerable time and patience, as well as courage to explore the problem, will be required.

## PROBABLE

## ■ Psychological Factors

With experience, sexual relationships expand to include more than intercourse alone, perhaps explaining why premature ejaculation is most common in young men. Psychological approaches encourage concentration on aspects of sexual behavior other than intercourse, for example, stroking and massaging. An aid to this is the "squeeze technique," when the partner, told that ejaculation is near, squeezes around the base of the penis for some seconds. This usually delays progress to orgasm without diminishing the erection. Further information should be sought from psychosexual therapists.

## BLISTERS ON OR AROUND THE GENITALIA

### PROBABLE

#### ■ Herpes

The same virus that causes cold sores can cause blisters on and around the genitalia.
• A few blisters crop up from time to time.
• Intensely painful when they appear, especially on the first occasion.
• May be accompanied by flu-like symptoms.
• Pain and difficulty passing urine in women.

Antiviral drugs may be helpful. It is especially important, if you are pregnant, to report any previous or current attacks of herpes to your doctor or midwife. This enables measures to be taken to diminish the risk of infecting the baby at birth.

## GENITAL LUMPS, ULCERS, AND SORES

Minor infections of the genitals are very common and are frequently obvious to an untrained eye. It is important to be alert to early symptoms of sexually transmitted infections, being especially careful if you have many sexual partners. You owe this not just to yourself but to your partners, too.

### PROBABLE

#### ■ Folliculitis or Boils

• Tiny pimples on the skin or at the base of pubic hairs.
• Tender, rapidly appearing lumps.
• Come to a yellow head.
• Discharge pus and blood, then disappear.

Severe cases may require a course of antibiotics.

Frequent or recurrent boils in the genital area can be caused by a skin condition called hidradenitis suppurativa, which is an acne-like condition; it also occurs in the armpits. Treatment is with long-term antibiotics or other anti-acne medications.

## ■ Scabies or Crab Lice

Scabies mites are too small to see with the naked eye; crab lice can usually be seen attached to the shaft of pubic hairs. Both bite the skin, causing;
• Itching with red pimples or burrows in the genital area or elsewhere on the body.
• Itch worse at night with scabies.
• Scabies commonly bite between the fingers and on the waist.

Treatment is with insecticidal shampoos and skin applications, plus careful decontamination of bedding and clothing. Partners and other close physical contacts need treatment as well. Consider the possibility of other sexually transmitted infections.

## ■ Warts

Fleshy growths that are a few millimeters in length, warts are fairly common and as harmless on the genitals as elsewhere.

Caused by the human papilloma virus but a different strain to the type associated with cancer of the cervix.

Warts respond to simple treatment but may recur. Can be sexually transmitted, so condoms may be helpful.

Quite different are masses of spreading warts, appearing like tiny, branching corals, often also found around the back passage. As these may be associated with syphilis, go to a specialist in sexually transmitted diseases.

## ■ Molluscum Contagiosum

Small, pearly lumps a few millimeters in diameter that appear in the genital area. Caused by a virus.
• The lumps have a solid feel to them and a central dimple.
• Painless unless they become infected.

Usually disappear spontaneously after a few months, although simple treatment can speed resolution. May accompany other sexually transmitted infections.

## POSSIBLE

## ■ Cysts

Women commonly develop Bartholin's cyst or labial cyst.
• Painless swelling in lip of the vagina.
• May cause no other problems.
• If infected, becomes very swollen and tender, sometimes with a fever.

Surgical drainage is needed.

## ■ AIDS

Suspected with homosexual practices, sexual promiscuity, sex with at-risk partners, or intravenous drug use. Symptoms, apart from the swelling of glands, include:

- Fever.
- Malaise.
- Headaches.
- Mouth ulcers.

Diagnosis requires blood tests over several months. There is now effective treatment, though as yet no cure.

## RARE

## ■ Syphilis

The symptoms of infection with syphilis appear two to four weeks after contact. Either partner may be infected. A painless ulcer appears on the genitals, subsequently turning into a firm lump. The ulcer, known as a chancre, may appear in or around the vagina or on the penis, in the mouth, or around the back passage, depending on the nature of the sexual activity. Local lymph nodes enlarge. It heals over several weeks. After a few months, secondary features appear, such as rashes on the palms and soles, joint pains, swollen lymph nodes, and genital warts. Years later, syphilis can rampage through the body, affecting just about every organ and causing dementia. Early disease is cured by penicillin.

## ■ Bechet's Disease

A combination of:

- Painful ulcers on the genitals and in the mouth.
- Red eyes, either conjunctivitis or iritis.

Symptoms tend to recur.

## ■ Tropical Venereal Diseases

Rare in Europe and the United States; sexually promiscuous travelers to the tropics are at risk. These diseases are chancroid, lymphogranuloma venereum, and granuloma inguinale (donovanosis). They all produce:

- Genital ulcer, within a few days of infection.
- May remain small or become very large.
- Usually very painful.
- Swollen local lymph glands.

The diagnosis is made on appearance and from results of swabs. Treatment with antibiotics usually leads to a cure.

## ■ Cancer

Skin cancer may be the reason for a persistent, ulcerated area on the penis or vagina—see a doctor.

# MISCELLANEOUS PROBLEMS FOUND IN MEN AND WOMEN

## LUMPS IN THE GROIN

The groin is the region at the top of the thighs, by the side of the genitals and in front of the hip joints. (Lumps of the genitals themselves are considered under specific headings.) Lumps in the groin are very common and are noticed early, being in such a visible part of the body. They are not usually serious. There are several different structures in the groin, so a lump in that region may have many causes. In practice, it is usually possible to make a confident diagnosis based on the appearance of the lump.

### PROBABLE

#### ■ Inguinal Hernia

An extremely common type of hernia, where the contents of the abdomen bulge through a weakness or defect in its muscle wall. Although typically a problem of adulthood, and made worse by lifting and straining, it may also be seen in children and very young babies. Typical features are:

• A soft bulge in the groin, which may be more noticeable on straining.

• Often completely disappears when lying flat.

• Slight aching or dragging sensation is common.

If it becomes painful and firm, bowel may be trapped within it. If this is the case, seek medical help immediately. Hernias in children should always be treated. Inguinal hernia in adults who are engaged in physical activity or lifting of weights (for example, laborers) can be extremely troublesome. In an elderly person who is not particularly active, repair may not be necessary.

#### ■ Enlarged Lymph Nodes

Just like the neck, the groin has groups of lymph glands, whose job is to protect against infection. It is normal to feel a few small glands in the groin, particularly in people of thin build; they are about half a centimeter in size, painless, and mobile under your finger. Minor scratches on the legs, or pimples around the groin, will cause these glands to enlarge for a few days, and it is best to keep an eye on these until they shrink again. Glands that remain swollen for longer, which are usually painful or unusually large, need to be thoroughly checked. There are so many possibilities that enlarged glands are treated as a separate topic (see Swollen Lymph Nodes, page 496).

Enlarged glands accompanied by any of the following symptoms should be taken seriously:

- Enlarged glands elsewhere, such as the neck or armpits.
- Sores on the genitals.
- Bleeding from the back passage.
- Fever, malaise.
- Anemia.
- Bruising.

## POSSIBLE

### ■ Varicose Veins

- Enlarged veins are often seen and felt in the groin.
- Swelling is very soft, easily squeezed by finger pressure.
- A bluish tinge may be noticeable.
- Usually, varicose veins further down the leg.
- Slight aching after standing.

### ■ Femoral Hernia

A femoral hernia arises from a weakness at the very top of the thigh and is different from an inguinal hernia. It carries a higher chance of strangulation, where the contents become dangerously trapped. Most common in older women.

- Often appears rapidly as a small, tender lump.
- Blockage causes a painful, hard lump, vomiting, and intestinal obstruction.

Femoral hernias almost always require surgical treatment.

### ■ Lipoma

A soft lump present for many weeks and growing slowly (if at all) is probably a lipoma, a benign fatty tumor.

- Painless.
- Often others elsewhere.

There is no need to remove the lump, unless there is any doubt about the diagnosis.

### ■ Undescended Testicle

*(See page 363)*

## RARE

### ■ Aneurysm of Blood Vessel

The large femoral artery, which carries blood to the leg, passes near to the surface in the groin. Its wall can weaken and it expands like a balloon, producing:

- A lump, pulsating in time with your heartbeat.
- Often tender.

Can be repaired surgically.

### ■ Tumors and Abscesses

As with lumps anywhere on the body, the possibility of a tumor or an abscess has to be kept in mind. Abscesses typically are rapidly swelling, painful tender lumps with redness and heat in the overlying skin; they may discharge pus or need surgical drainage. Tumors may be suggested if there is a hard, growing lump attached to surrounding tissues. There may be symptoms from tumors else- where or other symptoms of serious ill- ness, such as weight loss. In either case, seek medical advice right away.

## LOSS OF PUBIC HAIR

Although it is not a common problem, it is alarming to the individual when it happens. Thinning of the hair is a normal feature of aging, and it occurs as an ex- pected side effect of chemotherapy for cancer. Otherwise, it is probably caused by hormone disturbances.

### PROBABLE

#### ■ Alopecia

Alopecia is general term for hair loss of unknown cause occurring in both men and women. Typical features are:

• Thinning of hair, perhaps with some actual hairless patches.

• In severe cases, there is complete, generalized hair loss.

• Loss of eyebrows, armpit hair, and pubic hair.

Alopecia may resolve spontaneously, although some cases persist. Treatment is difficult and carries a low success rate.

### ■ Cirrhosis of the Liver

Usually due to alcoholism.

• Hair thins rather than disappears.

• Small, dilated veins appear on face and chest.

• Red palms.

• Impotence.

• Swollen ankles.

• Nausea, indigestion.

• Easy bruising.

### RARE

#### ■ Addison's Disease

A consequence of underactive adrenal glands, causing:

• Profound weakness.

• Dark patches in the mouth, on the gums, or on old scars.

• Weight loss.

• Nausea, vomiting, and stomach cramps.

• Fainting.

# THE BRAIN AND NERVOUS SYSTEM

The brain and the nervous system are unique among all the systems and parts of the body considered in this book as they are both the physical seat of the psyche and all that makes up thought, personality, and who we are and what we feel. In addition, they are physically the command and control centers for all the workings of the body. Ultimately, all symptoms are located in the brain, which in turn controls their perception and expression. Physical processes that affect the brain and nerves may cause symptoms—a brain hemorrhage, causing a stroke, may cause paralysis. Similarly, a person suffering from dissociation (hysteria) may present with an equally debilitating paralysis, but in this case the problem lies within the functioning of the mind and the realms of mental illness.

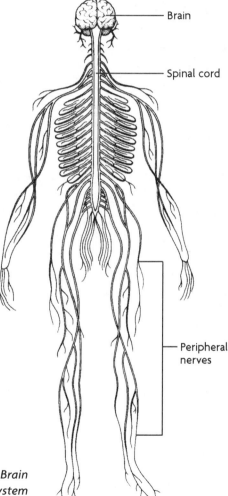

Brain

Spinal cord

Peripheral nerves

*The Brain and Nervous System*

383

This chapter describes a series of common symptoms that relate to the brain and nervous system. There is some overlap with symptoms described in other parts of the book. Topics are arranged alphabetically.

## ANXIETY

Anxiety can be defined as a state of worry and fear. It is universal and one might correctly identify it as part of the normal human experience. Mild degrees increase the body's readiness to deal with the problems of life, but it becomes abnormal when it is out of proportion to the situation or when one problem or event becomes the focus of severe worry and starts to interfere with daily life *(see Phobias and Obsessions, page 419)*. The symptoms are multiple and include:

• A feeling of tension mingled with apprehension and agitation.

• "Butterflies" in the stomach.

• Feeling of impending doom.

• Headache.

• Sweating—hands, armpits, and forehead are particularly affected.

• Insomnia.

• Palpitations.

• Dry mouth.

• Tremor.

But many other symptoms occur as well, such as overbreathing, impotence, dizzy turns, and restlessness. In children, there may be bed-wetting, nail biting, thumb sucking, and so on.

### PROBABLE

#### ■ Anxiety State

Worry comes naturally to human beings, to some more naturally than to others. Heredity plays a part. Every society has its own anxieties: the worry of choosing perfectly matched table decorations does not, on the face of it, compare with the worry of a saber-toothed tiger intent on repossessing your cave. But who are we to judge? Childhood experiences, repressed sexual urges, the depersonalization of modern society—all are, theoretically, reasonable explanations of anxiety. One thing is certain: there is more and more of it about.

Diagnosing anxiety is usually straightforward, based on the symptoms given above. Sympathetic discussion will usually reveal an underlying cause of stress. Physical symptoms as alarming as breathlessness may need investigating before the individual can accept the symptom is psychological in origin. Treatment ranges from drugs for acute, disabling anxiety to explanation via counseling or psychotherapy, such as cognitive behavioral therapy (CBT).

## POSSIBLE

### ■ Other Psychological Disease or Mental Illness

Possible when anxiety appears:

- In previously stable personality.
- Without an obvious source of stress.
- With other disturbance of mood, thought, or concentration.
- Accompanied by bizarre behavior or beliefs.
- Accompanied by severe memory problems or disorientation.

Possibilities, which are dealt with separately and should be followed up, include depression *(page 379)*, dementia *(page 376)*, and schizophrenia *(page 395)*.

### ■ Overactive Thyroid Gland

Gives all the symptoms of anxiety, but there are suggestive additional features:

- Fine tremor.
- Weight loss.
- Increased appetite.
- Intolerance to heat.
- Rapid pulse.
- Bulging eyes.
- Swelling in the neck.

The condition is easily confirmed with a blood test.

### ■ Drug and Alcohol Effects

Drugs such as amphetamines and cocaine commonly trigger anxiety. Similarly, withdrawal from many abused drugs (for instance, heroin and benzodiazepine tranquilizers) and from alcohol in alcoholics may cause:

- Coarse tremor.
- Anxiety.
- Sweating.
- Hallucinations.

There may be other features of drug abuse, such as:

- Neglected appearance.
- Needle marks on limbs.
- Social disintegration, crime, unemployment.

Specialized clinics are available to help with these problems.

## RARE

### ■ Low Blood Sugar

Usually occurs in a person with diabetes who is on treatment with tablets or insulin. The symptoms appear rapidly and consist of:

- Light-headedness.
- Sweating.
- Hunger.
- Drowsiness.

The condition is readily confirmed by testing of blood glucose levels and reverses quickly with glucose and carbohydrate supplements.

### ■ Pheochromocytoma

A very rare tumor that produces hormones leading to high blood pressure.

The level of hormones can rapidly increase, causing:

- Sudden anxiety, sweating, palpitations.
- Pallor or flushing.
- Headache.

When an attack is in progress, blood pressure will be very high.

## COMA

Coma is a precise medical term meaning a state of unrousability and unresponsiveness to stimuli. At its most severe, there is:

- No response to pain.
- No movement.
- No speech.

Stupor is less severe, as the individual can be roused by painful stimuli. The causes are the same. There are many stages in between the two, such as sleepiness and confusion, and there may be delirium as well.

Cases of coma require urgent hospital admission to treat and support vital body functions and in order to search for the many possible causes. You will be providing extremely useful information to the hospital if you can report on:

- A history of diabetes; any drowsiness and confusion in the preceding hours.

- Evidence of drug and alcohol abuse, such as bottles, syringes.

- Epilepsy, with details of previous fits and of medication.

- A head injury in the previous few weeks.

- Previous stroke; treatment for high blood pressure.

- Depression and suicidal intent; evidence such as empty pill containers.

### PROBABLE

### ■ Stroke

Usually in the elderly.
- Sudden collapse.
- One-sided paralysis.
- Loss of speech.

A very sudden severe headache at the back of the head, accompanied by vomiting and followed rapidly by loss of consciousness, suggests a particular type of stroke called a subarachnoid hemorrhage *(see page 110).*

### ■ Drugs or Alcohol

Diagnosis depends on knowledge of the person's habits and other pointers, such as the smell of alcohol. Opiate drug abuse is a strong possibility if there are:
• Needle marks (red marks on the arms or thickened hard veins).
• Pinpoint-sized pupils.
• Shallow breathing.

Deliberate overdose of prescription drugs as a suicide attempt may be suggested by:
• A history of depression or mental illness.
• Recent major life event or loss.
• Finding a suicide note or empty medication containers.

### ■ Injury

A head injury is the most common injury causing coma, usually following an accident. The diagnosis will be obvious. Recovery depends on the degree of brain trauma.

Stupor or coma occurring a few weeks after a serious head injury may be due to blood clot on the brain *(see Subdural Hematoma, page 391)* resulting from that injury; this condition is more common in the elderly, alcoholics, or those taking anticoagulants. Surgical removal of the blood clot usually allows for full recovery.

### ■ Metabolic Disease

Most probably diabetes, liver failure, or kidney failure, usually already known about.
• Hypoglycemia (low blood sugar) is suggested initially by light-headedness, hunger, shakiness, and confusion, followed by increasing drowsiness and unconsciousness.
• Hyperglycemia (high blood sugar) is often accompanied by another illness or missed insulin injections and suggested by thirst, vomiting, deep heavy breathing, and increased or reduced urine output, followed by increasing drowsiness and unconsciousness.
• Liver failure may be suggested by a history of previous alcoholism or other liver diseases and there may be jaundice or ascites (filling of the abdominal cavity with fluid).
• Kidney failure may be suggested by an alteration or loss of urine output, though frequently the diagnosis only comes to light after a blood test.

Treatment is aimed at correcting the metabolic disturbance, such as giving sugar to the diabetic patient with hypoglycemia.

■ **Epilepsy**

After a severe convulsion, someone suffering from epilepsy may be comatose for a few minutes or longer.

## POSSIBLE

■ **Infection**

Although any severe infection may cause coma through shock, meningitis is the most likely, especially in babies. It should be suspected in any infant showing otherwise unexplained:

- Irritability, drowsiness.
- Increasing drowsiness.
- Purple rash on body.
- In a baby, a bulging soft spot on the skull.

In older children, teenagers, and adults, there may also be:

- Severe headache.
- Neck stiffness.
- Aversion to bright lights.
- Vomiting.

Meningitis is a life-threatening emergency. Take the individual to a hospital without delay.

■ **Heart Attack**

Coma following:

- Severe chest pain.
- Breathlessness.
- Sweating and blue lips.
- May have known risk factors, including high blood pressure or high cholesterol, smoker, family history, and diabetes.

## RARE

■ **Hypothermia**

A profound drop in body temperature, most common in the elderly, in winter, or following a fall or a stroke.

■ **Other Causes**

A book could be written about the other causes of coma, since it can be the final scenario of any serious upset to the body's working. Rare causes can only be diagnosed after investigations, blood tests, and medical examination.

## CONCENTRATION, LACK OF

A person's attention span is very variable and depends on factors such as mood, conditions of work, and stress. There is rarely any serious reason for this symptom. Children have much shorter attention spans than adults, as measured scientifically by the "but you've only just had an ice cream" test.

## PROBABLE

### ■ Tiredness

May affect adults and children.
- Normally sound health and adequate concentration.
- Obvious lack of rest or overwork.

Concentration returns after rest. May be accompanied by insomnia or disturbed sleep.

### ■ Anxiety

*(See page 384)*

### ■ Depression

*(See page 379)*

### ■ Drugs and Alcohol

Alcohol intoxication produces obvious problems with concentration and behavior. Likewise, chronic alcoholism may damage the brain, leading to cognitive impairment and concentration difficulties.

Many prescription drugs, such as tranquilizers, reduce concentration. Similarly, drugs of abuse, such as cocaine and heroin, produce the same effect.

## POSSIBLE

### ■ Attention Deficit/Hyperactivity Disorder (ADHD)

Symptoms start in early childhood, progress through adolescence, and may persist into early adulthood. Typical features include:
- Constantly on the go.
- Constant movements and restlessness.
- Behind or in trouble at school.
- Impulsive or inconsiderate behavior.
- Disobedience and lack of discipline.
- Familial tendency.

Treatment is usually undertaken with the help of specialist services and may include the use of psychostimulant drugs such as methylphenidate, behavioral therapy, and special educational input.

## CONFUSION

Confusion is a combination of disorientation and emotional upset. Gradual onset of confusion over weeks and months is most likely to occur in the elderly and may be part of the natural aging process or degenerative brain disorders *(see also Dementia, page 396)*.

Sudden confusion at any age may have an immediate underlying medical cause and needs urgent investigation. It may be accompanied by drowsiness or altered consciousness, agitation, delusions, or hallucinations *(see also Delirium, page 394)*.

## PROBABLE

### ■ Senile Confusion

Seen in the elderly or very elderly. At its worst, it develops into dementia *(page 396)*, but for many elderly people, confusion is just a nuisance. Features that suggest senile confusion are:
• Memory for recent events becomes poor. Confusion follows and the individual may become disorientated in time and place.
• General health normal for age.
• No confusion or problems with familiar tasks and journeys.
• Can cope by using notes, lists.
• Social functioning unaffected or mildly impaired.
• Deterioration occurs only gradually, but major changes in lifestyle—for example, a vacation—may bring it on.

## POSSIBLE

### ■ Abnormal Blood Sugar Levels with Diabetes

• Hypoglycemia (low blood sugar) is suggested initially by light-headedness, hunger, shakiness, and confusion, followed by increasing drowsiness and unconsciousness.
• Hyperglycemia (high blood sugar) is often accompanied by another illness or missed insulin injections and suggested by thirst, vomiting, deep heavy breath-

ing, and increased or reduced urine output, followed by increasing drowsiness, confusion, and unconsciousness.

The condition is confirmed by measuring blood sugar levels. Diabetic patients should be taught how to recognize and treat hypoglycemia and hyperglycemia and to seek medical advice when it occurs.

### ■ Drugs or Alcohol

This diagnosis tends to rely on knowledge of a previous history of drug abuse or alcoholism. In alcoholics, an acute state of confusion may accompany alcohol withdrawal and needs urgent medical attention. Many prescription drugs (such as sleep aids), especially when used in the elderly patient, may potentially cause confusion.

### ■ Heart Failure

Confusion as a symptom of heart failure is most likely to affect the elderly, especially those with a known history of heart disease, high blood pressure, or diabetes. Suggested by:
• Shortness of breath on exercise.
• Swollen ankles.
• Breathlessness on lying flat in bed.
• Recent chest pain could indicate a heart attack or angina, which may accompany or be associated with heart failure.

### ■ Infections

In the elderly (and children), any infection may worsen a tendency to confusion. There may or may not be a fever. Common infections may present as:
• Cough and phlegm with a chest infection or pneumonia.
• Need to pass urine frequently suggests a bladder infection.
• A combination of confusion, headache, neck stiffness, and aversion to light suggests meningitis, needing emergency hospital care.

### ■ Minor Stroke

• Sudden confusion.
• Sudden slurring of speech or difficulty finding words.
• Face may droop on one side.
• Possibly loss of function or sensation in an arm and leg.

Recovery from such minor strokes is often rapid—always see a doctor for further assessment.

### ■ Respiratory Failure

Most likely in someone with chronic bronchitis or emphysema, usually a smoker.
• Long history of breathlessness, cough, and phlegm.
• A chest infection may be the trigger.
• Blue lips and tongue.
• Warm hands.

Needs hospital treatment.

### ■ Hypothermia

Confusion is a common early symptom of low body temperature. Usually affects the elderly living alone during winter months.

### ■ Underactive Thyroid Gland

*(See page 351)*

### ■ Metabolic Failure

This includes liver and kidney disease.
• Liver disease is suggested by previous history of alcoholism, jaundice, easy bruising, red palms, and swollen ankles.
• Kidney disease is suggested by either very high or very low urine output, anemia, malaise, or yellow tinge to skin.

Usually diagnosed on a blood test.

### ■ Subdural Hematoma

This is a collection of blood adjacent to the tissues wrapping the brain. Occurs following a head injury and later results in pressure on the brain. This condition is more common in the elderly, alcoholics, or those taking anticoagulants.
• Symptoms emerge over several weeks following a history of head injury or fall.
• A fluctuating degree of confusion and abnormal behavior.
• One-sided weakness of arm and leg may develop.

Diagnosed by computerized tomography (CT) or magnetic resonance imaging (MRI) scan. Small clots may resolve spontaneously, while larger ones require neurosurgery to remove them, usually with good recovery.

## CONVULSIONS

The features of a convulsion, also known as a fit or epileptic attack, are:

• Possibly a warning of an impending attack, called an aura—it may be a feeling, a visual disturbance, a smell, or a headache.

• The individual may cry out, then collapse unconscious.

• Remains stiff; may turn blue around the lips for about thirty seconds.

• Arms and legs then begin to jerk in a coordinated manner.

• Possibly incontinence of urine, frothing at the mouth, and cheek or tongue biting.

• Afterwards, drowsiness and confusion before a return to normal.

Not all convulsions are as dramatic. One form of convulsion is no more than a brief absence of consciousness, which may be misinterpreted as a blank look. A convulsion is different from a simple faint, where there is no aura, incontinence, or shaking of limbs. Investigations are needed if there is any doubt.

### PROBABLE

#### ■ Epilepsy

Epilepsy is caused by abnormal electrical discharges in the brain. Most cases are of unknown origin, but it can result from previous brain injury, for instance, a stroke or head injury. Alternatively, there may be a structural abnormality causing it, such as a brain tumor or an anomaly in the cerebral blood vessels. Anyone having a fit for the first time needs careful medical assessment, which would include blood tests, computerized tomography (CT) or magnetic resonance imaging (MRI) scan of the brain, and an electroencephalogram (a recording of the electrical brain activity).

Some patients with epilepsy are advised to avoid situations that would be dangerous if they had a fit, such as climbing ladders, driving, swimming, or using hazardous machinery. Treatment usually involves long-term medication with anticonvulsant drugs, though some people manage without if the condition resolves.

## ■ Febrile Fit

Febrile fits occur in children between the ages of six months and five years. They are fairly common, occurring in some 10 percent of all children, and do not mean that the child will grow up to become epileptic. Parents observing their child having a first fit frequently fear that death is occurring or is imminent, though this is not the case. Typical symptoms associated with a febrile convulsion are:

• Child is feverish, typically with a cold or ear infection.

• The fit usually occurs early on in the fever, as the temperature rises.

• Sudden stiffness, rolling of eyes, breathing stops, and the child may turn blue.

• Then, coordinated jerking of limbs and possibly incontinence.

• May last five to ten minutes.

• Child recovers and becomes responsive, but remains drowsy for a few hours.

A child having febrile fit for the first time needs immediate medical attention. Often, admission to a hospital will be advised, where the cause of the fever will be sought. Usually, this turns out to be a minor respiratory or viral infection, though meningitis is a rare possible cause.

Children who have recurrent febrile fits can be managed at home, as long as the parents know how to give an anti-convulsant if the fit becomes prolonged. Most febrile fits can be prevented by giving acetaminophen or ibuprofen at the first sign of a fever, which works by reducing body temperature; exposing and cooling the skin also helps.

In children below six months or older than five years, it is not safe to make a diagnosis of febrile fits, and other causes must be considered by a professional.

## POSSIBLE

## ■ Alcohol-Related

Convulsions are usually precipitated by sudden abstention from alcohol in a person with problematic drinking or alcoholism. They may be accompanied by withdrawal shakes or hallucinations. Long-term treatment should be aimed at addressing the problem drinking or alcoholism. Alcoholics are as likely as anyone else to develop true epilepsy, so the usual full assessment should be made.

## ■ Head Injury

A convulsion happening after a head injury should always be assessed in a hospital, as significant brain injury may have occurred

## ■ Stroke

A convulsion can sometimes accompany a stroke; hospital assessment is mandatory.

## ■ Meningitis

An infection around the brain that is possible at all ages, but is especially worrisome in childhood.

## ■ Metabolic Disorder

This usually means breakdown in the function of the kidneys or liver and should be detected on routine investigation of epilepsy. Low blood sugar (hypoglycemia) in diabetes is a possible cause of a convulsion.

## RARE

## ■ Eclampsia of Pregnancy

A risk of later pregnancy or following birth—the blood pressure suddenly rises too high and the mother has a convulsion. The situation should nearly always be avoidable by routine prenatal checks aimed at identifying preeclampsia, the condition which precedes it. Warning symptoms suggesting preeclampsia are:

- Fingers and feet swell rapidly.
- Sudden weight gain.
- Headache, flashing lights.
- Irritability.
- Abdominal or chest pain.

Tests will show high blood pressure, protein in the urine, and abnormal blood biochemistry. This is an emergency, calling for urgent specialist assessment. Treatment is aimed at safely delivering the baby at the earliest opportunity, while monitoring the mother for the complications of high blood pressure and the other bodily disturbances associated with the condition.

## DELIRIUM

Delirium is characterized by the rapid appearance of confusion, restlessness, hallucinations, and incoherent speech and thought. It is often worse at night. The confusion may fluctuate, with severe symptoms interspersed with relatively normal phases. The causes are those given under Confusion *(page 389)*, but with an added urgency because of the greater risk of serious underlying illness, and with a higher chance of an infection being the cause. The elderly are likely to become delirious during an otherwise moderately serious illness. In children, delirium frequently accompanies a feverish illness and should be treated by bringing the temperature down.

It is wise to seek medical advice if there is any suspicion of:

- Headache.
- Aversion to light.
- Neck stiffness.

Meningitis may be the cause, and immediate medical attention is needed.

## DELUSIONS

There is no reliable definition of a delusion. Conventionally, it is a belief that appears unfounded in reality—reality as judged by a reasonable group of people sharing the same cultural background. The difficulty in defining what constitutes a delusion gives scope for gross abuse of the term. It has, indeed, been a convenient way of labeling as mentally ill those who have held such "shocking" beliefs as liberty, democracy, and freedom. Nevertheless, there are individuals who hold beliefs that are so bizarre that they are taken as prime signs of mental illness. The unshakable conviction, for instance, that you are Napoleon Bonaparte or that if your left knee itches, then your wife is being unfaithful. The deluded person may then act on that belief, so that what appears to be a motiveless action proves to have been the logical outcome of a delusion. With appropriate caveats, psychiatrists therefore take delusions seriously.

### PROBABLE

■ Schizophrenia

This is a common mental illness in which the sufferer experiences a psychotic distortion of thinking and perception. The illness damages the thought processes that give a normal person their sense of individuality, personality, and self-direction. About 1 percent of the population suffers from this condition. A "schizoid state" is less serious condition and describes individuals who have an abnormal set of emotional responses and relationships with others and are frequently loners. Schizophrenia is not the "split personality" of popular myth. In fact the derivation of the word means "shattered mind," a description that very aptly describes the disorder. Most specialists believe that schizophrenia is the result an abnormality of brain chemistry.

Treatment based on this view is quite successful and may enable good social integration and functioning. Onset typically occurs in early adulthood and may endure long term. Specialist assessment and treatment with ongoing medication is usually advisable. Families and caregivers also need support.

Typical symptoms include:

• Delusions ranging from single ideas to whole networks of belief about the nature of reality. Typically, there is a complete lack of insight that the thoughts or delusions might be abnormal.
• Hallucinations, often hearing voices.
• Paranoia.
• Fragmentation in the train of thoughts, with bizarre or incoherent speech.

- Mood is often flat and emotionless.
- Apathy, self-neglect.
- Odd or abnormal behavior or movement.

## POSSIBLE

### ■ Early Dementia

*(See Dementia, below)* In the early stages, memory loss may result in giving delusional explanations for events, whose cause the individual has forgotten: for example, believing that a mislaid handbag has been stolen.

### ■ Depression

Those with severe depression may come to hold delusions about their own health or that of their families—for example, they may believe themselves or a loved one has an incurable disease. Delusions may also convince a sufferer that they are so worthless that suicide seems a logical option. Treatment with antidepressants and other measures are effective and may be lifesaving.

## DEMENTIA

With dementia, there is a general deterioration of intellectual capacity, together with impairment of memory. Dementia becomes more common with age. About 20 percent of those over eighty suffer from some degree of it. Once established, the condition inevitably deteriorates, though the progression occurs at very variable rates. Symptoms include:

- Memory loss—an early symptom, particularly of recent events or conversations, long-term memories are initially preserved.
- Disorientation—unable to identify correct current location and time.
- Slow thinking, muddled thought, and increasing confusion.

- Personality change.
- Self-neglect and loss of initiative.
- Depression and anxiety accompany early awareness of deterioration.
- Disturbed behavior.
- Delusions and hallucinations.
- Eventually incontinence, weight loss, and bedridden state.

Despite this picture, the individual appears fully conscious, with no drowsiness. Medical advice should be sought so that the cause of the dementia can be established. Investigations may include psychometric testing of mental state, physical examination, blood tests, and computerized tomography (CT) scanning.

Treatment depends on the cause of the dementia and presenting symptoms. Drug treatment may partially relieve some of the symptoms or at least slow progression, though the results may be disappointing. Social support and care are equally important to the sufferer and their caregiver or family, who often shoulder much of the burden.

## PROBABLE

### ■ Alzheimer's Disease

This is the most common cause of dementia, accounting for 65 percent of cases. The symptoms are listed above.

### ■ Vascular Dementia (Multi-Infarct Dementia)

This type of dementia accounts for a further 25 percent of cases. Essentially, it consists of damage to the brain resulting from multiple tiny strokes. Symptoms are listed above but also include:

• Onset sometimes sudden.

• Stepwise deterioration (corresponding to the occurrence of the multiple small strokes).

• Often accompanied by a history of high blood pressure or other vascular disease or other types of stroke.

Treatment of high blood pressure or the causes of the mini-strokes may help.

## POSSIBLE

### ■ Drug Effects

Might be suspected if:

• Dementia appears rapidly and fluctuates.

• The individual is on multiple treatments, especially common with tranquilizers and drugs to treat Parkinson's disease.

Condition improves when the offending drug is stopped.

### ■ Alcoholism

Gives rise to a distinct form of dementia due to lack of B vitamins.

• Profound loss of memory for recent events.

• A tendency to make up excuses to cover up for memory loss.

• Disorders of eye movements, for instance, jerking.

• Unsteady gait.

This condition is treatable with high-dose vitamin supplements.

### ■ Dementia with Lewy Bodies

This type of dementia includes the following specific, additional features:

• Pronounced "fluctuations" in alertness and attention, such as frequent drowsiness, lethargy, lengthy periods of time spent staring into space, or disorganized speech.

- Recurrent visual hallucinations.
- Symptoms mimicking Parkinson's disease, such as rigidity and the loss of spontaneous movement.
- May also cause depression.

## ■ HIV/AIDS

A symptom of AIDS in HIV-positive individuals. Most common in countries where HIV is widespread and where medical resources are scanty.

- May present with psychiatric symptoms and personality change initially.
- Clumsiness and difficulty walking are common accompaniments.

Dementia of this type is largely preventable with highly active antiretroviral therapy (HAART) given in the earlier stages of HIV disease. If it occurs, the dementia can improve dramatically with HAART treatment.

## RARE

### ■ Huntington's Chorea

- Family history (this disease has a known inheritance).
- Involuntary coarse movements and tremor of limbs may be the first symptom.
- Begins in one's thirties or forties.
- Physical and mental deterioration is progressive and inevitable.

## ■ Hypothyroidism

*(See page 351)* Treatment with thyroid hormone will reverse this condition.

## ■ Hydrocephalus

An uncommon condition of increased pressure and volume of fluid within the brain, usually found when a computerized tomography (CT) or magnetic resonance imaging (MRI) scan of the brain is done. Additional symptoms include:

- The degree of confusion fluctuates.
- Urinary incontinence.
- Unsteady gait.
- Clumsiness.

Treatments are available.

## ■ Liver and Kidney Disease

Should be detected on routine screening. *(See under Metabolic Failure, page 391)*

## ■ Meningioma

A very slow-growing brain tumor. Apart from dementia, dependent on its position, it may cause:

- Epilepsy.
- Weakness of an arm or a leg.
- Progressive headache.
- Loss of sense of smell.

Diagnosis will be confirmed by a brain scan.

## ■ Brain Hematoma

A blood clot on the brain, following a head injury. A possible cause of dementia of rapid onset. *(See Subdural Hematoma, page 391)*

## ■ Vitamin B$_{12}$ Deficiency

Another rare but treatable cause of dementia.

- Pernicious anemia.
- Tingling in the hands and feet.

## ■ Creutzfeldt-Jakob Disease (CJD) or Variant CJD

This is the human equivalent of mad cow disease (bovine spongiform encephalopathy or BSE). May be accompanied by fits, paralysis, or visual problems.

## ■ Syphilis

In its final stages, and many years after first infection, syphilis can cause dementia, plus:

- Unsteady gait.
- Drooping eyelids.
- Delusions, often of grandeur.
- Small, irregular pupils.

Blood tests will confirm the diagnosis and antibiotic treatment can then halt, though not reverse, the condition.

## DEPRESSION

When is depression an illness and when is it a natural response to life's trials? Nearly everyone experiences feelings of depression and unhappiness at some point in their lives. This becomes a problem when it is prolonged, severe, or starts to interfere with normal functioning. Everyone has a duty to be aware of depression as a significant illness in its own right. Growing out of unhappiness, or perhaps just from long-term "knocks," clinical depression goes beyond unhappiness and carries the real risk of suicide. Mood, appearance, and speech are usually enough to make a firm diagnosis of severe depression. The symptoms, not all of which may be present, are familiar to all and include:

- Low mood, sadness, tearfulness, feelings of despair and hopelessness.
- Often worse in the morning and improves through the day.
- Inability to enjoy things.
- Lack of energy and poor concentration.
- Feelings of anxiety.
- Negative thoughts about the future.
- Slowing down of thought, speech, and movement.
- Feelings of guilt.
- Poor sleep with early morning wakening.

- Loss of appetite and weight.
- Self-disgust, low self-esteem, sense of failure.
- Suicidal thoughts.
- Loss of sexual desire or impotence.
- Preoccupation or worry about the presence of a physical illness.
- Lack of energy and constant exhaustion.
- Difficulty making decisions.
- Feeling that you're forgetful.
- Loss of identity.
- Loneliness, even when around others.

Telling a depressed person to pull themselves together is as useless as telling someone with appendicitis to snap out of it. The elderly deserve particular attention, as does anyone who has attempted suicide; also, women experiencing severe depression after childbirth. Treatments range from counseling to antidepressants to hospital admission for electroconvulsive therapy. Exercise and alternative or complementary therapies are also useful. People suffering from depression frequently believe that they will never get better; in fact, quite the reverse is usually true.

## POSSIBLE

### ■ Other Physical Disease

Depression is an extremely common accompaniment to significant physical illness, for instance, cancer, heart disease, stroke, and diabetes. Often, this is overlooked in the quest to look after the physical body. So much more can be gained by simultaneously treating the psyche.

### ■ Post-Viral Syndrome and Chronic Fatigue Syndrome (CFS)

- Usually follows a physical illness with aches and pains.
- Profound weakness and tiredness are common.
- Muscle aches.
- Unrefreshing sleep.
- Impaired memory and concentration.
- Mild depression common.

The cause of post-viral syndrome and CFS is not understood. There are no precise tests to diagnose or monitor the condition. Treatment is difficult, though it often improves with time. A program of gradually increasing activity and exercise may help, as does psychological support and sometimes antidepressant medication. Complementary or alternative therapies are widespread.

### ■ Early Dementia

*(See Dementia, page 396)* In the late middle-aged or elderly.

### ■ Early Schizophrenia

*(See page 395)*

## RARE

### ■ Hypothyroidism

A severely underactive thyroid gland may give rise to a state simulating depression. Some other hormone disorders may do likewise.

### ■ Parkinson's Disease

Generally, in the elderly.
- Tremor of hands.
- Stiff, shuffling gait.
- Impassive appearance.

This can be helped by drugs.

## DIZZINESS

Dizziness is a common symptom, but rather difficult to define since it can mean different things. For some, it appears to be an inability to concentrate, with feelings of light-headedness; for others, it is true vertigo with giddiness. Your doctor will try hard to pin down just what you mean by dizziness.

## DIZZINESS WITH VERTIGO

There is giddiness, unsteadiness, and the room spins when you turn your head. Vertigo is the illusion of movement. A person with true vertigo will be able to tell you which way the room is moving.

### PROBABLE

### ■ Labyrinthitis

A harmless balance disorder of the inner ear, giving rise to:
- Abrupt onset of giddiness.
- Worse when turning head or changing position suddenly.
- No pain or ringing in ear.
- When lying flat, you feel completely well.

Though alarming, the symptoms fade over a few days, sometimes with the help of anti-nausea drugs. It may be caused by a viral infection.

### ■ Benign Positional Vertigo

A condition caused by movement of matter within the fluid in the inner ear. Sudden vertigo lasting thirty seconds or more is provoked by head turning. Usually self-limiting within a few months, but sometimes treated by a special repositioning technique (Epley maneuvers) done by a doctor.

## POSSIBLE

■ **Ménière's Syndrome**

A gradual process of degeneration in the ear, symptoms include:

• Ringing in the ear (tinnitus) is an early feature.

• Gradually worsening deafness.

• Can effect one or both ears.

• Sudden attacks of vertigo, in which the above symptoms worsen for a few minutes.

Treatments include drugs and devices to mask the tinnitus.

## RARE

■ **Disease of the Brain or Spinal Cord**

Although highly unlikely as a cause of a few episodes of sudden dizziness, there are several such diseases—for example, multiple sclerosis—which can cause dizziness in combination with:

• Unsteady gait.

• Tingling or numbness of hands or feet.

• Visual disturbances, such as double vision.

• Weakness of an arm or leg.

A neurologist's opinion will be needed.

## DIZZINESS WITHOUT VERTIGO

The crucial clues are in what circumstances the dizziness occurs, at what time of day, for how long, how often, and how you feel before and afterward.

## PROBABLE

■ **Cause Unknown**

This accounts for a great majority of cases. A safe conclusion as long as:

• You are otherwise well.

• Attacks of dizziness are not prolonged or recurrent.

A medical checkup may be reassuring; investigations are not needed.

■ **Emotional Factors**

Here dizziness is used to mean:

• Inability to concentrate.

• A "band" around the head.

• Muddled thinking.

• Difficulty in making decisions.

Try to review what in your life is giving rise to unusual degrees of stress and worry.

## POSSIBLE

■ **Anemia**

• Pallor.

• Tiredness.

- Breathlessness.
- A light-headed feeling when you stand up.

Unless the cause of the anemia is obvious, for instance, very heavy periods, a prudent doctor will probably recommend some investigations.

### ■ Low Blood Pressure

- Dizziness when you stand up.
- Passes off after a few seconds.

This is common in the elderly, whose circulation is less efficient at making the rather complex adjustments for standing up. Occasionally, it is because treatment for high blood pressure has been overly effective and sometimes medication must be changed. It is also common in pregnancy. Another increasingly recognized cause is vasovagal syncope, where emotion causes low blood pressure. Specialized tests are now available, such as the tilt-table test.

### ■ Low Blood Sugar

Most common in people with diabetes, especially if a meal is missed.

- Rapid onset.
- Difficulty concentrating.
- Irritability.
- Sweating.

Symptoms are quickly relieved by eating.

## RARE

### ■ Heart and Circulatory Problems

These can really only be confirmed by medical examination or hospital tests. They become more common with age, and pointers include:

- Palpitations.
- A pulse rate that feels unusually fast, unusually slow, or irregular.
- Breathlessness.
- Chest pains.
- Dizziness when looking up.
- Symptoms of minor stroke, with temporary limb weakness, disturbed speech or vision.

The underlying problem may be abnormal heart rhythms or narrowed valves of the heart, conditions which can be treated. Most likely, arteries to the brain have become "furred up."

### ■ Polycythemia

The opposite of anemia, in which there is an over-concentration of blood. Most common in those with chronic lung problems, such as bronchitis and emphysema.

- A red complexion.
- Headaches.
- Itchiness of skin.

Treatment depends on the underlying cause.

■ **Temporal Lobe Epilepsy**

Difficult to diagnose if dizziness is the only reported feature. Other symptoms may include:

• A warning sensation (an aura) preceding the dizziness.
• Associated drowsiness.

## DROWSINESS

Drowsiness caused simply by lack of sleep or by excess alcohol is not covered here. Drowsiness in someone otherwise expected to be alert is an important symptom, and in children unusual drowsiness is a warning symptom that always needs medical assessment.

### PROBABLE

■ **Drug Effects**

Most likely in the elderly.

• Commonly found in those on sleeping tablets or sedative medication.
• Drowsiness clears as the day goes on.

The dosage of medication may need adjustment or shorter-acting drugs may be appropriate.

■ **Infection**

Drowsiness commonly accompanies the early stages of many illnesses, especially viral infections. There may also be:

• Fever.
• Aching eyes.
• The infection soon shows itself, typi-

cally as a cough, sore throat, or flu-like illness.

More serious infections need medical attention.

### POSSIBLE

■ **Obstructive Sleep Apnea**

During sleep, the muscles at the back of the mouth and upper airway relax and breathing becomes obstructed. During this obstruction, which lasts for periods of more than ten seconds each time, there is no breathing (apnea); this pattern recurs many times per hour. The oxygen levels in the blood fall, causing the sufferer to wake briefly (often unconsciously) with a sudden loud snore or breath, followed by further sleep, and the cycle repeats. The consequence is that sleep quality is very poor. Common features include:

• Frequently drops off to sleep in the day.
• Daytime fatigue.
• Spouse or partner notices snoring or episodes of apnea.

- Much more common in the over-weight, especially those with large neck size.
- May accompany chronic bronchitis, emphysema, or heart disease.

Treatment involves weight reduction, stopping smoking, and various devices to reposition the jaw and airway. In severe cases, pressurized air delivered through a mask at night—continuous positive airway pressure (CPAP) devices—help to keep the airway open.

### ■ Encephalitis

A nonspecific irritation of the brain, commonly caused by viral infections, but which may accompany meningitis.

- Severe, persistent drowsiness.
- Confusion.
- Headache.
- Bright lights hurt the eyes.
- As it worsens, convulsions, coma, paralysis of limbs.

If you suspect encephalitis in a child, get medical advice at once. Adults should also see a doctor unless the above com-bination of symptoms is very mild.

### ■ Head Injury

Drowsiness occurring after a blow to the head may signify bleeding within the skull. Other warning signs are:

- Confusion.

- Nausea and vomiting.
- Loss of use of a limb.
- Double vision.
- Slow pulse.

Urgent hospital assessment is needed.

## Rare

### ■ Brain Tumor

Brain tumors really are rare, and when they do occur, they have usually spread to the brain from a tumor elsewhere, typically the lung or breast. The features of a brain tumor are:

- Consistent and progressively worsen-ing headache, especially on waking, and easing through the day.
- Change of personality.
- Double vision.
- Later, paralysis of one side of the body—symptoms similar to a stroke.

Treatment depends on the type of tumor and its location.

### ■ Narcolepsy

- Sudden sleepiness, totally out of the blue.
- For a while, the individual cannot be roused.
- This unusual illness tends to run in families.

It is treated with stimulant drugs.

## EMOTIONAL INSTABILITY

Feelings of emotion are part of the normal human experience. The range of such feelings is enormous and their expression likewise is diverse and variable. Cultural factors play an important part here. Emotional instability typically becomes a problem when it occurs in somebody who has not previously suffered from it or when it appears to be out of context with the person's situation. Likewise, it becomes a problem when it interferes with normal social and psychological functioning. Symptoms that might indicate there is an underlying problem include:

• Changes in personality.

• Persistent irritability.

• Mood swings.

• Inappropriate behavior.

• Poor judgment, with loss of insight.

In some highly strung people, apparent emotional instability is merely an exaggeration of the normal. They have abrupt mood swings, often intensified by alcohol. They are not "ill" as long as:

• Emotional states do not interfere with work or social and domestic life.

• The individual retains insight into his or her personality.

• General health and thought processes appear normal—for instance, no delusions.

However trying such people may be, they are often successful and creative. That leaves relatively few underlying causes of emotional instability, which are outlined below.

### PROBABLE

#### ■ Anxiety

Anyone, whatever their previous personality, will become emotional under conditions of stress and tension. However, they will be aware of the change and they will retain insight into their personality. *(See page 384)*

### POSSIBLE

#### ■ Mental Illness

When emotional instability really does appear to exceed the norm, psychiatrists will look for:
• Delusions.
• Hallucinations.
• Loss of insight into behavior.
• Severe depression.
• Manic, irresponsible behavior.

Underlying diagnoses include bipolar disorder, severe depression, and schizophrenia.

■ **Menopause**

*(See page 349)*

■ **After Childbirth**

Feeling "the blues" shortly after childbirth is very common and usually settles with time. This differs from postnatal depression, which is more serious and usually requires professional support or treatment.

■ **Early Dementia**

*(See page 396)*

■ **After a Stroke**

Mood swings or frequent and immediate weeping are common after a stroke, particularly in the elderly or in the types of strokes that affect the base of the brain.

## RARE

■ **Brain Tumor**

*(See page 417)*

■ **Brain Disease**

Numerous conditions can affect emotional control and are covered under Dementia *(see page 396)*.

---

## FAINTING

A momentary interruption in the flow of blood to the brain will cause lightheadedness; a longer pause is very likely to become a faint. Serious causes are unusual, unless fainting is recurrent or abrupt.

### PROBABLE

■ **Harmless Causes**

The great majority of causes are trivial: standing too long in the heat, missing a meal, overtiredness. Fainting is common in pregnancy, after emotional shock, and in reaction to severe pain.
• Recovery occurs within moments.
• No convulsions or incontinence.

Lying down and raising the legs helps with recovery.

### POSSIBLE

■ **Low Blood Pressure**

*(See page 403)*
• Recurrent light-headedness upon standing.
• Most likely if you have diabetes or if you take drugs that affect or control your blood pressure.

### RARE

■ **Heart Problems**

Worth considering if there is:
• Faintness on exertion.

- Palpitations.
- Slow, rapid, or irregular pulse rates.

Most of the heart problems that will lead to fainting are treatable.

### ■ Bleeding

Faintness, in combination with injury or pain, may be a symptom of serious blood loss.

- Sweating.
- Pallor.
- Thirst.

Sometimes, a small cut can produce the same effect, possibly through psychological triggering. Careful examination will reveal the source of bleeding. If you suspect internal bleeding—for example, after a car accident—seek medical help immediately.

### ■ Epilepsy

*(See page 392)*

### ■ Minor Stroke

Suggested also by temporary loss of speech or of the use of a limb.

## HALLUCINATIONS

A sensory experience—a vision, a sound, a sensation—without any basis in reality. Dreams are "normal" hallucinations. Likewise, many normal people (including children), in the twilight state before sleep begins, see things that aren't there. These are described as hypnagogic hallucinations. Another common hallucination phenomenon occurs following bereavement; typically, the bereaved person reports hearing or seeing a loved one who has recently died. This is normal and does not signify any sort of mental illness. Other hallucinations occurring in clear consciousness can be symptoms of a psychiatric disorder and appropriate medical help should be sought.

### ■ Delirium

*(See page 394)*

### ■ Schizophrenia

*(See page 395)*

### ■ Depression

Very severe depression may give rise to hallucinations, for instance, of abusive mocking voices.

### RARE

### ■ Temporal Lobe Epilepsy

Hallucinations of smell and taste are the most common; may also present with other features such as convulsions. *(See page 392)*

## HYPERACTIVITY

Typically, a childhood problem, combining:

- Constantly on the go.
- Frequent movements and restlessness.
- Behind or in trouble at school.
- Impulsive or inconsiderate behavior.
- Disobedience and lack of discipline.
- Familial tendency.

*(In adults, see Mania and Hypomania, page 412)*

### POSSIBLE

#### ■ Normal Child

Some parents have a low tolerance for normal childhood behavior.

#### ■ Attention Deficit/Hyperactivity Disorder (ADHD)

*(See page 389)*

#### ■ Psychological Conflict

A possible diagnosis where the immediate family displays:

- Emotional conflict.
- Alcoholism.
- Mental illness.

### RARE

#### ■ Food Allergy

A controversial diagnosis, which may be supported by experimenting with rotation diets.

#### ■ Minimal Brain Damage

Most likely if there is also:

- Clumsiness, difficulty in completing simple manual tasks.
- Severe learning difficulties.

Such children often need special schooling. This syndrome is new and not fully defined. Not all doctors agree on its cause or how best to manage affected individuals.

## HYSTERIA AND DISSOCIATION

The popular definition of hysteria is wild, reckless, exaggerated behavior. The (more precise) medical definition is: symptoms that have no physical basis, which appear to arise without a conscious desire to deceive. The term "hysteria" has a somewhat pejorative feel to it and the condition is now more properly known as dissociation. It can be difficult, if not impossible, to prove that the behavior is not motivated by a need to deceive. Women, usually between the ages of thirty and fifty, are more commonly affected than men. Dissociation symptoms include:

- Amnesia.
- Blindness.
- Paralysis of a limb.
- Lack of speech.
- Difficulty swallowing.

## PROBABLE

### ■ Psychological Factors

This diagnosis has some validity when physical disease has been excluded and is likely if:

- There is demonstrable psychological bonus from the behavior—typically, attention or enhanced status.
- The sufferer is indifferent to symptoms a "normal" person would find devastating, for instance, blindness.
- Sometimes follows a known trauma, such as the soldiers in World War One exposed to the horrors of trench warfare.

Treatment is extremely difficult. It requires the sufferer to recognize that the costs of his or her behavior outweighs the short-term psychological gain. In most cases, recovery occurs within a year or so.

## POSSIBLE

### ■ Undetected Physical Disease

About 5 percent of people diagnosed with dissociation are subsequently found to have an actual physical disorder. This emphasizes the need for very careful physical assessment before arriving at the diagnosis.

## RARE

### ■ Brain Disease

Dissociation may be an early symptom of dementia or other brain disorder. If symptoms specific to these diseases accompany the condition, seek medical advice. (See Dementia, page 396)

## INSOMNIA

Sleep is still a mystery—that we all need it is certain, but how much is astonishingly variable. Imagined insomnia is often a mismatch between how much sleep someone thinks they need and how much their body really needs. It is often worth asking the individual's partner how much sleep they are getting.

## PROBABLE

### ■ Temporary Disturbance of Sleep Patterns

Worries, pain, and life's stresses all cause insomnia, which frequently persists once these problems have passed. Stimulants such as coffee and alcohol may be to blame, as may daytime snoozes. A cause is usually obvious, after a little reflection. Associated symptoms include:

- Daytime drowsiness.
- Sleep eventually comes because you are exhausted.

Logically, the cause of the insomnia should be addressed by trying to sort out the cause of the stress. If this is not possible, then other measures may help—for instance, it is best to not go to bed until you feel tired, to avoid stimulants such as caffeine, and to follow a set routine leading to bed that produces suitable relaxation. Exercise may also help. Sleeping tablets have a role, but only in the short-term treatment of insomnia. Long-haul air travel, where time zones are crossed, may present short-term problems; judicious use of sleeping tablets and melatonin can help here.

## POSSIBLE

### ■ Reduced Need for Sleep

For many people, "eight hours sleep and a daily bowel movement" is life's Golden Rule. Some individuals often cannot accept that they need far less of either, and the rules of the institutions where they may find themselves may reinforce this opinion. The fact is that a lot of people function perfectly normally with, say, four to six hours of sleep. Symptoms suggesting reduced need for sleep are:

- No obvious worries.
- No daytime drowsiness.

People with reduced need for sleep do well to accept that they have gained extra hours in their day, and that nature is telling them to do the ironing at 3 A.M. and to leave the extra daylight hours for better things.

### ■ Depression

Insomnia is an important symptom of depression (see page 410).

---

## IRRITABILITY

Greater than normal anger and hostility. No one need be in any doubt about normal irritability—it is a simple response to the "F words" of workaday life:

- Fatigue.
- Frustration.
- Feeling fed-up.

Hunger and lack of sleep often makes irritability worse. The more sinister causes of irritability are the following.

## POSSIBLE

### ■ Anxiety State

*(See page 384)* Irritability out of proportion to circumstances.

### ■ Drugs and Alcohol

Drug and alcohol intoxication both lead to irritability and unreasonable behavior.

## RARE

### ■ Early Dementia

*(See page 396)*

### ■ Head Injury

An injury severe enough to cause unconsciousness is frequently followed by:
• Irritability.
• Difficulty in concentrating.
• Mood swings.

### ■ Overactive Thyroid Gland

*(See page 350)*

### ■ Meningitis

*(See page 428)*

## MANIA AND HYPOMANIA

Mania is the opposite of depression. Typical symptoms include:
• Euphoria and elevated mood.
• Irritability.
• Distractibility and poor concentration.
• Hyperactivity.
• Insomnia.
• Ideas spilling out, but barely connected.
• Grandiose thoughts.
• Rapid speech.
• Nervous jittery activity.
• Poor judgment with loss of insight.
• Hallucinations.

Full-blown cases of mania are rare. Hypomania, which is much more common, has the same symptoms but is less severe.

## PROBABLE

### ■ Bipolar Disorder

This disorder (also known as manic depression) consists of alternating periods of high (manic) and low (depression) moods. It is a long-term condition, typically starting before the age of twenty-five. Characterized by:
• Recurrent mania.
• Recurrent depression.
• A combination of both.
• Sometimes there is a family history of the condition.

Treatment of the highs and lows are with sedatives and antidepressants, respectively. Most sufferers with severe recurrent symptoms benefit from mood stabilizers such as lithium.

### ■ Drugs

Amphetamines or cocaine may precipitate mania. Prescription drugs, such as steroids and antidepressants, can also be responsible.

### ■ Emotional Stress

A severe anxiety state may mimic a hypomanic state, though typically there is preservation of insight and self-neglect is rare. The source of the anxiety is often obvious.

## POSSIBLE

### ■ Schizoaffective Disorder

Sometimes there is a blurring of symptoms between the major mental disorders involving psychosis. This overlap between schizophrenia and mania is sometimes referred to as schizoaffective disorder. *(See also under Schizophrenia, page 395)*

### ■ Overactive Thyroid Gland

*(See page 350)*

### ■ Dementia

Mania arises from the loss of inhibition, a distressing combination. *(See page 396)*

## MEMORY IS POOR

It is common to have an excellent memory for some types of information, such as names, but a poor memory for others, such as phone numbers.

### ■ Normal Aging Process

Every day, 10,000 of our brain cells die, more than 250 million die over a seventy-year lifetime. A dense web of additional cells and rich interconnections mask the effects of this loss, but eventually it catches up with us, and we notice our memory worsening. This normal process rarely produces more than passing irritation, differing from dementia in this respect. Typical symptoms include:

- Memory for long-past events remains good.
- Difficulty in learning new tasks.
- Personality generally unchanged.

### ■ Dementia

*(See page 396)*

### ■ Anxiety

Interferes with concentration and memory. *(See page 384)*

### ■ Head Injury

Following a head injury, there may be loss of memory for the time around the trauma. Later on, there may be difficulty with concentration and poor memory retention.

## Stroke

Sudden loss of memory, together with:
- Loss of use of a limb.
- Interference with speech.

There is often recovery from a minor stroke over several months.

*(See also Confusion, page 389)*

## Psychological Trauma and Dissociation

Severe psychological trauma can result in distortion or blocking of memory. One example is post-traumatic stress disorder.

*(See also Hysteria and Dissociation, page 409)*

---

# MENTAL IMPAIRMENT

A general lack of intellectual capacity, as shown by:
- Poor learning ability.
- Difficulty in coping with complex situations.
- Poor language skills.
- Clumsiness.

Past illness or injury may be to blame, but many cases remain unexplained.

## POSSIBLE

### Cerebral Palsy

Cerebral palsy refers to a group of disorders that involve loss of movement or loss of other nerve function. Often the cause is unknown, though it may involve a lack of oxygen resulting in brain damage around the time of birth. Many cerebral palsy sufferers have no mental impairment and merely suffer from movement or speech difficulties, though it can be part of the overall picture consisting of:
- Seizures.
- Muscle contractions.
- Difficulty sucking or feeding.
- Delayed development of motor skills, such as reaching, sitting, rolling, crawling, and walking.
- Mental impairment and learning disability.
- Speech problems.
- Visual problems.
- Hearing problems.
- Spasticity.
- Joint contractures that slowly get worse.
- Limited range of motion.

### ■ Congenital

A similar picture to that of cerebral palsy *(see page 414)*, but with specific features giving a recognized condition, such as Down syndrome.

### ■ Stroke

A reason for sudden deterioration in a previously normal intellect.

### POSSIBLE

### ■ Dementia

*(See page 396)*

### ■ Head Injury

Has much the same effect as a stroke.

### RARE

### ■ Degenerative Disorders of the Nervous System

This can happen in several ways. Possible if:

- Intellect was previously normal.
- Gradual deterioration of thought processes.
- Associated tremors, weakness, paralysis, and epilepsy.

Diagnosis is for a specialist.

### ■ Vitamin Deficiencies

Affects the growing child and is a tragic cause of impaired intellect in underdeveloped countries.

- Poor growth.
- Swollen belly, poor bone formation.
- Loss of hair, patchy pigmentation of skin.

Vitamin deficiencies are also found in alcoholics.

### ■ Metabolic Disorders

Such as liver and kidney disease.

## PARALYSIS, RAPID ONSET

Usually means the inability to use an arm or leg, but less commonly affecting muscles of the eyes, swallowing, and breathing. The manner of onset gives a clue to the cause. Urgent medical attention is always needed.

### PROBABLE

### ■ Stroke

This is by far the most likely cause. The mechanism is an interference in the blood flow to the brain, usually from a blood vessel blocked with a clot. A

thrombosis is where a clot forms within the brain circulation; an embolism is where a clot travels from outside of the head, typically the heart or arteries in the neck. Alternatively, a vessel bursts, causing a hemorrhage in the brain. Characteristic features and symptoms are:
• Normally in the middle-aged or elderly.
• Often a history of high blood pressure, high cholesterol, smoking, or diabetes.
• Paralysis affects one side of the body and face.
• Speech is slurred or lost.
• Confusion of variable degree, even coma.

Medical attention must be sought urgently. Investigations are initially designed to locate and define the cause of the stroke, usually by computerized tomography (CT) scanning. If a hemorrhage can be excluded, then drugs may be given to dissolve the clot (thrombolysis), although this can only be usefully done within six hours of the onset of the stroke. Otherwise, treatment consists of aspirin plus attention to underlying causes, such as high blood pressure or heart disease. A stroke caused by an embolism may be treated with an anticoagulant drug (warfarin). Good nursing care, intensive physiotherapy, and occupational therapy are also crucial. In many cases, a good return of function is achieved. Occasionally, investigations show a brain tumor or abscess.

### ■ Subarachnoid Hemorrhage

A special type of stroke, caused by a bleeding blood vessel on the surface of the brain. Relatively common in those aged fifty-five to sixty, but possible at any age.
• Sudden, severe headache, "like being hit on the back of the head."
• Vomiting.
• Collapse, neck stiffness, aversion to light.
• Sometimes coma and sudden death.

Surgical intervention is sometimes necessary to stop bleeding from the vessel and to prevent further occurrences.

### ■ Injury

A severe blow to the head.
• Probably coma and one-sided paralysis.

## POSSIBLE

### ■ Arterial Disease

Sudden paralysis of one leg, less commonly an arm, may be due to blockage of an artery with a blood clot (arterial embolus). Symptoms would include:
• Sudden pain in the affected limb.
• Sudden pallor of the limb, developing into blueness.

- The limb is extremely cold and looks lifeless.

To save the limb, the obstruction must be rapidly removed.

■ **Hysteria and Dissociation**

*(See page 409)*

## PARALYSIS, SLOW ONSET

### PROBABLE

■ **Compression of a Nerve**

Common sites are the neck (affecting the arms) or a slipped disc in the back (affecting a leg or foot).

- Persistent pain and tingling confined to one part of one limb.
- Partial weakness of the limb.
- Health otherwise sound.

Investigations will show a reason for the compression and exclude general disease of the nervous system. Treatment depends on the cause; for example, a slipped disc in the back may be treated by physiotherapy or chiropractic manipulation, or occasionally by surgery.

### POSSIBLE

■ **Multiple Sclerosis**

A slow degenerative disease of the young to middle-aged adults.

- Often begins with a sudden loss of vision in one eye.
- Numb patches, tingling, weakness of limbs, clumsiness.

- Symptoms come and go over months and years.
- Characteristically relapses occur with subsequent incomplete improvement.
- Bladder symptoms and infections are common.

The outlook is very variable, often with years of relatively good health. An unfortunate minority become severely disabled.

■ **Brain Tumor**

- Slow, progressive weakness of one side of the body.
- Headache.
- Change of personality.

The slow progression makes diagnosis difficult, but magnetic resonance imaging (MRI) or computerized tomography (CT) brain scans readily confirm the diagnosis.

■ **Vitamin B$_{12}$ Deficiency**

- Pallor.
- Tingling of hands and feet.
- Smooth, sore tongue.

- Stiff, weak legs.

The most common cause is pernicious anemia *(see page 494)*, easily treated with injections of vitamin $B_{12}$.

## RARE

### ■ Guillain-Barré Syndrome

A rare inflammation of the peripheral nerves that may follow a minor infection.
- Initially, tingling in the hands and feet.
- The condition worsens and paralysis of the limbs appears (may evolve over a few hours to as long as a few weeks).
- May spread to involve muscles of swallowing and breathing.

This serious condition needs intensive nursing care and sometimes assistance with breathing and feeding in an intensive care unit. Although recovery may take months, sufferers often recover completely or with only minor disability.

### ■ Motor Neuron Disease

An exceptionally rare, tragic disease causing deterioration of muscle function in middle age.
- Begins with loss of bulk of the muscles of the hands.
- Muscle-wasting spreads more generally, with resulting paralysis.
- Widespread twitching of the muscles.
- Mental function remains intact.

There is no known cure.

### ■ Poliomyelitis

Now almost eradicated, thanks to immunization programs. Symptoms include:
- Mild, viral symptoms of sore throat, diarrhea, muscle aches.
- Then symptoms of meningitis.
- Then increasing muscle ache.
- Followed by paralysis, especially of leg and shoulder muscles.

Recovery can take a year; residual paralysis is common.

## PERSONALITY CHANGE

### PROBABLE

### ■ Psychological Disorders

It is hardly surprising that psychological factors underlie most changes of personality, since personality is the sum of our emotional state, mood, and intellectual outlook and reflects our upbringing and experiences. Any psychological disease can affect personality. Noticeable features include:
- Anxiety.
- Emotional instability.
- Irritability.
- Aggression or passivity.

- Delusional thought.
- Self-neglect.

These symptoms have to be judged against the background of:

- General health.
- Relationships.
- Pressures at work and at home.
- Age.
- Drug and alcohol consumption.

The symptoms are covered under individual headings. Stress and minor anxiety states will most often be to blame.

## POSSIBLE

### ■ Alcohol or Drug Abuse

Usually a self-evident diagnosis, suggested by:

- Self-neglect.
- Tremor.
- Emotional instability.
- Drunken or drug-intoxicated behavior.
- Needle marks or drug-taking equipment evident.

- Smell of alcohol at inappropriate times.
- Social, employment, and criminal problems.

### ■ Head Injury

Personality change after severe head trauma is common, together with:

- Irritability.
- Poor memory.

### ■ Stroke

*(See page 415)* The resulting brain damage can cause erratic behavior, irritability, and emotional instability.

## RARE

### ■ Brain Tumor

Although a rare reason for personality change, doctors bear it in mind if rapid change in personality is combined with other symptoms of a brain tumor *(see page 417)*. Tumors affecting the frontal lobe typically cause personality change.

## PHOBIAS AND OBSESSIONS

Meaning morbid fears or a recurrent train of thought. Mild obsessions are common; for example, a fear of spiders or checking that you have locked the back door three times before leaving on vacation. Severe forms can dominate your life, such as agoraphobia, the fear of experiencing a difficult or embarrassing situation from which you cannot escape. Probably these symptoms reflect an inner insecurity, although often there is no obvious cause. Obsessions and phobias feed on themselves—what you have avoided in the past, you fear to meet in the future.

Sufferers commonly develop avoidance behavior. Psychological treatment and medication can prove very effective.

## ■ Psychological Factors

In this situation, external factors cause stress, which leads to exaggerated feelings. These then become an obsession or phobia.

• Rest of personality and thought is normal.

• The individual retains insight into the problem but feels powerless to control it.

It is only when the particular phobia starts to make life unnecessarily difficult or impossible that you need professional help.

## POSSIBLE

### ■ Schizophrenia

*(See page 395)*

## SHOCK

In medical language, "shock" means a massive and rapid fall in blood pressure with its accompanying effects; a very serious condition that requires rapid treatment. This is very different from the layperson's use of the term, in which "shock" is the emotional reaction to a serious psychological blow, such as awful news or witnessing a serious accident. Nonetheless, the symptom is considered here in the context of the brain and nervous system because shock can appear to be a nervous reaction. Indeed, the nervous system is in part responsible for its occurrence.

Anyone thought to be in "medical" as opposed to emotional shock needs emergency help as quickly as possible. *(See also Bluish Skin—Cyanosis, page 438, and Collapse with Shock or Coma, page 480)*

Critical features of medical shock are the rapid appearance of:

• Collapse.
• Sweating.
• Pallor.
• Weak, rapid pulse.
• Confusion.

## PROBABLE

### ■ Blood Loss

The source may be obvious; for example, after a stab wound. Less obvious sources are:

• Bleeding into the stomach—may vomit fresh blood or altered blood looking like coffee grounds.
• Black, tarry-looking stools following a bleed into the gut.

- Ruptured ectopic pregnancy *(see page 479)*.
- Severe chest or abdominal pain going through to the back with a ruptured aortic aneurysm *(see page 162)*.

## ■ Heart Attack

A combination of:
- Chest pain.
- Collapse.
- Breathlessness.

*(See page 231)*

## POSSIBLE

### ■ Serious Infection

Danger arises when infection spreads into the bloodstream. Most common in babies or the elderly.
- Usually a preexisting illness, commonly of the chest or of the skin.
- Fever, sweats, and rigors.
- Rapid collapse.
- Purple spots may appear on the skin.

### ■ Dehydration

Extreme loss of fluid from the body, such as from severe diarrhea and vomiting, eventually causes:
- Thirst.
- Restlessness.
- Dry mouth, lax skin.
- Reduced output of urine.

Those especially at risk are babies and diabetics.

## RARE

### ■ Allergic Shock

Medical term, anaphylaxis. This is an unpredictable reaction that occurs in some people to a bee sting, an injection, or some foods.
- Face and lips swell within minutes.
- Breathing rapidly becomes wheezy.
- Collapse, possibly within a few minutes.

Those who know that they are at risk should carry an adrenaline injection to self-administer. This can be lifesaving.

## SHOCK, EMOTIONAL

Features following emotional shock from a severe "fright reaction" include:
- Pallor.
- Numbness of thought.
- Difficulty in concentrating.
- Life seems trivial.
- Nothing matters except the event.
- Tearfulness.
- Feelings of guilt.
- Loss of confidence.

Continuous support from relatives and friends is important. Talking about the event and emotional release are helpful and necessary.

# "GENERAL" SYMPTOMS

## LOW BIRTH WEIGHT BABY

Defined as less than 5 pounds (2.5 kg) birth weight or very low birth weight—less than 3.3 pounds (1.5 kg). Generally, the smaller the baby, the more risk of problems, which include:

• Breathing problems immediately after birth.

• Difficulty feeding.

• Jaundice.

• Bleeding in the brain.

• Heart problems (patent ductus).

• Bowel problems (necrotizing enterocolitis).

• Eye problems.

There are two main reasons for babies being born with low birth weight: premature birth, that is, birth before thirty-seven weeks gestation (about two-thirds of cases), and small-for-date babies, whose growth has become restricted de-spite normal gestation (about one-third of cases). Sometimes both causes co-exist. Routine prenatal care aims to detect and control problems in the mother, such as high blood pressure or smoking, that might result in a premature or a low birth weight baby. Estimates of fetal growth can be made by measuring the enlargement of the womb (fundal height measurement) or serial ultrasound scanning to directly measure fetal dimensions. Low birth weight babies often need sophisticated monitoring and support after birth in special care baby units. Frequently, the reason for low birth weight is unknown and the baby goes on to develop into a normal child.

No one can be certain of the long-term consequences of low birth weight, but there is some evidence that babies born small can remain smaller than average at least up to puberty, and sometimes into adult life. There may be an association with the development of type 2 diabetes in later life.

## PROBABLE

### ■ Prematurity

That is, a baby born before thirty-seven weeks gestation, for any reason. Sometimes, doctors find it difficult to judge whether a baby is premature or has a low birth weight. The diagnosis depends on the overall appearance and behavior of the baby.

### ■ Socioeconomic Disadvantage

The birth weight of a baby is linked to the mother's standard of living, presumably reflecting her general nutrition and self-care during pregnancy.

### ■ Smoking, Alcohol, or Illicit Drugs

Babies born to mothers who smoke are, on average, about a half pound (0.25 kg) lighter than babies of mothers of similar social class who are nonsmokers. Similarly, alcohol and illicit drugs can cause problems.

## POSSIBLE

### ■ Multiple Pregnancy

Twin pregnancies tend to produce smaller babies and are more at risk of premature birth.

### ■ Maternal Illness in Pregnancy

The most common in developed countries is high blood pressure (preeclampsia). Other possibilities are heart, lung, or kidney disease. Worldwide, severe malnutrition is the major scourge.

### ■ Abnormalities of the Baby

Many congenital abnormalities and genetic defects cause low birth weight.

### ■ Inadequate Maternal Weight Gain

Women who gain less than the normal twenty-five to thirty-five pounds in pregnancy have a higher risk.

## RARE

### ■ Infection in the Mother During Pregnancy

Genital infections in the mother, such as *Chlamydia,* can cause premature birth. Rubella, which is completely preventable through immunization, can harm the baby. Other maternal infections such as cytomegalovirus, toxoplasmosis, and chicken pox are also dangerous.

## BABY OR CHILD UNABLE TO PUT ON WEIGHT OR TO GROW ADEQUATELY

The medical term for this symptom is "failure to thrive" and applies to babies and young children who fail to reach the accepted milestones of growth and development for their age. Growth can be readily assessed by measuring height and weight and comparing them to the expected norms on a chart. It is especially significant if a previously normally growing child fails to put on weight at the expected rate. The search would be on for physical reasons, but it is well recognized that emotional neglect can also contribute to failure to thrive.

### PROBABLE

■ **Feeding Problems**

No neglect is implied, but simple problems such as:
• Breastfeeding difficulties.
• Bottle feeds prepared or given incorrectly.
• An overrigid feeding schedule.

The baby rapidly catches up once the problem is identified.

### POSSIBLE

■ Vomiting

All babies vomit, some more than others. It is usually a passing feature and the baby's weight soon catches up. Gastroesophageal reflux is common in small babies and may result in repeated vomiting.

Pyloric stenosis is a rare reason for persistent vomiting. It is caused by a blockage in the stomach outlet and relieved by a minor operation.
• Much more common in boys than in girls.
• Vomiting begins after the first few weeks of life, typically at six weeks of age.
• The baby feeds normally, then vomits forcefully, so-called projectile vomiting.
• The baby is ravenous.

■ Malabsorption

The child has a normal intake of food, yet fails to grow. Suspicious symptoms would include:
• Chronic diarrhea, especially with bulky, greasy, smelly stools.
• Recurrent chest infections.

The most common causes of malabsorption in developed countries are cystic fibrosis *(page 144)* and celiac disease *(page 144)*.

■ Infection

Repeated infection over time slows down growth. The most common culprit is a urinary infection, causing fevers and abdominal pain. However, urinary infections may cause no symptoms at all, other than poor growth. Recurrent chest infections and gastrointestinal infections are other causes. They need to be individually investigated.

### ■ Anemia

Anemia can be a symptom or a cause of failure to thrive. The most common cause is poor dietary intake of iron.

### ■ Low Birth Weight

Severely premature babies, with low birth weight, may not grow as well as normal babies at first. Babies born small but at term can be expected to grow at a normal rate, although they may remain smaller compared to other children.

### ■ Neglect

This includes emotional neglect as well as food deprivation.
- A withdrawn, unresponsive child.
- Fearful of strangers.
- Other signs of neglect such as injuries, bruising, dirtiness.

### ■ Cow's Milk (Lactose) Intolerance or Allergy

Symptoms include:
- Persistent diarrhea.
- Sometimes skin problems or wheeze.

Resolves with elimination of lactose in the diet—substitution of cow's milk formula with soy milk.

## RARE

### ■ Hypothyroidism

This should be avoided by early heel-prick blood testing for the condition and, if identified, it is easily treatable. If it goes undetected, symptoms could include:
- Prolonged jaundice in the days after birth.
- A lethargic baby, tending to constipation and poor feeding.
- Later, developmental delay and learning disability.

## BIRTH ABNORMALITY PLUS FAILURE TO GROW

If the causes of failure to grow, as listed above, have been excluded, malformation might be suspected. Specialists will test for: interference with swallowing, perhaps due to a cleft palate; cerebral palsy; heart disease; a chromosomal abnormality (see Chromosomal or Genetic Disorder, page 429); or (rarely) a metabolic disorder or kidney failure. See relevant sections for further details.

## DISTRESSED OR CRYING BABY

First, know your child. All mothers know that a child will cry in different ways, depending on whether he or she is hungry, angry, or in pain. Daily experience of your child qualifies you to recognize when the child is crying in an unusual way. When this happens, check through the common causes below. Remember also that a usually placid baby or child can become irritable in response to your own mood or even to the way you handle him or her.

### PROBABLE

#### ■ Hunger or Thirst

• Due for a feed.
• Roots for the breast or bottle.
• Sucks eagerly and settles when fed.

#### ■ Discomfort

• A soiled diaper.
• Too hot—look for flushed appearance and sweating.
• Too cold—blue hands, cold to the touch.
• Noise, bright lights, smoke.

#### ■ Desire for Comfort

• Excited when you appear.
• Crying stops when cuddled, recurs when put down.

### POSSIBLE

#### ■ Colic

After a feed or in the evening:
• Draws up legs, whimpers.
• Relieved by burping or, in the case of evening colic, the problem simply stops after a few weeks.

#### ■ Infection

• Snuffles, a cold *(see page 466)*, or a cough.
• Other signs of infection: fever, off feeds, vomiting or diarrhea, increased sleepiness, flushed appearance, or rash.

#### ■ Pain

• Rubbing ear; teething.
• More of a scream than a cry.
• Only briefly relieved by comforting.

May respond to simple painkillers such as acetaminophen.

#### ■ Injury

Usually a fall or accident that has been witnessed or heard by a parent; sometimes if the accident occurs out of sight, the only sign may be a cut or a bruise. More serious injuries may cause fractures—look for swelling of the limbs or joints and the child "not using" the injured part.

## RARE

### ■ Meningitis

A serious infection of the brain and its coverings; meningitis can appear in hours in a previously well baby or child. It is rare, but potentially so serious that anxiety is understandable.

- The baby or child is initially irritable.
- Increasingly drowsy, lethargic.
- Vomiting.

- Soft spot of skull may be bulging.
- High-pitched, animal cry.
- Fine, purple skin rash.

Difficult to diagnose in very young babies—much depends on how ill the child looks. Because of the difficulty of diagnosis, see a doctor immediately if you suspect meningitis. The child may need admission to a hospital for investigation.

## SHORT STATURE IN CHILDREN

This is generally defined as height that is in the lowest 3 percent of the population for age. Although parents worry about it, regular measurements at quarterly intervals will show whether a child is small but growing at a normal rate, in which case the child is almost certainly short because he or she is made that way.

## PROBABLE

### ■ Family Pattern

Short parents have children who will be short, although genetic mechanisms ensure that, on average, the children end up taller than the parents. There are formulas, based on parental height, which can help to predict the final height of a child.

### ■ Constitutional Growth Delay

A term used to describe children who are small for their age but who have a normal growth rate. Also known as "late bloomers," these children often have:

- A close relative who displayed constitutional growth delay.
- In girls, periods may start at a later age.
- Growth may continue longer.
- Adult height may not be reached until after the age of eighteen.
- Eventual height in keeping with size of rest of family.

## POSSIBLE

### ■ Chronic Disease

Any long-term disease will stunt growth. Common culprits are kidney disease, heart disease, and respiratory disease.

### ■ Malnutrition

Worldwide, this is the most common

cause, associated with poverty and socioeconomic factors.

### ■ Chromosomal or Genetic Disorder

Common disorders include Down syndrome with characteristic flat face, large hands, fold of skin on inner part of eyeball, and other abnormalities. Another is Turner's syndrome *(page 274);* two symptoms of this condition are:

• Webbed neck.
• Infertility in later life.

Another example of a genetic disorder is achondroplasia, in which there is an alteration of body proportions, typically:

• Very short limbs.
• Head and trunk are normal size.

### ■ Hypothyroidism

An underactive thyroid gland *(see page 426)* is another possibility.

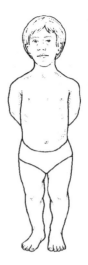

*Child with Achondroplasia.*

### RARE

### ■ Growth Hormone Deficiency

This unusual condition is now treatable by giving injections of the missing hormone.

• The child is normal, but grows slowly.
• Tendency to be overweight around the waist.

## BRUISING

A bruise is an area of skin discoloration that occurs when small blood vessels break and leak their contents into the soft tissue beneath the skin. Medical attention should be sought if the size of the bruise is large or disproportionate to the supposed cause.

*(See also Bleeding—Spontaneous and General, page 440)*

## PROBABLE

### ■ Accident or Trauma

Bruises on exposed areas, such as shins or elbows, which come and go.

### ■ Drug Side Effect

Typically seen after minor or trivial trauma in people taking anticoagulants, such as warfarin. Aspirin has a similar but weaker effect.

## POSSIBLE

### ■ Senile Purpura

Purple bruise-like marks occurring without obvious trauma, commonly seen in elderly people (on the arms and backs of the hands). These need no treatment and are not dangerous.

### ■ Blood Disorder

Severe anemia and serious blood disorders.

• Purple spots or patches appear on skin.
• Spontaneous bleeding from gums, nose.
• Rapid onset in an already ill person.

A blood test is essential and should be taken as soon as possible.

### ■ Physical Abuse

Suggested in particular if there is a history of family difficulties.
• Multiple bruises of varying ages, some old, some fresh.
• Inadequate explanation.
• Appearance of neglect—dirty, ill-fed.
• Bruising around ankles or wrists.
• The characteristic bruising of bite marks is not unusual on abused children.

## RARE

### ■ Scurvy

Caused by lack of vitamin C.

---

## PALE APPEARANCE (PALLOR), SLOW ONSET

Some people are naturally pale, so the best way to check for pallor is to look at the areas where blood flows close to the surface, for example, beneath the fingernails and under the eyelids. Pallor alone, even if the cause can be narrowed down to anemia, invariably requires medical assessment and detailed investigation.

This section refers to pallor coming on over weeks or months.

### PROBABLE

### ■ Anemia

(See also Looking Pale and Anemic, page 433)

General features include:

- Tiredness; being easily fatigued.
- Breathlessness, gradual onset.
- Dizziness, especially on standing up.

In addition, there may be symptoms suggesting the underlying cause, such as:

- Weight loss.
- Self-neglect.
- Sores on skin and bruising.
- Heavy periods.
- Jaundice.

It is essential to determine the cause of the anemia in order to treat it fully.

## POSSIBLE

### ■ Hypothyroidism

An underactive thyroid gland causes a slowdown in all aspects of body function over several months. As well as pallor, which is due both to a mild anemia and to changes in the skin, you may notice:

- Sensitivity to the cold.
- Gruff voice, coarse skin, thinning hair.
- Constipation.
- Slowness of thought.

This condition is readily treatable by taking thyroid hormone tablets once the diagnosis has been established by a doctor.

## RARE

### ■ Hypopituitarism

A failure of the pituitary gland in the brain, crucial to controlling many hormones (the body's chemical messengers). Pallor can be a striking feature of this condition, plus other symptoms, such as:

- Hypothyroidism.
- In women, periods cease; loss of sexual drive.
- Reduction of pubic hair, and hair in armpits.
- Lack of stamina.

This condition requires specialist medical assessment and management.

## PALE APPEARANCE (PALLOR), RAPID ONSET

This section refers to pallor coming on over days, hours, or minutes. Unless the individual has simply fainted, this may signify a problem that requires urgent medical attention. The likeliest reason is blood loss.

## PROBABLE

### ■ Fainting

The many well-recognized causes of fainting include missing a meal, emotional shock, prolonged standing, excessive heat, and pregnancy.

- Otherwise sound health.
- Initial light-headedness, sweating, dizziness.
- Collapse to ground or onto furniture.
- Cold, clammy skin.
- Thin, slow pulse.

It is essential to leave someone who has fainted lying flat until they recover, which generally takes just a few minutes.

### ■ Internal Bleeding

Often, there is a previous history of abdominal discomfort. The blood loss may be obvious:

- Bloody or black stools.
- Vomit containing blood or with specks looking like coffee grounds.
- Excessive vaginal bleeding, especially after a delayed period.
- Blood in urine.

Early symptoms are similar to those of anemia but of more rapid onset. As blood loss increases, there will be:

- Severe giddiness or faintness.
- A feeling of being cold; plus cold, clammy extremities.
- Low urine output.
- Rapid breathing.
- Eventually, drowsiness and unconsciousness.

There will probably be pointers to the cause of the bleeding. Previous dyspepsia (indigestion) suggests a duodenal or gastric problem. Bowel disturbance may signify inflammation of the bowel, a tumor, or a perforation (hole) in the intestine. Aspirin and other antiarthritic drugs can also cause bleeding into the stomach or gut. Previous alcoholism may suggest bleeding esophageal veins (varices).

## POSSIBLE

### ■ Hypoglycemia

A problem for diabetics, especially those on insulin, who must learn to recognize the early symptoms:

- Hunger, irritability, light-headedness. Progressing to:
- Sweating, confusion, slurring of speech, unconsciousness.

Taking glucose or glucagon gives relief in minutes.

### ■ Heart Rhythm Disorder

Very rapid, slow, or irregular heart rhythms mean that blood is pumped around the body with reduced efficiency. Most common in those over fifty years old.

- You may be aware of a thumping or a fluttering in your chest.
- Onset is usually abrupt; symptoms often end abruptly, too.
- Pallor, breathlessness, dizziness.

## ■ Stomach Upset

The early stages of a severe attack of gastroenteritis may be ushered in with:

• Nausea, vomiting, sweating, griping abdominal discomfort.

• Pallor.

• Diarrhea follows within a few hours.

## ■ Heart Attack

Pallor will probably not be the only, or even the main, symptom. The classic picture is:

• Crushing pain in the central chest, going into the left arm or neck; arising suddenly.

• Breathlessness, sweating, pallor.

Heart attacks, especially in the elderly, may not be so clear-cut, causing just pallor, fatigue, and breathlessness. Always seek urgent medical help.

## RARE

## ■ Acute Blood Disorder

Including leukemia and any breakdown in the blood's clotting mechanism. Most common in children and young adults. Suggested by:

• Pallor.

• Nose bleeds, bleeding gums, blood in stool or urine.

• Spontaneous bruising.

Medical assessment is essential.

## LOOKING PALE OR ANEMIC

The red blood cells in the body last on average ninety days. They are in constant production, while those cells coming to the end of their lives are broken down and their constituents recycled. When the number of red blood cells fall below the necessary level—either through inadequate production or excessive loss, or if hemoglobin (the oxygen-carrier in red blood cells) is somehow impaired or reduced—anemia develops. It results in:

• Paleness or pallor—an important sign of anemia but often a misleading one, since many people are naturally pale.

Best judged by looking at parts of the body where the blood runs close to the surface, typically the undersurface of the eyelids or under the fingernails, and confirmed by a blood test.

• Feeling tired much of the time.

• Fatigue on exertion.

• Faintness (in severe cases).

• Breathlessness.

There are a vast range of possible causes for anemia, but in practice a blood test, together with the patient's history and an examination, usually help narrow down the possibilities and assist with the diagnosis.

## PROBABLE

### ■ Menstrual Blood Loss

The 70 to 80 milliliters of blood lost in normal menstruation is replaced by the body within a day or two. If more blood is lost, then anemia becomes a possibility. This is suggested if periods are:

• Very heavy with clots.
• Very frequent.
• Prolonged, or there is bleeding between periods.
• If you have a poor diet.

### ■ Pregnancy

Anemia in pregnancy should be detected by routine blood tests. In fact, it is so common in pregnancy that some degree of anemia is considered normal. Iron supplements are not always given to pregnant women—your doctor will advise you if it is necessary. If it is needed, iron is commonly given together with folic acid, another important vitamin for blood production. Further blood loss occurs during birth and may require treatment with iron.

### ■ Poor Diet

That is, a diet deficient in iron or in the vitamins needed to make hemoglobin (the oxygen-carrying protein in blood). The elderly, alcoholics, or those on low incomes are at risk. Similarly people with restricted diets, such as vegans, can become anemic. The chief source of iron in the diet is red meat; green vegetables contain lesser amounts.

## POSSIBLE

### ■ Cancer or Other Chronic Disease

Anemia is unlikely to be the only symptom, except for cancers causing internal bleeding (mainly, cancer of the colon). The same is true of chronic diseases such as kidney failure or rheumatoid arthritis. There are numerous possibilities, and the management is generally directed at controlling the underlying disease and giving drugs to facilitate blood production; occasionally, blood transfusion is helpful.

### ■ Chronic Bleeding

Caused by disease, such as a bleeding peptic ulcer, or by drugs, of which aspirin, anti-inflammatory agents, and steroids are the most common culprits. Also, don't underestimate the effect of chronically bleeding hemorrhoids. Symptoms of chronic bleeding include:

• Passage of bloody or black stools.
• Blood in vomit.
• Excessive or prolonged menstrual bleeding (see left).

• Features of underlying disease, weight loss, loss of appetite, alteration of bowel habits.

### ■ Thalassemia and Sickle-Cell Disease

Both of these conditions are genetically inherited disorders of hemoglobin production, the oxygen-carrying protein in blood. Thalassemia is most common among people of Mediterranean extraction, while sickle-cell disease affects African Americans. A mild form of sickle-cell or thalassemia causes no problems, while the severe form of each disease can result in major debility.

### RARE

### ■ Pernicious Anemia

Caused by lack of vitamin $B_{12}$, because of failure to absorb the vitamin.

• Gradual onset, sometimes leading to very low levels of hemoglobin.
• Often, a family history.
• Sore, smooth tongue.
• Tingling, numbness of limbs.
• Unsteady walk.

### ■ Worm Infestations

For example, hookworm. Unlikely in developed countries, but common causes of anemia in tropical countries. Detected from stool samples.

---

## LOOKING PALE OR ANEMIC, PLUS SKIN PROBLEMS

Rashes, sores, and skin changes can be a feature of anemia, but usually only if the anemia is especially severe or if it is one of the rare types that are a side effect of some other underlying disease. Full medical evaluation is advised.

### PROBABLE

### ■ Iron Deficiency Anemia

General features of anemia, plus:
• Painful, cracked skin at corners of mouth.
• Sore, smooth tongue.

Common causes include poor dietary intake of iron or abnormal blood loss from the gut or female genital system.

### POSSIBLE

### ■ Pernicious Anemia

• Can cause a sore, smooth tongue.

### RARE

### ■ Drug Side Effect

Any drug that causes anemia may also cause skin rashes, blotches, bruises, and a sore mouth.

■ **Autoimmune Disease**

A range of diseases in which the body attacks its own components, resulting in general effects of malaise, rashes, and joint pains.

• A butterfly-shaped rash across the cheeks is characteristic of systemic lupus erythematosis (SLE, *see page 460*).

## LOOKING PALE OR ANEMIC, PLUS LOSING WEIGHT

This is a worrying combination, especially in the middle-aged and elderly. There is the possibility of underlying disease causing internal bleeding or possibly affecting the ability of the body to absorb the food, iron, and vitamins needed to make red blood cells. In children, the combination is more likely to suggest poor food intake or a malabsorption condition. Medical advice should always be sought.

### PROBABLE

■ **Neglect**

Typically self-neglect, with a diet so poor that individuals are literally starving themselves. In developed countries, it is usually only seen in those who are either very poor, living alone, or too frail to provide adequately for themselves. It is sometimes found in alcoholics, drug abusers, and people suffering from depression or dementia. In children, there may be other signs of neglect by their guardians, such as:

• Unexplained bruising.
• Dirty appearance.
• Withdrawn behavior.
• No food in the house.

■ **Malabsorption**

The term covers a range of conditions that undermine the digestive tract's ability to absorb nutrients. The possibilities are wide and what is probable in children is rare in adults. Some clues that suggest malabsorption as the underlying cause of anemia and weight loss are:

• Gradual appearance of symptoms.
• Change in bowel habit, with persistent, loose stools or diarrhea; sometimes the stools float and are difficult to flush away.
• An apparently adequate intake of food.
• Appetite healthy until later stages of the illness.
• Coexisting, recurrent chest infections in patients with cystic fibrosis.

## POSSIBLE

### ■ Bowel Cancer

Bowel cancer is common. In the United States, routine, annual bowel examinations are increasingly used to test for cancer. A simpler screening test consists of a stool examination to detect the presence of hidden blood, which, if positive, is followed by a more detailed examination of the bowel (by colonoscopy, barium x-rays, or computerized tomography scanning). A family history of bowel cancer means that you run a significantly increased risk of developing the condition. Besides anemia and weight loss, the other warning signs are:

• Persistent change of bowel habit from the normal known pattern for the individual in question. Alternating diarrhea and constipation is often a suspicious pattern.

• Blood in stools.

• Mucus or slime from back passage.

• A feeling of not completely emptying the bowel.

This common cancer has an excellent outlook if diagnosed sufficiently early.

### ■ Inflammatory Bowel Disease

Consists of either ulcerative colitis or Crohn's disease. Symptoms consist of:

• Diarrhea, often with blood.

• Weight loss.

• Abdominal pain.

### ■ Chronic Disease

Several chronic diseases, such as tuberculosis or long-term infection, can cause this combination of symptoms. HIV/AIDS is another possibility. The nature of the underlying disease will require full investigation. Seek help from your doctor.

### ■ Stomach Cancer

The earlier this is diagnosed, the better the outlook. In addition to weight loss and sometimes anemia, symptoms include:

• Indigestion and acidity as a new symptom in middle-age or old age.

• Loss of appetite.

• Persistent pains in upper abdomen.

• Vomiting of blood or passage of black stools.

### ■ Anorexia Nervosa

Although associated with young women, it is sometimes seen in men. Those with anorexia are often good athletes or high achievers at school. The signs are:

• Obsession with body image—the individual is convinced that he or she is obese.

• Appearance may vary from very slim to outright starved.

• In women, monthly periods cease.

• An excess of fine body hair may appear.

- Bouts of binge eating (bulimia).
- Excessive exercising.
- Self-induced vomiting or laxative abuse.

### RARE

■ **Chronic Myeloid Leukemia**

A disease of gradual onset in middle-age, which may present with anemia and weight loss. May also cause:

- Susceptibility to infections.
- Bruising or bleeding.
- Enlarged spleen.

Diagnosis made on blood tests.

## BLUISH SKIN (CYANOSIS)

Otherwise known as cyanosis, a bluish-purple coloring, visible especially where blood flows close to the surface (for example, the lips, the tongue, and under the fingernails). It arises when blood becomes deoxygenated, unable to discharge carbon dioxide waste or to take on fresh oxygen from the lungs. Fingers commonly show cyanosis in cold weather due to sluggish blood flow. In more serious cases, the lips and tongue also become blue.

### PROBABLE

■ **Temporarily Poor Circulation**

Common at any age:

- Results from a drop in temperature.
- A slight degree of cyanosis confined to fingers and toes, which feel cold and numb.
- Disappears rapidly on warming the limb.
- Worse in winter, better in summer.

Sometimes seen in Raynaud's syndrome, where there is spasm of the blood vessels in the fingers reducing circulation temporarily. Raynaud's may also produce whiteness in the fingers.

Occasionally, a blood clot may block the circulation to part of a limb, usually the lower leg or toes. This gives a quite different set of symptoms, typically found in an elderly person with preexisting circulatory disease or an irregular heartbeat (atrial fibrillation).

- Sudden onset of pain, coldness, numbness, and paralysis of the limb.
- Limb may at first look pale, cyanosis setting in over a few hours.

This is an emergency—seek urgent medical help at once.

### POSSIBLE

■ **Chronic Obstructive Pulmonary Disease (COPD)**

Chiefly caused by chronic bronchitis

and emphysema in smokers; these lung diseases cause persistent cough with phlegm, wheeze, and breathlessness. It is only after many years of disease that cyanosis becomes a regular feature, by which time the sufferer has long suffered breathlessness on the slightest exertion.

- Cyanosed nail beds, tongue, and lips.
- Hands and feet can feel surprisingly warm.

Caused by high concentrations of carbon dioxide in the blood. There are a number of other rare lung diseases that may cause cyanosis.

### ■ Heart Failure

Mild heart failure caused usually by diseased coronary arteries does not cause cyanosis. It is readily and effectively treatable. Only in severe cases is cyanosis a prominent symptom, together with:

- Constant breathlessness.
- Swollen legs.
- Breathlessness on lying flat.
- Coughing frothy fluid.

There may be coexistent COPD *(see page 438)*, a condition called cor pulmonale, or disease of the heart valves.

### ■ Lung Infections and Asthma

Severe pneumonia or asthma can produce cyanosis—this is a very grave sign, indicating life-threatening illness. Similarly a child with symptoms of croup or epiglottitis *(see pages 209 and 229)* who becomes blue is in serious danger of suffocation—call an ambulance or doctor at once.

## RARE

### ■ Congenital Heart Disease (Children)

Following conception, the human embryo's heart and great blood vessels develop via a complex process open to error at all points, and it is remarkable that so few serious congenital heart conditions occur. If they do, the result may be a "blue" or cyanosed baby, in whom the blood is not pumped properly through the lungs. Symptoms show at or very soon after birth.

- Breathlessness on feeding.
- The baby fails to gain weight normally during the first few weeks and months of life.
- Dizziness, headache, and fatigue.
- Thromboses (blood clots).

### ■ Drug Overdose

Suspected in an otherwise well young person who is:

- Unconscious.
- Breathing reduced to a point at which cyanosis appears.
- Pinpoint pupils suggest a heroin or opiate overdose.

## ■ Inhaled Foreign Body

The rapid appearance of cyanosis in someone who is suddenly breathless suggests an immediate obstruction to airflow. In children, it may be caused by inhaling a small object or item of food, such as a peanut.

- Typically occurs when eating steak or similar chunky food, or in children, nuts.
- Clutching at the throat, trying to gasp; clearly very distressed.
- Collapse.

The Heimlich Maneuver *(see page 206)* is a useful first aid procedure designed to relieve such obstructions.

## BLEEDING—SPONTANEOUS AND GENERAL

Everyone experiences surprise bleeding from time to time: a nosebleed or perhaps bleeding from the back passage. Follow up these symptoms in detail under the relevant sections for the part of the body involved. Covered here is spontaneous bleeding from the gums or the nose, and blood in the urine, in stools, and from the vagina. It will almost certainly be accompanied by widespread bruising. The symptoms point to a general breakdown of the blood-clotting process. Lesser degrees of all the causes listed below will give rise to prolongation of clotting time after an injury or easy bruising.

### PROBABLE

#### ■ Anticoagulant Treatment

The drug warfarin is widely used for certain heart disorders and also for thrombosis in a limb. Regular blood tests help to check that the dose is correct. At a therapeutic dose, blood takes longer to clot and spontaneous bleeding is more likely, but in overdosage bleeding can be catastrophic. See your doctor immediately if you begin bleeding unexpectedly while taking warfarin. Nosebleeds can be the first sign of excessive dosage.

#### ■ Thrombocytopenia

A general term for a reduction in the numbers of platelets in the bloodstream. Platelets are crucial to blood clotting, so if they are in short supply, widespread bleeding or bruising occurs. Many serious general illnesses can cause thrombocytopenia, the cause usually being obvious after just a few investigations, for example:

- Aplastic anemia—with rapid appearance of weakness, pallor, and malaise.
- Childhood leukemia—symptoms as with aplastic anemia, but also sore throat.

• Adult leukemias—a slower onset than childhood leukemia, enlarged lymph nodes, sweats.

• Bone cancer—with pain, malaise, weight loss.

Thrombocytopenia can also be drug-induced. There is also a benign form, affecting children, which cures itself spontaneously.

Treatment is aimed at the underlying cause, if known.

## POSSIBLE

### ■ Hemophilia

A bleeding disorder caused by a genetically controlled deficiency in the blood factors necessary in the normal clotting mechanism. It is found almost exclusively in males.

• A family history is common: two-thirds of cases are hereditary.

• Early symptoms are prolonged bleeding from, say, a small cut; spontaneous bruising; or bleeding into joints, giving joint pain and swelling.

### ■ Severe Infection

Many serious infectious diseases cause chaos in the blood-clotting system. These include septicemia (blood poisoning), malaria, and typhoid fever.

• Sweats and chills.

• Generally very ill.

## RARE

### ■ Scurvy

Results from a diet lacking in vitamin C, which is contained in fresh fruits and vegetables. So, the problem is usually one of the elderly or malnourished.

• Chronic feeling of being ill.

• Bleeding, especially from between the teeth.

• Sore gums, loose teeth.

• Easy bruising.

Readily treated by vitamin C supplements.

---

## TALLNESS

Meaning (for a given age) height greater than that of the tallest 3 percent of the population. Only rarely is tallness due to disease.

## PROBABLE

### ■ Natural Tendency

Tall parents have tall children. There are scientific formulas that can predict a child's height, based on the heights of the parents.

■ **Early Puberty**

The complex hormonal changes of an early puberty can make a child leap up in height. As puberty progresses, growth slows, so the child who was unusually tall with an early puberty may eventually finish smaller than his or her peers. The familiar signs of puberty are:
• Growth of body hair around genitalia, armpits.
• Breast development.
• Deepening voice.

### RARE

■ **Hyperthyroidism**

This will enhance growth in childhood.

■ **Genetic Abnormality**

The most common (it affects one in 500 males) is Klinefelter's syndrome.
• Tall and thin with a female body shape, small testicles, and breast development.

• Usually infertile.

■ **Excess Growth Hormone**

In children, this causes excessive height and size. In adults, it causes acromegaly with progressively coarse, heavy features.
• Enlargement of hands and feet.
• Protrusion of lower jaw.
• Possibly heavy sweating and diabetic symptoms.

■ **Marfan Syndrome**

This interesting hereditary condition affects about two people per 100,000. It causes:
• Long, thin bones; spider-like fingers and toes.
• An unusually high arch to the palate.
• Heart valve problems, which may cause breathlessness.
• Visual disturbance through dislocation of the lens of the eye.

## BODY SWOLLEN WITH EXCESS FLUID (EDEMA)

Three categories of disorder cause generalized body swelling with excess fluid, known as edema: heart failure, kidney disease, and low protein states. The mechanics of swelling are complex. Because fluid sinks to the lowest level of the body, the early signs are swollen ankles or a puffy face in the morning. This is easy to test for in the ankles by applying gentle pressure with a finger tip to the swollen ankle—when the finger is removed an indentation remains, confirming the presence of edema. As more fluid accumulates, swelling spreads up the legs and builds up inside the abdomen and chest.

## PROBABLE

### ■ Premenstrual Swelling

Hormone changes in the few days before a period cause a mild degree of fluid retention.

• A regular pattern each month; health otherwise normal.

• Breasts, abdomen, ankles all become slightly enlarged.

• Weight gain of a few pounds.

• Disappears within days of the period beginning.

### ■ Heart Failure

A common cause of persistent swelling of the legs in later life.

• Often, high blood pressure, angina, or other heart disease.

• At first, swelling of ankles, tiredness.

• Later, breathlessness on exertion or when lying down (causing inability to lie down).

• Paroxysms of breathlessness at night, coughing frothy sputum.

Modern drugs can usually provide effective treatment, although the swelling may not clear completely.

## POSSIBLE

### ■ Liver Disease

One of the liver's many functions is to make proteins. These circulate in the bloodstream, and if their levels fall, edema follows.

• Often, a history of alcohol abuse, hepatitis, drugs toxic to the liver.

• Easy bruising, blood-stained vomit.

• Tiredness, loss of sexual drive, clubbed fingers.

• Tiny, spider-like red veins on the face, upper body.

• Red palms.

• Swelling of the abdomen with fluid.

• Jaundice is a late symptom, as is confusion, coma.

### ■ Preeclampsia

A condition causing edema, high blood pressure. and loss of protein in the urine in pregnant women. *(See page 394)*

### ■ Malnutrition

Globally, this is a major cause of edema in children.

• Swollen abdomen.

• Patchy pigmentation of the body.

• Apathy, coarse skin, lack of resistance to infection.

### ■ Malabsorption

A possibility in those with chronic bowel disease, such as celiac disease or ulcerative colitis, which interfere with the absorption of nutrients. Some general symptoms include:

• Failure to thrive (children).

- Diarrhea; smelly, greasy stools.
- Bleeding from the bowel.
- Chronic abdominal pain.
- Recurrent, severe chest infections.
- Clubbing of fingernails.

### ■ Glomerulonephritis and Nephrotic Syndrome

Glomerulonephritis is actually a group of diseases, all of which involve some degree of inflammation of the kidneys. This can cause edema, partly due to loss of protein in the urine and partly due to failure to excrete sufficient urine. Nephrotic syndrome, which may de due to glomerulonephritis, refers to the edematous state of the body in combination with loss of protein in the urine. In children, glomerulonephritis and nephrotic syndrome present with:

- Sudden onset, often after a minor throat infection.
- Low urine output.
- Blood in urine.
- Puffiness, especially of the face.

The outlook for recovery is good. In adults, it tends to present more slowly, with:

- Progressive swelling of the legs.

Assessment involves blood tests and biopsy of the kidney, after which the outlook can be judged, depending on the type of glomerulonephritis. Often, the outlook is good with full recovery, though some cases progress to kidney failure.

### RARE

### ■ Thiamine Deficiency

Otherwise called beri-beri. Thiamine is found in whole-grain cereals, including rice, and in liver. In developed countries, the deficiency is likely only through severe deprivation, as thiamine is routinely added to many manufactured foods.

- Early symptoms are tender calves and vague weakness.
- Then swelling of the legs, palpitations.
- Eventually, general swelling, exhaustion, rapid pulse.

## SWOLLEN PART OF BODY

### PROBABLE

### ■ Injury

Tissue swelling is the normal reaction to any modest injury, together with reddened, warm skin.

### ■ Infection

Including insect bites and minor cuts.

- Throbbing pain, redness.
- Swelling of local lymph glands.
- Pus may be visible.

# ■ Dependant Edema

Older people who are inactive frequently notice this condition, one of the most common reasons for a mild degree of ankle swelling. No need for treatment unless it is a nuisance. Care should be taken to distinguish this condition from other causes of edema *(see page 442)* requiring medical treatment. It is best to ask a doctor to help with this distinction. With dependant edema:

- General health good.
- Swelling lessens if activity is increased.

## POSSIBLE

# ■ Deep Vein Thrombosis (DVT)

Sudden swelling of a limb, nearly always a leg, suggests thrombosis. It occurs when clotted blood obstructs a vein. Risk factors include the contraceptive pill, long-haul air travel, and certain blood disorders.

- Acute onset of pain in calf.
- Swelling and warmth of calf.

If confirmed, DVT needs anticoagulants to reduce the risk of a pulmonary embolus *(see page 227).*

# ■ Allergy

In reaction to an insect bite or injection.
- Limb swells dramatically in a few seconds.

- Swelling may spread to body, lips, and throat.
- At worst, difficulty breathing, collapse.

# ■ Lymphatic Obstruction

Also known as lymphedema. Results from interference with the lymphatic channels, which drain away tissue fluid. Most common after surgery in the groin or armpit (typically to treat breast cancer). In rare cases, it can be congenital.
- Gross swelling of limb.
- Swelling becomes hard; does not easily indent when pressed.

## RARE

# ■ Cancer

Suspected in otherwise unexplained swelling of a limb. Long bones are the likeliest sites.
- Persistent pain, tenderness.
- Enlarged local lymph nodes.

Cancer may also obstruct the drainage of lymphatic fluid or blood from a limb; for example, pelvic cancers may cause swelling in the legs.

# ■ Filariasis

A tropical worm infestation capable of causing massive swelling of limbs (elephantiasis).

## WEIGHT LOSS—PROGRESSIVE

Persistent, progressive weight loss ranks as one of the major symptoms of disease. People with weight loss usually seek help at an early stage, when other features of disease may not be prominent. Obtaining the individual's full background story usually reveals other symptoms—for example, abdominal pain —and these may lead to a tentative diagnosis. The following are some of the possibilities for which there are few other symptoms to point the way. Many of these possibilities are considered in more detail elsewhere in the book.

### POSSIBLE

#### ■ Diabetes

In young adults and children, the onset of diabetes tends to be dramatic: rapid weight loss is prominent, along with thirst and excessive urine output. *(See page 492)*

#### ■ Anxiety and Depression

A modest, slow weight loss could reasonably be put down to anxiety or depression in the absence of other symptoms and where there is no other clear cause for concern. Generally, it is prudent to exclude physical causes of weight loss first.

#### ■ Chronic Infection

This includes chronic abscesses and chronic chest conditions such as cystic fibrosis *(see page 216)*.

#### ■ Anorexia Nervosa

Excessive dieting, usually in young women who have a distorted image of their true size. *(See page 437)*

#### ■ Overactive Thyroid Gland

Weight loss alone is unusual, unless the accompanying tremor and sweating have been overlooked. *(See page 437)*

#### ■ Tuberculosis

The poor, alcoholics, and people from underdeveloped countries might have this serious but curable infection. *(See page 472)*

#### ■ Cancer

Cancer might explain weight loss in the forty-plus age group. It is by no means the only explanation, yet it remains true that, occasionally, an advanced cancer that has spread around the body produces only vague symptoms until a late stage. So, be aware of your body and report to your doctor any unusual changes, such as bleeding, swellings, weight loss, pain, or prolonged cough.

### ■ HIV/AIDS

Needs to be considered in any case of vague ill-health, weight loss, fevers, and cough. HIV/AIDS is widespread in certain parts of the world. Transmitted by sexual contact or blood-to-blood contact.

## RARE

### ■ Malabsorption

This causes weight loss by preventing the absorption of food. Associated symptoms are:

- Difficulty in swallowing.
- Anemia.
- Recurrent abdominal pains, intermittent diarrhea, greasy stools.
- Blood in stools.

Underlying causes include cancer of the esophagus, which causes very rapid weight loss, ulcerative colitis, Crohn's disease, celiac disease, and chronic pancreatitis.

### ■ Parasite Infection

Not a usual cause of weight loss except in Third World countries, where it is very common. Diagnosis is confirmed by stool tests.

### ■ Kidney Disease

At the early stage of causing weight loss, this needs to be confirmed by blood tests. *(See page 387)*

### ■ Pyloric Stenosis

A childhood condition. Part of the intestine is obstructed, causing profuse vomiting and rapid weight loss a few weeks after birth. Occasionally seen in adults with stomach cancer. *(See page 163)*

## LOSING WEIGHT PLUS JAUNDICE

The combination of weight loss and jaundice points to disease of the liver and related parts of the digestive system. Its appearance in adults must trigger a careful search for a primary cancer (such as bowel cancer), which may have spread to involve the liver. The jaundice results from obstruction to bile flow from the liver.

## PROBABLE

### ■ Cancer of the Pancreas

The pancreas lies at the back of the abdomen, partly surrounding the bile duct. The tumor blocks the bile duct, producing jaundice.

- Initially, vague upper abdominal pain.
- Weight loss.
- Painless jaundice.

### ■ Secondary Cancer of the Liver

Cancers of many kinds can spread around the body from their original site. The liver is a common secondary site. The primary cancer is likely to have shown itself already, with symptoms such as:
• Weight loss.
• Pain.
• Swelling.
• Unusual bleeding.

### Possible

### ■ Cancer of Stomach

*(See Stomach Disease, page 163)*

### ■ Primary Cancer of the Liver

A complication of liver cirrhosis in an alcoholic or hepatitis B or C infection.

### ■ Pernicious Anemia

The combination of anemia and a yellow tinge to the skin gives an impression of jaundice. The diagnosis is based on blood tests. Treatment reverses symptoms. *(See page 494)*

### Rare

### ■ Cancer of the Gallbladder

A disease of the elderly, causing symptoms similar to gallstones.
• Recurrent pains in the right upper abdomen.
• Jaundice.

## POSTURE APPEARS STIFF AND HUNCHED

### Probable

### ■ Aging and Osteoporosis

With age, bone density is lost and there is shrinkage of the discs between the vertebrae, the bones which link together to form the spine. Rapid thinning of bone (osteoporosis) takes place, leaving the vertebrae somewhat delicate and liable to collapse.
• Posture becomes hunched over several years.

• Collapse of a vertebra causes a sudden change of posture plus pain.

Osteoporosis is treatable with bisphosphonate drugs, calcium and vitamin D supplements, or other medications. Some bone repair can take place with these treatments, but lost height and deformity persist.

### Possible

### ■ Ankylosing Spondylitis

A disease that begins in early adult life,

especially affecting men. Over many years, the normal joints and ligaments of the spine are replaced by inflexible bone. A blood test for the tissue type HLA-B27 is generally positive.

- Initially just back pain, and morning stiffness of the spine.
- The back becomes increasingly rigid, with a stooped posture.
- Eventually, spine movements are severely restricted.

The stooped posture, though not totally avoidable, need not be as severe a problem as in the past, thanks to improvements in treatment.

### ■ Kyphoscoliosis

This is a twisting of the spine, often starting during the teenage years for no apparent reason. Treatable surgically.

### ■ Parkinson's Disease

*(See page 451)* A neurological disease rarely present before the age of fifty. The main symptoms are:

- Tremor of the hands at rest.
- Stooped, inflexible posture.
- Shuffling gait.
- Immobile facial expression.

### ■ Paget's Disease

A disorder of bone formation, quite common in a mild form in later life and frequently causing no symptoms.

- Pain in the bones.
- Legs becomes bowed, back stoops; head may enlarge (hat size may increase).
- Deafness.

Advanced cases are generally easy to recognize, but usually x-rays and blood tests are needed to confirm the diagnosis.

## RARE

### ■ Tuberculosis (TB) of the Spine

This used to be common. The infection destroys the bone.

- Increasing pain and stiffness in part of the spine.
- Other features of TB include malaise, weight loss, cough, night sweats.

---

## LOOKING OLD BEFORE YOUR TIME

### POSSIBLE

### ■ Smoking

This is known to accelerate lining of the face and coarsening of the skin.

### ■ Underactive Thyroid Gland

*(See page 351)* This common condition makes the skin thicken and coarsen.

### ■ Sun Damage

In hot, sunny climates, such as that of Australasia, sun damage is the most common cause of a prematurely aged appearance.

## RARE

### ■ Hereditary Causes

With one exceptionally rare condition, progeria, in which growth ceases by about three years of age and the child becomes mentally retarded, bald, and develops a beaked nose.

## BODY SIZE, SHRINKING

## PROBABLE

### ■ Osteoporosis

*(See page 282)*

## RARE

### ■ Paget's Disease

Also known as osteitis deformans. Abnormal turnover of bone, causing thickening and deformity of bones, particularly the skull and the long bones. The bone, despite appearing thicker, is weaker than normal bone. The disease affects men and women equally, but rarely affects people from Asia, Africa, and the Middle East. It normally appears after the age of forty. Although often symptom-free, there may be:

• Bony deformities—the skull may appear large; often, only one bone is affected.

• Fractures.

• Kyphosis *(see page 295),* causing apparent height loss.

• Heart failure, due to increased workload on the heart.

• Vision and hearing deteriorate as deformed bone damages nerves.

Diseased bone can, very rarely, develop into a malignant bone tumor (osteosarcoma). Diagnosis is confirmed by blood tests.

## TREMBLING OR SHAKING

## PROBABLE

### ■ Normal Variation

How steady are your hands? Everyone has tremor to a greater or lesser degree.

• Mostly causes no interference with delicate manual activities.

• Worsened by anxiety, alcohol, stimulants such as coffee, some illicit drugs.

## ■ Benign Essential Tremor

An exaggerated form of normal tremor and an embarrassment rather than a disease.

• Hereditary.
• Slow tremor, affecting upper limbs and head.
• Gradually worsens with age.

### POSSIBLE

## ■ Overactive Thyroid Gland

*(See page 350)* An overactive thyroid gland causes an exaggeration of normal tremor.

## ■ Parkinson's Disease

Trembling movements of the thumb and forefinger.

• An early symptom is loss of normal swinging motion of arms when walking.
• Limbs held rigid; slowing of all movements.
• Tremor at rest, diminishing on activity.
• Immobile, "mask-like" facial appearance.

• Handwriting becomes increasingly smaller.
• Dribbling.

There are now many useful treatments for this common disorder.

## ■ Drug Side Effect

Some drugs, especially major tranquilizers used in the treatment of mental illness, cause tremor.

### RARE

## ■ Brain Disease

Brain tumors, strokes, multiple sclerosis, and head injuries may all cause tremors. Associated symptoms might include:

• Paralysis of one side of the body.
• Progressive headache, blurring of vision.
• Change of personality.
• Deterioration of memory, slurring of speech.
• Noticeable flicking movements of the eyes.
• Difficulty in walking.

## TWITCHING

Uncontrollable, short-lived muscle jerks. The gulf between the common twitches and those with a serious cause is so wide that there should rarely be any reason to suspect disease in the absence of other symptoms.

### PROBABLE

## ■ Habit or Nervous Tic

Blinking and similar grimaces, normal in everyone to a degree, may sometimes become excessive. Deserves sympathy

even in twitching schoolboys, in whom it disappears gradually.
• Typically, young boys or nervous adults.
• Frequency increases under stress.

No satisfactory treatment and, please remember, sufferers really cannot help it.

### ■ Spasmodic Torticollis

Recurrent jerking of the neck to one side.
• A disorder of the middle-aged.
• The individual is otherwise perfectly well.

Treatment with botulinum toxin (Botox) helps.

## POSSIBLE

### ■ Benign Fibrillation or Fasciculation

A part of a muscle that twitches spontaneously; the thigh or around the eye are common sites, probably because it is easily noticed.
• Other muscles unaffected.
• Muscle strength normal.
• Disappears after a few days.

Tiredness is a common cause.

### ■ Epilepsy

Spasmodic jerking of limbs is a feature of most forms of epilepsy.
• Same limb is affected each time.

• Brief warning before the jerking episode starts.
• May progress to a generalized fit, with loss of consciousness, incontinence, foaming at mouth. There is usually very little doubt that epilepsy is the cause.

## RARE

### ■ Chorea

Irregular, involuntary flailing movements of limbs. Rheumatic fever was once a common cause. Other neurological conditions with twitching as a feature include Huntington's chorea.
• A strong family history.
• Disintegration of personality in middle-age.
• Eventually dementia, epilepsy, paralysis.

### ■ Tourette Syndrome

A disorder with a reputation out of all proportion to its rarity.
• Onset in adolescence.
• Multiple tics.
• Abrupt swearing or obscenities, grunting.
• Echoing other people's words.

### ■ Motor Neuron Disease

Exceptionally rare disease causing deterioration of muscle function in middle-age.

- Begins with loss of bulk of muscles in hands.
- Muscle-wasting spreads generally.
- Widespread twitching of muscles may be seen.
- Mental function remains intact.
- Eventually, paralysis.

### ■ Kidney Failure

A late symptom in someone already known to have kidney disease.

- Nausea, vomiting.
- Twitching of muscles.
- Clouded consciousness.
- Spontaneous bleeding.
- Low urine output.

## FEVER

Just why the body produces fever in response to illness is still not fully understood. Presumably, it helps in some way to fight illness, but exactly how is still surprisingly controversial. Since ancient times, fever has been recognized as a key signal that someone is unwell. Fevers tell us much about the illness itself: not only is it important to take account of its severity, but also of its variation during the day and over the course of the illness. Modern medicine offers diagnosis and treatment of most prolonged fevers, replacing the long, anxious period of observation until the fever breaks.

With the decline of serious infections, at least in developed countries, the onset of fever should not cause alarm. In the very young and in the elderly, fever still calls for a careful assessment of health. But in older children and for much of adult life, a day or two of raised

### Taking Temperature

An adult's normal temperature is conventionally taken to be 98.6°F (37°C), based on an oral reading. You may have a temperature half a degree either way and be perfectly well. In children, temperature can be measured under the armpit, in which case 97.7°F (36.5°C) is the norm.

Take into account:

- Mouth breathers, whose mouth temperature is lower than normal.
- The amount of clothing worn may raise or lower temperature.
- Warm or cold drinks alter temperature in the mouth for about fifteen minutes.

Feeling the brow offers comfort, but is not very reliable, especially if there is a low-level fever with sweat on the forehead that cools the skin.

temperature will usually be the prelude to one of the minor illnesses considered in the following pages. Of course, there are more sinister causes, but they are rare, and fever alone is unlikely to raise even the professional's suspicions. Before worrying about serious disease, look at the individual's overall condition, assessing:

• Risk factors for unusual disease, such as foreign travel, poor sanitation, epidemics.

• Rapid onset of a high fever, greater than 104°F (40°C).

• Severe headache or delirium.

• Pain.

• Night sweats.

• A rapid pulse or fast breathing, remembering that pulse rate rises by about ten beats per minute for every degree Celsius rise in temperature. A baby's normal pulse rate is about 120 per minute, even at one year of age.

To list all the hundreds of possible reasons for fever would simply be confusing. Instead, we look on the following pages at fevers of different durations. We believe that this is how you will usually meet the problem. The possibilities listed are those expected in a developed country. There is a separate section on tropical diseases. We remind you again that fever in the very young and very old demands special attention and that, in any case, concern about a person's overall condition means you must get professional advice, even if the fever itself is minor.

## FEVER—THE FIRST FORTY-EIGHT HOURS

Along with the fever, there will be some combination of chills, muscular aches, sweating, a mild headache, and fatigue.

### PROBABLE

■ **Viral Illness**

Including the buildup to a common cold or flu.

• Mild sore throat.

• Headache and muscle and joint aches.

• Symptoms oscillate between mild and irritating within hours.

• Sniffing and sneezing begins after a couple of days.

• Or the illness fades away leaving you, and your doctor, none the wiser.

■ **Ear Infection**

Very common in children, sometimes with no other symptoms.

• Typically, the child already has a cold.

- Abrupt onset of pain in ear.
- Babies just begin crying and will not settle, even with comforting. They may shake their head or rub an ear.

Occasionally progresses to a burst eardrum, causing a green or yellow (possibly bloodstained) discharge for a few days. Healing over a couple of weeks is the norm. Painkillers will help the symptoms. The role of antibiotics is controversial.

### ■ Tonsillitis

The picture presented is usually unmistakable:
- Pain in the throat, worse on swallowing.
- Swollen neck glands.
- Nasal twang to speech.
- Breath smells foul.
- White spots on the tonsils.

### ■ Chest Infection

The symptom picture is usually clear:
- Cough.
- Phlegm.
- Shortness of breath or wheeze.
- Chest pain when breathing deeply.

### ■ Urinary Infection

Common in women, unusual in men.
- Pain or burning sensation when passing urine.
- A need to pass urine frequently.
- Aching over the kidneys or bladder.

- In severe cases, rigors, blood in the urine.
- In babies, there may be no symptoms other than fever and irritability, hence the need to test urine in a feverish infant.

## Possible

### ■ Chicken Pox

A viral illness causing small fluid- or pus-filled blisters over the body, in the mouth, and on the scalp. Usually occurs in epidemics. Incubates for about eleven to twenty-one days after contact with another carrier.
- Itchy rash appears within forty-eight hours of fever.
- Rash lasts for two or three weeks.

The rash consists of spots, which tend to appear in crops and soon become blisters; they then dry out and become scabs. Usually a mild, though miserable, illness, calling for plenty of care and attention.

## Rare

### ■ Rubella (German Measles)

Rubella is mild in itself but notorious because of the risk it poses to the developing baby if the mother catches it during early pregnancy. For this reason, there are public health immunization programs, which have made this disease very infrequent.

• A fine, red-brown rash appearing after twenty-four to forty-eight hours of fever.

• Rash with no particular pattern to its spread appears all at once.

• Swollen, tender glands at the back of the skull.

• In adults, commonly accompanied by mild arthritis lasting for some weeks.

## ▪ Mumps

An infection of the salivary glands uncommon thanks to vaccination programs. The incubation period is two to three weeks.

• Nonspecific fever and chills for twenty-four to forty-eight hours.

• Then, the salivary glands (parotid and submandibular) enlarge at the angles of the jaw and just in front of the ears.

• The illness resolves in five to ten days.

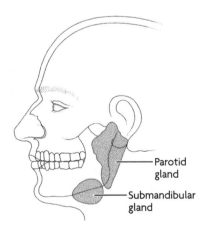

*Parotid and Submandibular Glands*

Complications can include pain in the testicles and the abdomen or may cause deafness, but these are rare.

## ▪ Scarlet Fever

• Onset is sudden with high fever, sore throat, or tonsillitis.

• A very fine, generalized red rash after twenty-four to forty-eight hours.

• The rash spares the area around the mouth, giving it a contrasting, white appearance.

• Furred tongue goes from whitish to raw over a few days.

Scarlet fever was once much feared because it could cause rheumatic fever and glomerulonephritis *(see page 444)*. These complications are now extremely rare. However, penicillin is still necessary if scarlet fever is diagnosed.

## ▪ Meningitis

Mentioned here as a reminder that it should be considered in any feverish child, especially if the child shows:

• Drowsiness.

• Stiff neck.

• A wish to avoid bright lights.

• Sudden appearance of a fine, purple rash.

• And, in a baby, a bulging soft spot (fontanelle) on the top of the head.

If suspected, this is a medical emergency and help must be sought.

## FEVER—THREE TO FOURTEEN DAYS

Minor viral illness is still likely to underlie this symptom, just as with fever lasting forty-eight hours. However, the need to consider less common illnesses arises.

### PROBABLE

#### ■ Viral Illness

No rash, no progression, and no other symptoms apart from sweats, aches, and generally feeling unwell. But although the cause is probably a virus, it is prudent to review the diagnosis every few days, considering the possibility of any of the following.

### POSSIBLE

#### ■ Glandular Fever

• Bad sore throat or tonsillitis.
• Enlarged lymph glands.
• Sometimes, abdominal pain or jaundice with inflammation of the liver or spleen.
• Fatigue persisting for weeks or months.

A blood test will confirm the diagnosis.

#### ■ Pneumonia

Certain forms of pneumonia are known for causing fever alone, without the other, more dramatic symptoms of pneumonia.
• Slight cough.

• Feeling vaguely unwell; fatigue, night sweats.

A chest x-ray confirms the diagnosis and treatment is straightforward.

#### ■ Abdominal Infection

Suspect this if fever starts soon after abdominal surgery or after abdominal pain. Prolonged fever can signal an abscess in any of the abdominal organs, the more common ones being:
• The appendix—preceded by a few days of pain, which may start centrally but then settles down low on the right side.
• The large intestine—pain in the lower left side, possibly bleeding from the back passage, intermittent diarrhea.
• Infected ovaries or fallopian tubes—lower abdominal pain, vaginal discharge.
• Gallbladder infection—typically, with pain in the upper right abdomen, usually in the presence of gallstones.

#### ■ Infectious Hepatitis

Caused by several different viruses, with hepatitis A, B, or C being the usual culprits. Hepatitis B and the less common hepatitis C are the dangerous forms, which can lead to long-term liver complications. The virus is spread by shared needles used for intravenous drug abuse and unprotected sexual intercourse. Hepatitis B can also be passed from mother to baby in pregnancy. The incubation period of hepatitis A is a few weeks, and of hepatitis B a few months. Both hepatitis A and B are preventable by immunization.

- Fever, chills, joint pains, backaches; generally feeling unwell for a week.
- Jaundice (yellowish discoloration of the skin) first spotted in the whites of the eyes; then the skin turns yellow.
- Darkening of urine, light stool color.

### ■ Roseola

A fairly common, harmless viral illness that can fool doctors into suspecting measles.

- High fever for three to four days; the child is snuffly.
- A pinkish rash appears over the body.
- The fever stops, and the child perks up.

## RARE

### ■ Measles

"Measles is misery" sums up this childhood illness, which is very infrequent now due to immunization programs. There is an incubation period of ten to fourteen days after being infected by another carrier.

- A miserable, snuffly, coughing child with bloodshot eyes who wants to avoid bright lights.

- Delirium at night is common.
- White spots may be seen in the mouth by the back teeth.
- A blotchy, red rash appears after four days of fever, spreading downward from the face via the chest to the limbs.
- The child continues feverish for several more days as the illness subsides.

Measles is a serious problem in underdeveloped countries, but in developed countries its complications, such as pneumonia or encephalitis, are rare.

### ■ Typhoid or Paratyphoid Fever

Infections spread via food and water in conditions of poor sanitation. Profuse diarrhea is a major feature.

- Fever, gradually rising to a peak over a couple of weeks.
- Cough, headache, limb pains.
- After a week, a non-itchy rash appears on the stomach, chest, and lower back. In typhoid, it is sparse and rapidly fading; in paratyphoid, it is more widespread.
- Diarrhea begins after a week or so, becoming profuse.

Typhoid is still a very serious illness, despite modern antibiotic treatment. Paratyphoid, though less serious, is nevertheless very unpleasant. Immunization is recommended for many parts of the world.

## ■ Septicemia

Infection spreading in the bloodstream. It is usually a rapidly developing illness, causing chills and collapse.

## ■ Endocarditis

*(See page 471)* An infection of the valves of the heart, causing chronic illness, including fever, anemia, and clubbed fingernails.

# FEVER LASTING TWO WEEKS OR MORE

By now, fever is a diagnostic challenge. It is likely that someone who is ill as well as feverish for as long as this would be admitted to a hospital for investigation. However, in some people, fever shows itself only with the feeling of being vaguely unwell (malaise), together with night sweats and other symptoms pointing to nothing in particular. Causes now include not only infections, but also rheumatic diseases, connective tissue disease, cancers, and drug side effects. But remember that many of the illnesses noted above could still be suspected, along with the following.

## PROBABLE

## ■ Chronic Infection

This is still the likeliest reason for prolonged fever. Recent surgery, together with abdominal pain, could be pointers. Less common causes might include:
• Prostatitis in men—pain between the legs, burning urine.
• Osteomyelitis—pain and tenderness

in a bone; usually in children. The long bones, typically of the leg, are most commonly involved.
• Bronchiectasis—causing persistent cough, sweats, possibly breathlessness, finger clubbing.

## ■ Tuberculosis

A significant possibility, causing chronic illness, weakness, and infection.
• A low-grade fever.
• Weight loss.
• Cough.
• Night sweats.
• Possibly blood-stained sputum.

## POSSIBLE

## ■ Ulcerative Colitis

A chronic inflammation of the bowel. The early symptoms may be limited to:
• Persistent diarrhea.
• Low-grade fever.
• Vague malaise.

Once suspicion is aroused, this illness can be rapidly confirmed and treated.

## ■ Cancer or Leukemia

Fever that is otherwise unexplained and lasts for months brings these conditions to mind. There may be other suspicious symptoms, such as:

• Weight loss.
• Unusual pains.
• Unusual bleeding from the bowel, bladder, vagina, stomach.
• Chronic cough.

These symptoms may allow the cancer to be tracked down. Blood tests will screen for leukemia. Cancer of the kidney is one tumor known to cause persistent fever.

## ■ Hodgkin's Disease and Other Lymphomas

These are malignant diseases of the lymphatic tissues. Hodgkin's disease mostly affects young adults. The treatment is usually chemotherapy and radiotherapy —in the case of Hodgkin's disease, the chances of a cure are good.

• Persistently swollen, painless glands in the neck, groin, or armpits.
• Night sweats.
• Anemia.

## ■ HIV/AIDS

Human immunodeficiency virus (HIV) acquired through sexual or blood contact can produce a flu-like illness early on (days or weeks after contact). This occurs as the body seroconverts, the point at which HIV antibodies develop in the blood (shown by the HIV-antibody blood test becoming positive). Months or years after seroconversion, an untreated sufferer develops impaired immunity, which may present as odd opportunistic infections or malignancies. Symptoms of opportunistic infection include fever, with:

• Diarrhea.
• Enlargement of lymph nodes.
• Cough.
• Headache or confusion.
• Thrush in the mouth.
• Rashes.
• Loss of weight.

Many other symptoms are possible. Tell your doctor if you think you might be at risk of HIV infection.

## ■ Rheumatoid Arthritis

Usually there will be joint pain, swelling, and deformity. Persistent fever and vague malaise can continue for several weeks. *(See page 285)*

## ■ Systemic Lupus Erythematosis (SLE)

One of a group of connective tissue disorders in which the body reacts against its own tissues. It can be a very vague illness at first. Most common in women aged thirty to fifty.

• Rashes, joint pains, malaise.

• A butterfly rash across the cheeks is typical.

Early diagnosis is important to prevent progression to the kidneys or the brain.

## Rare

### ■ Syphilis

Characteristically, six to twelve weeks after the initial infection, syphilis causes:
• A rash over hands and feet, including the palms and soles.
• Malaise, fever, enlarged lymph nodes.
• Aching joints.
• Wart-like swellings around genitalia and back passage.

Readily treatable.

### ■ Drug Side Effect

When all else fails, drugs may be suspected as the cause of a persistent fever.

### ■ Brucellosis

A disease spread through cow's and goat's milk, and therefore a risk for workers in the dairy industry.
• Gradual onset, with fevers, joint pains, cough, anorexia, night sweats.
• Bouts of fever every few days or few weeks.

Often cures itself.

## FEVER, RECURRENT ATTACKS

Apart from brucellosis, most of these infections are somewhat unusual in developed countries. Their symptoms return after a period of apparent recovery. This is in contrast to the far more conventional pattern of infections, in which there is fever by day or by night, whose disappearance can be taken as a reliable sign of recovery.

## Possible

### ■ Malaria

*(See page 465)* Anyone who has returned from a trip abroad to an area where malaria is present, and who develops a high temperature and chills, should be suspected of having this dangerous illness, particularly if they have not been taking anti-malaria tablets. Depending on the type of malaria, the episodes of fever and shaking return every three or four days. The fever may recur some months after foreign travel.

### ■ Brucellosis

*(See above)* It gives rise to bouts of fever for days at a time, which appear to settle, only to recur after weeks or months.

## ■ Typhoid

*(See page 458)* A feverish illness causing severe diarrhea, typhoid is spread through poor sanitation or contaminated water or food (mainly, shellfish products). The illness takes three to four weeks to run its course.

## RARE

Meaning rare in developed countries. Elsewhere, these are fairly common diseases, but they pose a relatively small risk for tourists. Inquire locally about areas where these diseases might be a hazard. If you develop feverish illness soon after returning from a danger area, report it to a doctor without delay, being ready with details of where you have been.

## ■ Dengue Fever

A mosquito-borne infection of Southeast Asia and Africa.
• Begins with sudden fever, aches, and rash.
• Severe pains in back and bones are particularly characteristic.
• Improvement over about a week.
• Relapse after another few days, with a more widespread rash.

Recovery takes several weeks.

## ■ Relapsing Fever

Spread by ticks. Common in Africa, India, South America, and parts of the Mediterranean.
• Abrupt high fever and confusion lasting for about a week.
• Then, apparent recovery, followed by relapse after another week or so.
• Several further relapses may occur.

Effective treatment exists.

## ■ Trypanosomiasis

Sleeping sickness. Different forms exist in Africa and South America. After an insect bite, there is typically:
• Painful swelling at the site of the bite.
• Then, relapsing fevers, enlarged lymph nodes.
• Eventually, after months or years, lethargy, continuous mild confusion, headaches, drowsiness.

Treatment, started early, is quite effective.

## ■ Yellow Fever

Especially prevalent in Africa and Central and South America.
• Abrupt fever, rigors, jaundice.
• Signs of improvement by the fourth or fifth day.
• Relapse during the next week, with more fever, jaundice.

There is no specific treatment for this serious illness, but vaccination is effective.

## FEVER IN OR AFTER VISITING THE TROPICS

Tropical disease should always be considered in someone who becomes feverish soon after returning from a Third World country or, indeed, certain developed countries where they are a known risk. The following are the more common examples, rather than an exhaustive catalog, of these many dangerous diseases.

If suspected, seek help urgently—you will probably be sent to a specialist. Protective measures and vaccinations exist for many of these diseases and anyone likely to be at risk should see their doctor to arrange for these before traveling. Some of the measures require time to become effective. The most likely tropical disease is malaria, common in Africa, India, and the Far East. Symptoms include high fever, drenching sweats, and rigors *(see page 461)*.

Among the rarities are:

• Plague—Far East, Africa, India, South America. It is a flea-borne illness, with dramatic onset, high fever, delirium, and tender, swollen lymph nodes (glands) in the groin.

• Relapsing Fever—South America, Africa, India, Near East. Sudden high fever, rigors, delirium. Liver and spleen enlarge.

• Sleeping Sickness—tropical Africa. Spread by the tse-tse fly. At first fever, enlarged lymph nodes, anemia. Later (months, years), drowsiness, tremors, fits.

• Typhus Fever—a term covering several diseases, named for the areas where they are found, for example, Rocky Mountain spotted fever. Fever increasing over several days, with headache, red eyes, rash, delirium.

• Yellow Fever—Africa (especially West Africa) and South America. Fever with rigors and jaundice. Effective vaccination exists.

## ABNORMALLY LOW TEMPERATURE

Defined as a fall in core body temperature to below about 95°F (35°C) when measured via the rectum (rear passage). Technical term: hypothermia. Below about 89.6°F (32°C), there will be drowsiness, apathy, coma, and eventually death.

Those at risk are the elderly without adequate heating and the newborn. Cold newborn babies do not shiver: they become lethargic, with cold limbs. Elderly people who suddenly become confused in the winter may be suffering from hypothermia. It is not advisable to give alcohol to an elderly person whom you suspect is suffering from hypothermia, as it may worsen their condition.

Hypothermia is an emergency, requiring immediate warmth and warm fluids. Severe hypothermia requires gradual, carefully monitored rewarming. Rapid heating up can be dangerous.

## PROBABLE

### ■ Exposure to Cold

- Shivering, feeling cold.
- Then apathy, slurred speech, difficulty in concentrating.
- Finally confusion, coma.

Remember, babies cannot control their temperatures as adults do. They are at risk in low temperatures, unless kept warm.

## POSSIBLE

### ■ Excess Alcohol

By dilating blood vessels, alcohol increases heat loss. Add confusion (if not unconsciousness) following a heavy drinking bout, plus cold conditions, and there is potential for serious danger.

## RARE

### ■ Underactive Thyroid

A grossly underactive thyroid gland can cause severe hypothermia. It is rare nowadays for this degree of underactivity to not be noticed.

### ■ Drug Side Effect

Antidepressants and tranquilizers can make temperature drop. Usually, this is a trivial effect, unless the drugs are taken in overdose or combined with self-neglect, alcohol, and exposure to the elements.

## SHIVERS OR CHILLS PLUS FEVER AND HEADACHE

In adults, this combination of symptoms, in a mild form, is not unusual and is often the earliest sign of a viral illness. In children, viral illness is also by far the most likely reason, but other possibilities need to be considered, especially if the headache seems to be the major feature.

### PROBABLE

### ■ Common Cold
*(See page 466)*

### ■ Influenza
*(See Viral Illness, page 454)*

## Possible

### ■ Chest Infection

These three symptoms in combination can be a feature of severe chest infections.

### ■ Infection Elsewhere

Any infection in the body may give this combination of symptoms. Parts of the body that might give rise to them when infected range from the joints, through internal organs, to the skin. Consider whether you have any other noticeable symptoms and look those up too.

## Rare

The possibilities below are the rarities that someone in a developed country might occasionally encounter.

### ■ Meningitis

An infection of the brain and surrounding tissues. Meningitis is mainly a disease of childhood. The condition is checked for as a matter of routine if a baby appears to be seriously ill.

• The illness may develop rapidly over a few hours.
• Light hurts the eyes.
• Pain or stiffness in the neck on trying to lift the head.
• Nausea and vomiting.
• Drowsiness, delirium, or coma.

Meningitis in the very young can occur in outbreaks and on the face of it

can seem identical to a simple viral illness. So, if you hear of meningitis in your locality, be on the lookout for:

• Excessive irritability, or worsening of an existing condition.
• Temperature rises higher than expected.
• Pain on being moved about.
• Inability to feed or drink adequately.
• Fine, purple rash.

Always seek help or advice at an early stage. If later still in doubt, check again with your doctor. If suspected, immediate medical attention is required.

### ■ Weil's Disease (Leptospirosis)

Rats spread this disease by infecting lakes, canals, sewers, and mines. Swimmers and boaters should be aware of this, as should sewage workers, miners, or anyone working in a rat-infested area.

• Rapid onset of fever, headache, and backache.
• Red eyes.
• A mild degree of jaundice is usual.
• Spontaneous bleeding from mouth or nose may occur.

### ■ Malaria

Caused by a parasite spread by mosquitoes. A major risk in the tropics, where mosquitoes enjoy long periods of warmth and humidity. Modern air travel means that malaria can spread anywhere in the world, so the possibility is worth considering in someone recently returned from Africa, Asia, or India, even if they have been taking anti-malaria tablets.

• Attacks every two or three days.
• Attack begins with an hour or two of severe shivering and headache.
• High temperature starts as shivering finishes, and lasts for several hours.
• Heavy sweating.
• In between attacks, the infected person may feel quite well.

If malaria is suspected, seek medical help urgently.

### ■ Other Tropical Disease

If someone recently returned from the tropics becomes ill with high fever, it is safest to suspect tropical disease first.

Which specific one it is will depend on where they have been staying and on the features of their illness. Seek medical help urgently.

### ■ Typhus

A general term for a variety of diseases spread by fleas and lice. Found not only in the Third World, but also in parts of the United States (Rocky Mountain spotted fever) and in Britain (Lyme disease).

• Illness develops over seven to fourteen days.
• Tenderness and redness of the eyes is typical.
• A rash eventually appears.
• Joints may be painful.

The illness varies from mild to severe, depending on the cause.

## COLD

Runny nose, itching eyes, and aching across the face? Statistics say that you will suffer from this miserable, though trivial, illness two or three times a year. It is usually caused by an infection of the upper respiratory tract, which includes the nose, larynx, and pharynx. Hence, the medical term for a common cold—upper respiratory tract infection (URTI). Any of more than 100 different viruses may be responsible. However, a cold might be

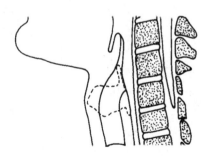

*Pharynx/Larynx*

more than just a cold if the symptoms are recurrent or persistent.

## PROBABLE

### ■ Common Cold

A Nobel Prize awaits the medical researcher who finds a cure for this condition.
• Begins with a sore or raw throat.
• Increasingly runny nose and sneezing with clear mucus.
• Mucus may turn yellow or green.
• Two or three days of loss of smell and taste.
• Occasionally progresses to a chest infection.

The illness runs its course over five to seven days, usually requiring no more than fluids, rest, and warmth. Antibiotics are not needed unless complicated by a chest infection.

## POSSIBLE

### ■ Hay Fever

An allergic reaction of the lining of the nose in response to pollens, grass, and other irritants.
• Sneezing in specific locales or at certain times of the year.
• Persistent sniff and blocked nose.
• Tickly feeling in throat and palate.
• Itching, watery eyes.
• Sufferers frequently also have eczema or asthma.

### ■ Allergic Rhinitis

A general term that includes hay fever and perennial rhinitis ("allergic" runny or streaming nose).
• Reactions as for hay fever.
• Provoked by certain environments; occurring throughout the year.

### ■ Sinusitis

• Persisting common cold symptoms.
• Passage of large quantities of yellow or green mucus through the nose or dripping down the back of the throat; sometimes bloodstained.
• Aching across face, above and below the eyes, especially on leaning forward.
• Nasal tone of voice.

### ■ Nasal Polyps

Common in people who suffer from allergic rhinitis.
• Visible as fleshy, gray lumps inside the nostrils; easily removed surgically but they frequently recur.
• Constant feeling of blocked nose.
• A persistent sniff with clear nasal discharge.

### ■ Foreign Body in the Nose

Peculiar to small children for whom small, round objects and body openings have a compelling interest.
• Persistent infected discharge from one nostril.

- Discharge may be blood streaked.
- The foreign body, typically a bead, is often visible.

## RARE

### ■ Head Injury Complication

Leakage of cerebrospinal fluid, the liquid that surrounds the brain, might be suspected if, after a head injury, there is a persistent, clear watery discharge from the nose.

### ■ Nasal Tumor

Persistent, one-sided bloody or foul-smelling discharge.

## SWEATING

Sweating is one of the body's ways of balancing heat loss against heat gain, an unglamorous but nonetheless sophisticated mechanism. Normally, it goes on as a background activity with barely noticeable perspiration. Even apparently heavy sweating may not be abnormal if it is serving to regulate temperature.

## PROBABLE

### ■ Exercise

It is, of course, normal that one should sweat when taking vigorous exercise. If you haven't exercised for a long time and you are also overweight, you may be unpleasantly surprised at how much sweat you produce, but it is normal.
- Perspiration from brow, armpits, and back.
- Clearly related to increased levels of exertion.
- Diminishes over a few minutes once exercise is stopped.

### ■ Fever

Most fevers are accompanied by sweating. There will be the familiar symptoms of feverish illness, such as:
- Aching muscles, headache, malaise, shivering.
- Commonly progressing to a sore throat, cough, earache.

Sweating as part of a feverish illness is less noticeable in the very old and the very young, whose temperature control mechanisms are less efficient than those of adults.

### ■ Stress

Anxiety is included as well, which can be described as a long-term form of stress.
- Sweaty palms, but dry mouth.
- Rapid heartbeat.
- Tension in neck muscles and across forehead.

Those who are prone to chronic anxiety may suffer chronic sweating.

## POSSIBLE

### ■ Excess Alcohol

Strong drink dilates the blood vessels, and this often causes sweating across the brow.

### ■ Pain

Any severe pain causes sweating through nervous reflexes that also cause:

- Pallor, restlessness.
- Rapid pulse.
- Collapse in severe cases.

Thus, sweating would be expected in any of the conditions causing collapse *(see page 475)*, including heart attacks and severe abdominal pain. But if there has been so much blood loss that the circulation is beginning to fail, clamminess replaces sweating.

## RARE

### ■ Drug Related

Reactions due to abrupt withdrawal from alcohol or narcotic drugs cause sweating, plus:

- Restlessness, muscle pains, drowsiness.
- Runny nose, dilated pupils, abdominal pains (narcotics).
- Tremor, disorientation, hallucinations (alcohol withdrawal).

Several other drugs, including antidepressants, can cause unusual sweating and need to be considered in otherwise unexplained cases.

### ■ Tuberculosis

Frequent night sweats may well be the first indicator of this serious infection. You should seek a doctor's advice as soon as possible.

### ■ HIV/AIDS

Sweating is a common symptom in acquired immunodeficiency syndrome (AIDS), sometimes in association with AIDS-related opportunistic infections.

## HEAVY SWEATING

Covered here are causes of sweating *other* than infectious diseases *(see Fever, page 453)*.

## PROBABLE

### ■ Natural Tendency

In other words, the way you are made.

Though frequently just a nuisance, it becomes a significant problem if it ruins clothes, causes unpleasant body odor, or interferes with manual activities. The problem starts after puberty.

- Hands, armpits, or feet pour sweat.

• Symptoms tend to be unrelated to exertion, temperature.

Several effective roll-on and lotion treatments are available. As a last resort, it is possible to cut the nerves near the spinal cord that control sweating of the hands or feet.

## POSSIBLE

### ■ Overactive Thyroid Gland

*(See page 350)* The thyroid gland could be described as the body's thermostat. Overactivity "turns up" all aspects of body function. Profuse sweating, plus:

• Hyperactivity, jitteriness.

• Prominent staring eyes.

• Weight loss, hunger, diarrhea.

• Trembling hands.

### ■ Menopause

Even before periods cease, women may be aware of flushes and sweating. Blamed, perhaps unfairly, for a wide range of middle-age symptoms.

• Usually in the forty to fifty-five age range.

• Periods become infrequent, then cease.

• Associated with increased wrinkling (loss of elasticity) of skin, irritability, or mild depression.

• Hot flashes.

• Sudden sweats at any time, especially at night.

• Tiredness, headache, palpitations.

## RARE

### ■ Carcinoid Syndrome

Another hormone disorder caused by a hormone-secreting tumor in the intestine or liver. The full picture may take years to develop.

• Bouts of profuse watery diarrhea with excessive bowel sounds.

• Facial flushing and sweating, especially after alcohol.

• Asthma.

### ■ Pheochromocytoma

A tumor that may occur near the kidneys, although not exclusively. Causes high blood pressure and sudden, severe bursts of anxiety. It is curable, and though relatively rare, doctors quite often run tests for it if there is:

• High blood pressure, sometimes highly variable.

• Abrupt episodes of headache, sweating, pallor, palpitations.

Tracking the tumor down can be like detective work. Removed by surgery.

### ■ Acromegaly

*(See page 96)*

## NIGHT SWEATS

If this goes on for a few days in an otherwise well person, don't worry. It is, however, a different matter if the symptoms are prolonged, especially if there has been recent illness, surgery, or debility. Possibilities revolve around infectious diseases or collections of pus in the body.

### PROBABLE

#### ■ Flu-like Illness

• Muscle aches.
• Mild headache.
• Sweating can be profuse.

After a few days, symptoms die away, with the possible emergence of a sore throat, cough, or similar mild illness.

### POSSIBLE

#### ■ Abscess

An abscess is a collection of pus; it can form anywhere in the body and can cause a variety of symptoms. Most commonly, pain at the site of the abscess should help localize the problem. Recent surgery can sometimes be followed by abscess formation near the operation. Blood tests, ultrasound, or computerized tomography (CT) scanning may give further information. Treatment consists of surgical drainage of the infection and antibiotics.

#### ■ Subphrenic Abscess

A collection of pus underneath the diaphragm. Could be a possibility after abdominal surgery or peritonitis. There may be no more than nonspecific features, such as:

• Malaise, sweats, anemia.
• Recurrent fever.
• Shoulder tip pain is a more tell-tale sign, caused by irritation of the diaphragm.

Treatment involves drainage and intensive antibiotic therapy.

#### ■ Endocarditis

Infection of the valves of the heart. There is usually a previous history of heart valve problems. May occur after minor surgery or dental procedures—hence, the need for at-risk patients with known valve problems to take prophylactic antibiotics before dental or surgical treatment. Onset can be gradual, with:

• Anemia.
• Malaise, recurrent sweats.
• Eventually, clubbed fingernails, enlarged spleen.

- Splinter-like marks under the finger-nails.

Treatment with intravenous antibiotics takes several weeks, with monitoring of the heart valves by echocardiography.

## RARE

### ■ Tuberculosis

Although previously a disease of under-developed countries, low-income groups, and alcoholics, tuberculosis is increasing again after many years. All ages and all income groups can be affected.

- Cough, which may be bloodstained.
- General malaise, weight loss, debility.

Modern treatments cure the disease, if continued over several months.

### ■ Brucellosis

*(See page 461)*

### ■ Hodgkin's Disease

*(See page 496)*

### ■ HIV/AIDS

*(See page 460)*

## TIREDNESS

This symptom is so common one might consider it part of normality. When tiredness becomes a burden or does not have a simple explanation, then medical advice can be helpful. In most cases, no serious medical cause is found.

## PROBABLE

### ■ Overexertion

A few remarkable people never need relief from constant pressure and stress and can make do with short periods of sleep. But even they usually have some compensatory mechanism. The rest of us suffer from fatigue, which commonly goes with:

- Irritability.

- Tense feelings in neck and head.
- Diminished enthusiasm for life.

### ■ Anxiety

One expert has described this universal symptom as "fear spread thin." As well as the symptoms given above for over-exertion, there may be:

- Palpitations, muscle tremors.
- Sweating.
- A constant fear that something unpleasant is going to happen.

At worst, anxiety is a truly disabling disorder needing treatment with a combination of psychological counseling and medication.

## POSSIBLE

### ■ Anemia

*(See page 217)*

### ■ Pregnancy and Childbirth

The birth and the physical process of looking after a newborn baby will challenge even the strongest parent. There is some comfort in knowing that night feeding usually ceases after a few weeks or months. Tiredness associated with early pregnancy can be a puzzle, since it can pre-date the first missed period, when diagnosis is easy.

- Tender breasts.
- Desire to pass urine frequently.

### ■ Viral Infection and Post-Viral Fatigue

Common viral infections such as colds or flu typically cause a feeling of tiredness or weakness. Usually this will resolve as the illness subsides, but sometimes tiredness persists longer. Glandular fever caused by the Epstein-Barr virus is well-known for causing a prolonged period of tiredness, perhaps lasting weeks or months. Psychological support and an undemanding lifestyle are the best advice that doctors can offer at present.

### ■ Depression

*(See page 399)* Most common in adult life, appearing over several weeks.

- Low mood.
- No enjoyment of anything, lack of motivation.
- Sleep disturbance.
- Changes in body weight.
- Poor concentration.

### ■ Diabetes

Fatigue can be an early symptom of diabetes when there are no other obvious features. As diabetes is such a common disease, anyone with unusual fatigue should be tested for it. *(See page 494)*

### ■ Underactive Thyroid

A disease of middle and later life, progressing so slowly that even the close family may not spot anything wrong, sometimes putting the symptoms down to aging.

- The skin becomes dry and rough.
- You "feel the cold."
- Your voice becomes gruff, your features coarse.
- Weight gain, constipation, slow speech, slow thought.

It is important to recognize this combination of symptoms because the disorder is so easily treated.

### ■ Overactive Thyroid Gland

Surprisingly, an overactive thyroid gland can also cause tiredness. This is usually a rather dramatic disease, appearing over a few weeks with:

- Nervousness, fine tremor of the hands.
- Sweating, weight loss, increased appetite.
- Muscle ache.
- Staring eyes.
- Diarrhea.
- Rapid heart rate or palpitations.

Again, treated easily.

## RARE

### ■ Heart Disease

In heart failure, especially in the elderly, fatigue may be the only early symptom. Look also for:

- Breathlessness on mild effort and when lying flat.
- Swollen ankles.

### ■ Cancer

Fatigue is worrying if found together with other symptoms suggesting cancer, such as:

- Weight loss, loss of appetite.
- Unusual pains.
- Unusual swellings.
- Blood in phlegm, vomit, urine, stools, or from the vagina.

*(See under individual entries for these symptoms)*

### ■ Malnutrition

Common worldwide but rare in the developed world. The fatigue is due to lack of vitamins, protein, and energy supplies. In developed countries, this may be seen in those with malabsorption *(see page 436)* or alcoholics who eat poorly.

### ■ Kidney Disease

A symptom of kidney failure, which is usually diagnosed on a blood test.

### ■ Neurological Disease

Diagnosis is a matter for specialists, since early changes are subtle and nonspecific. Neurological disease might be suspected if there is:

- Progressive weakness of a group of muscles.
- Tingling, numbness, or tremors of limbs.
- Unsteady gait.

Fatigue is a common symptom in multiple sclerosis.

### ■ Other Disorders

Severe, unexplained fatigue also raises the possibility of two rare disorders: adrenal insufficiency and myasthenia gravis, a disease of gradual onset in which muscles seem to work normally but rapidly tire, with exceptional weakness. Drooping eyelids are typical.

## FEELING WEAK OR FEEBLE

Weakness is such an unspecific symptom that few medical textbooks even recognize it as a topic in its own right. Nonetheless, people often go to their doctors saying that they feel weak and expecting the doctor to discover associated symptoms that will point to a diagnosis. Usually, no medical cause is found and the explanation lies in an imbalance between the physical and psychological capabilities of our bodies and the expectations of modern life. Sometimes there will be a medical explanation. The possibilities are broadly similar to the causes listed under Tiredness *(page 472)*.

## COLLAPSE

The term "collapse" means different things to different people. Common to most views is the picture of a person who was either upright or capable of being upright suddenly lying in a heap on the ground. Prostration is another description of the collapsed person. Often, there is a transient disturbance of consciousness. Broadly speaking, the causes of collapse depend on the age of the sufferer (with some degree of overlap)—these are summarized below.

First-aid treatment is the same for all groups: put the collapsed person in the "recovery position" and get medical help fast. Recovery position: anyone who collapses should be laid on their side, leaning forwards. Make sure their airway (neck and throat) is not obstructed. If possible, keep their head lower than, or at the same level as, their heart. Always seek professional medical help immediately when anybody collapses.

## COLLAPSE IN A YOUNG ADULT UP TO FORTY YEARS OLD

### PROBABLE

■ Faint

Short-lived unconsciousness, caused by temporary reduction in blood supply to the brain. Caused typically by standing upright in warm or hot conditions. Lying flat will lead quickly to recovery.

■ Epilepsy

• Often a known previous history of epilepsy.

- Aura or warning before a fit.
- Convulsive shaking of limbs.
- Tongue biting or frothing at the mouth.

Recovery accompanied by an initial period of confusion or sleep.

### ■ Drug or Alcohol Abuse

- Usually, a known history of alcohol or drug misuse.
- Smells of alcohol.
- Neglected appearance.
- Pupils may be widely dilated or pinpoint sized.
- Inflamed veins or puncture marks on skin made by a needle, usually at the front of the elbow, forearm, or on the back of the hand.
- Empty pill packets or psychiatric history suggesting drug overdose.

## POSSIBLE

### ■ Severe Infection

The possibilities are considered in detail in Fever *(page 453)*.

### ■ Pulmonary Embolus

*(See page 227)* A blood clot settles in the lung, cutting off blood flow. May be a rare but serious side effect of oral contraceptive use.

### ■ Dehydration

*(See page 490)*

## RARE

### ■ Pseudoseizure

Looks like a seizure but is in fact enacted by the patient. A form of dissociation *(see page 409)*.

### ■ Addison's Disease

Progressive, generalized weakness until some stress causes collapse. *(See page 495)*

### ■ Other Causes

The other causes of collapse will normally be accompanied by another symptom *(see Collapse with Abdominal Pain, page 478, and Collapse with Shock or Coma, page 480)*.

## COLLAPSE IN A MIDDLE-AGED ADULT

### PROBABLE

#### ■ Alcohol Related

- Usually a history of alcoholism or problem drinking.
- Collapse occurs when intoxicated.
- Alternatively, abrupt withdrawal of alcohol results in a seizure.

## POSSIBLE

### ■ Heart Rhythm Disturbance

The heart beats abnormally fast or irregularly and circulation to the brain becomes insufficient, leading to the person collapsing. Warning symptoms include:

- Palpitations.
- Chest pain or shortness of breath.
- Family history of heart disease.
- History of high blood pressure or high cholesterol.

An electrocardiogram (ECG) will identify the abnormal rhythm and appropriate treatment is given.

### ■ Drop Attack

This is usually a harmless condition, typically occurring in middle-aged women, in which the legs suddenly give way; there is no loss of consciousness. No treatment other than reassurance is needed.

### ■ Partial Seizures Due to Cerebrovascular Disease

Usually occurs in a person with a history or risk factor, such as smoking, high blood pressure, diabetes, or high cholesterol. The collapse is a form of epileptic seizure, but may not involve unconsciousness. Part of the brain malfunctions and the person collapses. Treatment is aimed at the underlying cause, often with the addition of anti-epileptic medication.

### ■ Other Causes

The other causes of collapse will normally be accompanied by another symptom (see Collapse with Abdominal Pain, page 478, and Collapse with Shock or Coma, page 480).

## COLLAPSE IN THE ELDERLY

### PROBABLE

### ■ Sudden Drop in Blood Pressure on Standing

Also known as orthostatic hypotension. The elderly person is normally taking medication for high blood pressure or their heart; when they stand up, their blood pressure falls further with gravity and they collapse. Treatment usually requires an adjustment or withdrawal of medication.

### ■ Slow Heartbeat

Known medically as bradycardia. There are various patterns in which the heart rate slows down or misses beats to the point where the brain is receiving an inadequate blood supply. An electrocardiogram (ECG) or twenty-four-hour ECG recording usually identifies the problem. Treatment may involve medication or sometimes the insertion of a pacemaker.

## POSSIBLE

### ■ Other Causes

The other causes of collapse will normally be accompanied by another symptom (see Collapse with Abdominal Pain, below, and Collapse with Shock or Coma, page 480).

## COLLAPSE WITH ABDOMINAL PAIN

Often hard to diagnose, because the reasons for abdominal pain differ with age. The following is the obvious, but not an exhaustive, list of illnesses that can cause collapse in adults. Get medical help at once, otherwise shock and coma will follow.

### PROBABLE

The possibilities below all involve inflammation of internal organs, which can progress to rupture of the organ. It is frequently impossible to differentiate these causes without tests or surgery.

### ■ Perforated Peptic Ulcer

There is erosion of the lining of the stomach or of the duodenum, forming an ulcer. The condition is almost always associated with infection with a bacteria called *Helicobacter pylori*. If the ulcer perforates, acid, food, and blood gush into the abdomen.

- Most common in middle-age.
- A history of upper abdominal discomfort or indigestion.
- Dyspepsia; may be waking at night.
- Severe pain in the upper abdomen, apparently radiating into the back.
- Vomit containing blood or particles looking like coffee grounds.
- Stools may be black, tarry-looking, or bloody.
- A sudden severe worsening of pain, with collapse, suggests perforation.

### ■ Pancreatitis

The pancreas lies at the back of the upper abdomen. There is usually existing gallbladder disease or a history of heavy drinking.

- Excruciating upper abdominal pain, worsening over a few hours.
- Pain in the back.
- Vomiting.
- Collapse.

### ■ Gallbladder Disease

Inflammation or obstruction of the gallbladder, usually connected with gallstones and most common in middle-aged women.
• Pain felt in the upper right abdomen, under the ribs.
• Often, a long history of discomfort on that side.
• Excruciating pain for hours at a time.
• Fever.

### ■ Ectopic Pregnancy

If a fertilized egg lodges in a fallopian tube, it can grow for a few weeks, eventually rupturing the tube and causing serious internal bleeding. This possibility should not be ignored in any fertile woman, even if there are no symptoms of pregnancy.
• A missed period, tender breasts, nausea.
• Rapidly increasing lower abdominal pain, usually one-sided.
• Vaginal bleeding.

Precise diagnosis is now relatively easy, thanks to sensitive pregnancy tests and ultrasound scanning.

### POSSIBLE

### ■ Gastroenteritis

An infection of the bowels, which, if severe, causes rapid dehydration as well as toxic effects from the actual infection.
• Cramping abdominal pains.
• Vomiting.
• Diarrhea immediately or after a few hours.

### ■ Inflammatory Bowel Disease

Typically, ulcerative colitis or Crohn's disease. Associated with:
• A long history of recurrent abdominal pains, diarrhea.
• Bleeding or mucus in stools.

### RARE

### ■ Intestinal Obstruction

Most often due to a trapped hernia or a growth in the intestine.
• A trapped hernia gives a tender swelling in the groin.
• At first, cramping abdominal pains.

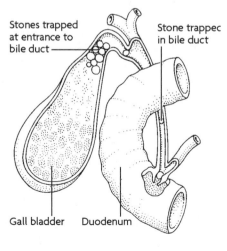

Stones trapped at entrance to bile duct

Stone trappec in bile duct

Gall bladder    Duodenum

*Gallbladder*

- Vomiting, swelling of the abdomen, and constipation.
- Within hours, fever, generalized abdominal pains.

### ■ Intestinal Ischemia

A clot blocks blood supply to the intestines. Most likely in the elderly with preexisting heart disease.

- Sudden abdominal pain.
- Diarrhea, vomiting, blood in stool.
- Rapid progression to collapse.

Surgical removal of the clot can be successful, but it ought to be done early.

## COLLAPSE WITH SHOCK OR COMA

This is an emergency. Making a precise diagnosis is less important than resuscitating the individual. As a medical term, "shock" strictly means drastic reduction in blood flow around the tissues. Here, the term is used in a less technical sense, so as to include a wider range of symptoms:

- Skin is clammy, cold, pale.
- Thready, weak pulse.
- Cyanosis.
- Individual reaction can vary from confusion to coma.

Coma may here be taken to mean unconsciousness. In trying to work out the cause of collapse with shock or coma, also consider the possibilities in the two preceding sections.

### PROBABLE

### ■ Stroke

Mainly affects the elderly. Caused by a blood clot or bleeding in the brain.

- Loss of consciousness.
- Paralysis of one side of the body.
- "Sighing" rough breathing.

The diagnosis is usually confirmed by computerized tomography (CT) scan. The outlook depends on the reason for the stroke and the individual's overall health. The longer the period of unconsciousness, the worse the outlook.

### ■ Heart Attack

A risk in the middle-aged and elderly.

- Sudden, crushing, central chest pain.
- Pain radiates up into jaws or down the left arm.
- Breathlessness, sweating.

Collapse with coma in a heart attack victim usually means that the heart is severely compromised, and the outlook is generally poor.

### ■ Heart Rhythm Abnormality

Very rapid, very slow, or irregular heart rhythms reduce the blood output from the heart. You may notice:

- Abrupt onset of thumping or fluttering in chest.
- Breathlessness.
- Shock.

## ■ Blood Loss

*(See also Dehydration, page 490)* Not always obvious, but easy to recognize if the blood loss is visible, for example, in vomit, stool, or from the vagina. A risk after injury, especially trauma to the abdomen, which can rupture the spleen, or a fractured thigh bone with severe bleeding into muscle.

## ■ Overwhelming Infection

For complex reasons, a major infection that gets into the bloodstream causes collapse via a drop in blood pressure. There will be the general symptoms of infection, such as:

- Fever, rigors, headache.
- Spontaneous bleeding and bruising.

## ■ Severe Pain

Severe pain from any source can cause collapse and coma as reflex actions.

## POSSIBLE

## ■ Diabetic Coma

Diabetics can have two types of coma. Collapse due to low blood sugar gives:

- Sweating, light-headedness, irritability.

- Rapid progression to confusion, then collapse.

If blood sugar remains high for long, a less sudden form of collapse (ketoacidosis) can occur:

- Usually during another mild illness.
- Onset over a few hours or days.
- Dehydration, intense thirst, vomiting.
- Sweet smell on breath.

Both these conditions respond rapidly to the appropriate treatment.

## ■ Alcohol/Drug Excess

*(See Drug Overdose, page 439)*

## ■ Leaking Aortic Aneurysm

The aorta is the major artery leading from the heart and carries its whole blood output. After years of service, its walls can swell out, weaken, and then split, just like a car tire may bulge and blow out. A not uncommon cause of sudden death, but there are sometimes warning symptoms:

- Unusual pulsation in the abdomen, in time with the heartbeat.
- A lump you can feel in the abdomen.
- Onset of backache as the aorta starts to leak.

Surgery is successful in early cases.

## ■ Burns

Loss of body fluids invariably accompanies serious burns, with shock resulting both from this loss and from pain.

## RARE

### ■ Anaphylaxis

This term describes the worst form of severe allergic reaction. It is an unpredictable risk to be kept in mind whenever someone is given an injection, but anaphylaxis can happen in response to foods and insect stings/bites. Minor warning signs of allergic reaction are:

• Swelling of the lips.
• Itchy, raised skin wheals that come and go.

In anaphylaxis, there is:
• Abrupt wheezing, progressing to cyanosis.
• Difficulty in swallowing, from swelling of the throat.
• Collapse.

Those fortunate enough to know that they are at risk should carry the appropriate medication or a warning bracelet.

## NO APPETITE OR VERY POOR APPETITE

Brief episodes of loss of appetite accompany our changing moods and minor infections. Indeed the regaining of appetite is among the earliest signs of recovery from these minor upsets, as is the disappearance of fever. If loss of appetite is accompanied by abdominal pain or weight loss *(see these symptoms)*, then more unusual disease is a possibility.

## PROBABLE

### ■ Minor Feverish Illness

• Fever, muscle aches, sore throat, or cough.
• Appetite disappears suddenly.
• The return of appetite lags a day or two behind the disappearance of fever.

### ■ Stress

Or worry. This all-too-standard ingredient of modern life can either stimulate or reduce appetite.
• Tense feelings in head, neck, shoulders.
• Irritability; mild depression.

Mood and appetite recover rapidly when the source of stress is absent.

## POSSIBLE

### ■ Depression

*(See page 399)* Suggested by prolonged loss of appetite, as well as:
• Low mood.
• Loss of enjoyment.
• Expressions of despair, crying, poor self-image.

• Early morning wakening (or disturbed sleep pattern).

## ■ Alcoholism

The high carbohydrate content of alcohol satisfies hunger and causes loss of appetite for normal solid food. Of course, drink is not at all nutritious, and eventually symptoms of vitamin deficiency appear, as well as those of alcoholism:

• Self-neglect, smell of drink.
• Memory disturbance, mood swings.
• Sore mouth, cracks at corners of lips, recurrent infections.
• Dilated veins over the face.

## ■ Hepatitis A

The combination of loss of appetite, fever for five to seven days, plus muscular aches and abdominal pains should arouse suspicion.

• Jaundice appears with yellowed eyes, dark urine.

As the jaundice clears up, you begin to feel better.

## RARE

## ■ Cancer of the Stomach

For reasons not understood, early cancer, especially of the stomach, can cause loss of appetite before other features appear. However, it is rare for loss of appetite alone to continue for long without the other symptoms *(see under No Appetite, Losing Weight, page 484, and No Appetite, Losing Weight and Chest Pain, page 485).*

• Most common in those over age forty-five.
• Persistent, otherwise unexplained loss of appetite.
• Feeling of fullness very soon after eating a small amount.
• Otherwise unexplained symptoms, such as generally feeling unwell, tiredness, unusual bleeding, or unusual pains.

## ■ Heart Failure

In certain forms of heart failure, loss of appetite is a noticeable symptom, probably related to congestion of blood in the liver. Among the many other symptoms that appear over days or weeks are:

• Breathlessness on exertion; tiredness.
• Breathlessness when attempting to lie flat.
• Preexisting chest disease, such as chronic bronchitis, bronchiectasis, or heart disease (typically, angina).
• An early feature is swollen ankles, and eventually a swollen abdomen.
• Tenderness over the liver, reduction in the volume of urine.

## NO APPETITE, LOSING WEIGHT

This is a worrying combination. In those under forty, the cause is usually a prolonged feverish illness or a psychological upset. In the middle-aged and elderly, more serious disease must be carefully considered. If you have noticed loss of appetite and weight loss, check whether you have any of the symptoms in the lists below. Then, look them up elsewhere in the book, where they are featured under a heading of their own.

### PROBABLE

#### ■ Prolonged Feverish Illness

In children and young adults, loss of appetite and weight loss will accompany any moderately extended illness, such as a bad chest infection or prolonged gastroenteritis. Both appetite and weight are rapidly regained after a couple of weeks. In adults, a wider net has to be cast in order to look for:

• Chills or night sweats.

• Recent abdominal surgery.

• Prolonged cough, diarrhea, abdominal pains.

• Unusual bleeding.

• Changes in amount of urine.

Follow up these symptoms individually, looking at other sections in this book where they are discussed in detail.

#### ■ Duodenal Ulcer

Painless ulcers, though a little unusual, can cause:

• Hunger.

• Bleeding (from the ulcer), seen in vomit or revealed by your stools turning black.

#### ■ Anorexia Nervosa

*(See page 437)*

### POSSIBLE

#### ■ Emotional Upset

If severe enough, self-neglect may follow. Usually there is an obvious cause of stress.

• Other symptoms of emotional upset, such as swings of mood, irritability, crying, depression.

#### ■ Cancer

In those over forty, these symptoms also require a careful check for other features suggestive of cancer, such as:

• Unusual pains.

• Unusual bleeding from the mouth, vagina, bowel, in phlegm, in urine.

• Swellings, lumps, enlarged lymph nodes.

• Malaise, tiredness.

## NO APPETITE, LOSING WEIGHT, AND CHEST PAIN

Though worrying, this combination is a little less so than simple *No Appetite, Losing Weight (see page 484)*. Of course, any adult with these symptoms still needs careful assessment by a doctor, but there are relatively innocent causes.

### PROBABLE

■ **Peptic Ulcer**

The lining of the stomach and duodenum is washed by highly corrosive acid and salts. The digestive system has mechanisms to cope with this, but if the mechanisms break down, inflammation and eventually ulceration occurs. Smoking, drinking, worry, and most antirheumatic drugs predispose to peptic ulcers. A high proportion are associated with bacterial infection in the stomach and gut—namely, *Helicobacter pylori*. Successful treatment includes eradication of *H. pylori* with antibiotics and a drug (proton pump inhibitor) to stop acid production.

• Burning pains behind the breastbone and in the upper abdomen.

• Food may help or worsen the pain.

• If it worsens pain, food is avoided, causing weight loss.

• You may be awakened at night by the pain.

• Simple antacids give temporary relief.

The treatment of peptic ulcers is one of the outstanding successes of modern medicine, making surgery, which used to be the only long-term cure, unnecessary. Two types of peptic ulcer exist: duodenal and gastric ulcers. Duodenal ulcers are four times more common than gastric ulcers. Duodenal ulcers do not turn into cancers; gastric ulcers may become cancerous, though there is debate about this. Twice as many men as women have ulcers.

■ **Hiatus Hernia**

A failure of the one-way valve mechanism that keeps stomach contents from regurgitating up into the esophagus. Often just a nuisance, but if long-standing, it can cause scarring of the esophagus and interfere with normal swallowing of food. Weight loss then results. A condition of middle to later life, especially in the overweight.

• Burning pains.

• Belching, especially on bending over or lying flat.

• Very commonly, the symptoms are worse during pregnancy.

■ **Esophagitis**

Inflammation of the esophagus usually due to acid reflux from the stomach. The condition often co-exists with hiatus hernia *(above)*.

- Burning pain behind the breastbone (heartburn).
- Worse after hot or acidic food.
- Pain may seem to spread across the chest and up to the jaw.

Improves with antacids or drugs that stop acid production.

## POSSIBLE

### ■ Gallbladder Disease

This usually means gallstones, causing pain in the upper abdomen after eating and resulting in disinclination to eat. *(See Gallbladder, page 479)*

### ■ Cancer of the Stomach

*(See page 467)* This has to be checked for in anyone over the age of forty who develops these symptoms, especially for the first time. The stomach is examined by endoscopy (passing a flexible tele-scope or camera into the stomach). The earlier such symptoms are reported, the earlier the diagnosis and the better the chance of successful treatment.

## RARE

### ■ Lung Cancer

Ninety percent of lung cancers occur in smokers. In addition to the three main symptoms, there may also be:

- Breathlessness.
- Coughing of blood.

*(See page 226)*

### ■ Tuberculosis

Weight loss and loss of appetite, and sweating, are general features of this disease. Chest pain results from swelling of glands inside the chest. Cough is usually present, sometimes with bloodstained phlegm. *(See page 472)*

---

## ABNORMAL HUNGER

## PROBABLE

### ■ Indigestion

Food reduces the feelings of pain or emptiness caused by the excess acid present in indigestion. You feel like taking frequent snacks to relieve the discomfort.

- Burning sensation behind the breastbone.
- Burping, belching, or other signs of wind.

Persistent symptoms may signify a peptic ulcer.

### ■ Low Blood Sugar

Very common in a mild form if you miss a meal. Diabetics, especially those on insulin, must be alert to the early symptoms.

• At first, you feel light-headed and have difficulty concentrating; also, irritability, headache.
• As it worsens, sweating, confusion, drowsiness.

Symptoms rapidly eased by taking sugar.

## POSSIBLE

### ■ Overactive Thyroid

• Weight loss, sweating, tremor of the hands.
• Often, bulging eyes.
• Hyperactivity, restlessness, nervousness.

## RARE

### ■ Intestinal Worms

Very unlikely unless living in or having traveled in underdeveloped countries.

The worm infects humans via beef, pork, or fish.
• Usually, no other symptoms until segments of worm appear in stools.

### ■ Bulimia

Bulimia is binge eating, associated with anorexia nervosa *(see page 437)*.
• Typically, in young women worried about their weight.
• Excess dieting, interrupted by bouts of voracious feeding to the point of vomiting.

### ■ Hypothalamic Disease

Disease of the hypothalamus gland in the brain can gradually cause excess appetite and:
• Passage of enormous amounts of urine.
• Drowsiness, narrowing of visual field.

## PUTTING ON WEIGHT

The "glands" so often blamed are rarely the culprits.

## PROBABLE

### ■ Eating Too Much

This is not the same as overeating. Some individuals really do eat very little, yet gain weight. The reason is unknown. Overweight is a major cause of ill health, if not outright disease, including osteoarthritis, heart disease, and diabetes.

• Worsens with age.
• Fat is generally spread around the body.

Honest, purposeful dieting achieves weight loss.

## POSSIBLE

### ■ Underactive Thyroid Gland

Slow, progressive weight gain. *(See page 351)*

### ■ Drug Related

Most commonly complained about is the contraceptive pill. Typically, the pill results in less than 10 percent increase in weight, often increasing mainly breast and hip size. Careful attention to healthy eating and using the lowest effective dosage of the pill are the cornerstones of management. The other common culprit is steroid treatment, widely used in chest and rheumatic diseases, eventually causing the same symptoms as Cushing's syndrome *(see right)*.

## RARE

### ■ Hormonal Causes

Several unusual hormonal disorders, mainly in boys, cause obesity.

• Obese child is unusually small or unusually tall.
• Delayed puberty.
• Underdevelopment of penis and testicles.

### ■ Cushing's Syndrome

Results from overproduction of natural steroids by the body.
• Gross obesity of body, with prominent purple stretch marks.
• Thin, stick-like limbs.
• "Moon" face.
• Pronounced hump of fat on the back.
• Symptoms of diabetes.
• Thin skin, easy bruising.

There are sophisticated treatments, depending on the cause.

## RAGING THIRST

This is the counterpart to Craving for Water, Feeling Dehydrated *(see page 490)* and should be read in conjunction with that topic.

## PROBABLE

### ■ Poor Fluid Intake

Circumstances that could make this a possibility are:
• Prolonged vomiting.
• Disabled individual (for example, a stroke victim who must rely on others for drinks).
• Hot climate or excess exercise.
• Conditions that make swallowing difficult.

The symptoms are:
• Dry mouth, low output of concentrated, dark urine.
• Skin becomes lax and loses its elasticity; eyes appear to sink.

- In babies, the soft spot on the skull becomes sunken.
- In extremes, apathy, confusion.

### ■ Sweating

The fluid lost in sweat has to be replaced, otherwise thirst will follow. Fever, heavy exercise, and hot weather might all cause profuse sweating. The symptoms are the same as for poor fluid intake.

### ■ Diarrhea

The body can cope with brief episodes of diarrhea, but if it is prolonged, dehydration and thirst will follow. Babies are particularly susceptible to the effects of diarrhea, which is also often accompanied by vomiting at that age. A careful watch must be kept for signs of dehydration.

## POSSIBLE

### ■ Excess of Diuretic Drugs

These medications are widely used to treat heart disease. They rid the body of fluid, but even so, thirst is not often a problem, unless doses are excessive, when you may see:

- Passage of large quantities of urine for hours after taking the diuretic.
- Increasing weakness over several days or weeks.
- Constipation.

### ■ Bleeding

This has to be heavy and sustained to cause thirst. External bleeding is usually obvious, but internal bleeding may be another matter.

- Pallor, rapid pulse, collapse, and thirst.

   Suspicious circumstances include:
- Recent abdominal injury (for example, a ruptured spleen).
- Recent severe abdominal pain (from, say, a perforated ulcer).
- Fractured thigh.
- Abdominal distension.

## RARE

### ■ Drug Side Effect

Many drugs cause a dry mouth; not, strictly speaking, true thirst, but the remedy is sips of fluid. Common drugs with this side effect are antidepressants and drugs for urinary incontinence.

## RAGING THIRST, HIGH URINE OUTPUT

### PROBABLE

#### ■ Diabetes

*(See page 492)* This combination of symptoms is the classical presentation of diabetes.

#### ■ Psychological

A vicious circle of drinking to excess followed by urinating to excess. Surprisingly common, especially in children, where consuming sweet drinks becomes their main source of comfort. To diagnose, a doctor must exclude other causes.

### POSSIBLE

#### ■ Chronic Kidney Failure

The passage of large quantities of dilute urine is an early sign of this problem. Often, the sufferer is unaware of this; other symptoms are rather vague and may be completely unnoticed.
- Excessive urine day and night.
- Malaise.

- As it worsens, thirst, mild anemia, fatigue.

Usually diagnosed on a blood test. The outcome depends on the underlying cause, of which there are many.

### RARE

#### ■ Hyperparathyroidism

The parathyroid glands lie in the thyroid gland in the throat; they control calcium balance. Too much calcium in the blood gives:
- Excessive thirst and urine output.
- Pains in bones.
- Constipation.
- Kidney stones that may be painful.
- Depression, malaise.

Summed up by generations of medical students as "Moans, bones, and abdominal groans."

#### ■ Diabetes Insipidus

*(See page 493)*

## CRAVING FOR WATER, FEELING DEHYDRATED

Dehydration is the result of water loss exceeding water intake, remembering that water is lost not just in urine but in feces (especially in diarrhea), sweat (especially in heat exhaustion), blood (especially in hemorrhage), and via

breathing. Thirst is frequently a symptom of dehydration; other signs, in order of severity, are:

- Dry tongue (but be aware of mouth breathers, whose tongues are dry anyway).

- Reduced output of urine, the urine being dark and strong-smelling.

- Dry, lax skin.

- Sunken eyes.

- In babies, a sunken soft spot in the skull.

- Eventually apathy, confusion, collapse.

Depending on the cause, dehydration can develop over any length of time, from days to weeks, unless there has been a large and sudden loss of fluid. It is important to realize that babies and elderly people can dehydrate in a matter of hours, typically from diarrhea and vomiting, and may not show any symptoms apart from restlessness until the fluid loss is extreme.

## PROBABLE

### ■ Vomiting

Whatever the reason for the vomiting, eventually dehydration results simply because insufficient water is being kept down. In both children and adults, the usual cause is gastroenteritis, otherwise known as gastric flu or tummy upset, with:

- Abrupt onset of vomiting.
- Chills; muscular aches.
- Diarrhea may accompany these or begin a few hours later.

Provided adequate fluids are taken frequently in small amounts, there will usu-ally be enough fluid retained within the body to prevent dehydration. Proprietary glucose and electrolyte rehydration solutions are very useful in helping to avoid dehydration, especially in babies and small children. In practice, dehydration is an uncommon risk except in babies, who should be carefully watched.

### ■ Diarrhea

A few episodes of diarrhea cause no harm. Profuse, watery diarrhea is a different matter, because if that continues for more than a few days, dehydration becomes a real risk, especially in the very old and the very young.

### ■ Sweating

In a hot, dry atmosphere, it is possible to lose large amounts of fluid by sweating without noticing it. Those who run for pleasure should also remember this and take fluids regularly, even when on the move. Early features would be:

- Muscle cramps.
- Thirst, but not as a prominent symptom.
- Weakness, vomiting.

### ■ Decreased Fluid Intake

If disease interferes with swallowing, dehydration, and indeed starvation, are a risk unless arrangements are made to enable food to be taken some other way.

Similarly, one should be concerned with anyone unable to take sufficient fluid because of confusion, stroke, or unconsciousness. The symptoms of dehydration can become confused with the symptoms of their disease, leading to a vicious circle. Look for:

- Low urine output.
- Increasingly lax skin.
- A tongue so dry it begins to crack.
- Increasing confusion.

## POSSIBLE

### ■ Overuse of Diuretics

These invaluable and widely used drugs cause an increased output of urine. They are used to treat heart failure or high blood pressure. When they are used over long periods, they can cause a slow dehydration. You may come to accept as normal a dry mouth or increased thirst. It is rare for diuretics to cause rapid dehydration, except through deliberate overdose—for instance, if used as a slimming aid or when used in high dosage to relieve serious heart failure, when it is normal to monitor their effect with blood tests. The symptoms would be those of dehydration, as listed above, with:

- General weakness, also muscle weakness.
- If very severe, apathy and vomiting.

### ■ Diabetes

In this condition, excess sugar in the bloodstream starts to "leak" through the kidneys, dragging large quantities of water with it. Water laden with sugar leaves the body in the form of large quantities of urine, day and night, giving the combination of thirst and dehydration. Other features might include:

- Tiredness or weakness.
- Vague feeling of ill-health.
- Weight loss.
- A sweet smell on the breath.
- Eventually, confusion and coma.

This would be the typical presentation of type 1 diabetes in a child or young adult (the type that requires insulin to treat). In middle-aged or elderly people, type 2 diabetes (usually managed with diet and initially tablets) is much more common. The onset is usually less dramatic and slower, sometimes with rather vague symptoms or no symptoms at all. In both cases, a blood test rapidly confirms the diagnosis.

## RARE

### ■ High Blood Calcium

Occurs mainly in association with diseases that affect the bones and tends to be part of a rather vague, gradually developing picture that might include:

- Weakness, drowsiness, nausea, vomiting.
- Pains in the abdomen; constipation.

Diagnosis of this condition constitutes a medical detective story.

### ■ Diabetes Insipidus

This results from damage—typically, as a result of head injury, tumors, or meningi-tis—to the part of the brain (pituitary gland) that controls water balance.

- Passage of gallons of urine a day.
- A huge compensating thirst.

If you have this condition, now readily treatable, every medical school for miles around will be asking you to appear as a case in their students' examinations.

## HICCUPS

Hiccups result from a sudden contraction of the diaphragm, the sheet of muscle that separates the chest from the abdomen. It is an uncontrollable reflex action, like blinking. The chance of hiccups being the only symptom of illness is remote, even if hiccups are unusually persistent.

## PAINS IN VARIOUS PARTS OF THE BODY

A precise definition is essential. Considered here is *recurrent, generalized pain* as opposed to pain in a specific part of the body. Such generalized pains can include the vague aches and pains that plague most people from time to time and which may well have a psychological origin. Generally speaking, pain as a symptom of serious underlying disease is obvious when it strikes.

### PROBABLE

### ■ Depression

The pains tend to be the same minor ones everyone experiences, but they take on an exaggerated significance for the depressed person, who has a lower tolerance of irritation.

- Low mood.
- Loss of enjoyment.
- Disturbed sleep, poor appetite, and weight loss.
- Crying, negative feelings.

### ■ Hypochondria

If you have bought a copy of this book, you probably need no one to define for you the agonies of occasional hypochondria. It is a universal human condition, and if you automatically think the worst of every symptom, this book ought to give you some relief. Persistent hypochondriacs—the ones who see their doctors as often as once a week—are another matter, characterized by:

- Lack of insight.
- Resistance to reasoned explanation or proof, after investigation, that they are healthy.
- Often, a long history of neurotic behavior.

Hypochondria is sometimes not as benign as it seems. Those who constantly complain of sundry symptoms can be so preoccupied that they neglect the early symptoms of true disease. Everybody eventually dies of something, the hypochondriac included.

## POSSIBLE

### ■ Diabetes

Diabetes affects the working of nerves all over the body and can cause widespread nerve disturbance. Sometimes, neuropathic pain (pain derived from damage to nerves) can be the presenting symptom of diabetes.

- Pain, tingling of lower limbs, especially the feet.
- Pain worse at night.

- Other symptoms of diabetes.

Neuropathic pain is more common with poor blood glucose control. Once established, the symptoms are difficult to control, though they often give way to loss of sensation (anesthesia). Early attention to improving blood glucose control is therefore crucial.

### ■ Polymyalgia Rheumatica

A disease affecting the elderly. It comes on over a period of a few weeks, giving pains in any muscles, but particularly:

- Pain across the shoulders.
- Tenderness at the temples.
- Vague malaise, occasional fever.
- Weight loss.

Diagnosis is confirmed with a simple blood test. The symptoms rapidly improve with steroid medication, which usually needs to be continued for two years or more.

### ■ Pernicious Anemia

General features of anemia (see page 430), plus:

- Tingling, numbness of limbs, hands, or feet.
- Unsteady walking.
- Sore tongue.
- A hint of jaundice or yellowed skin.

Vitamin $B_{12}$ injections treat both the anemia and the pains.

## RARE

### ■ Sickle-Cell Disease

In which hemoglobin, the blood's oxygen carrier, is abnormal. Found in African Americans.

• Normal, pain-free existence interrupted by bouts of pain in limbs, abdomen.

• Pains set off by infection, surgery under anesthetic, pregnancy.

Screening is simple.

## FEELING THE COLD

## PROBABLE

### ■ Natural Tendency

In the great majority of cases, sensitivity to cold is a natural feature of your constitution: you may well have always suffered from numb and/or bluish fingers and toes *(see also Bluish Skin, page 438)*. The elderly often find that they "feel the cold." Similarly, babies have a reduced ability to compensate for low temperature, making adequate room temperature and warm clothing essential.

## POSSIBLE

### ■ Raynaud's Phenomenon and Disease

Common conditions in which the circulation of the fingers and toes overreacts to changes in temperature.

• Fingers and toes always feel cold; go white or blue easily.

• Pain and redness are evident as they warm up.

Severe forms of Raynaud's can cause ulceration of the fingers and toes. The problem may occasionally arise as a side effect of taking beta-blockers for high blood pressure or of working with vibrating equipment. It might also be a complication of a connective tissue disorder, such as systemic lupus erythematosis *(see page 460)*.

### ■ Underactive Thyroid Gland

Slowly increasing sensitivity to the cold is one of the classic features of this easily treated disorder. *(See page 351)*

## RARE

### ■ Addison's Disease

A gradually developing hormone deficiency causing generalized weakness and lack of resistance to physical stress, including low temperature. People with Addison's look strikingly pale.

## SWOLLEN LYMPH NODES

The lymphatic system, which includes the lymph nodes, liver, and spleen, is in the front line of defense against infection and, indeed, other threats to the system. Temporary swelling for a week or two is, therefore, of little significance, being a feature of many minor viral illnesses and injuries. However, there is no escaping the fact that prolonged swelling of lymph nodes can be a sign of several serious conditions. Frequently, these conditions are treatable, especially at an early stage, making it essential to report persistently swollen lymph nodes. Blood tests and lymph node biopsy are usually needed to confirm the diagnosis.

### PROBABLE

#### ■ Glandular Fever

An extremely common infection in teenagers or young adults, with a combination of severe sore throat, swollen glands, and tiredness. A blood test confirms the diagnosis. No specific treatment but be reassured that you will eventually make a full recovery.

#### ■ Tonsillitis

Just a sore throat can cause massive swelling of lymph glands below the chin. This can be particularly dramatic in children. *(See page 135)*

### POSSIBLE

In most of the following conditions, the lymph nodes gradually enlarge and remain enlarged.

#### ■ Hodgkin's Disease

A particular type of cancerous condition of the lymphatic system and lymph glands (lymphoma). Typically occurs in young adults.
• Painless.
• Rubbery feel to lymph nodes.
• Lymph nodes grow steadily over a few weeks or months.
• Tiredness, sweats at night.

Swelling of the neck glands is the most likely symptom to be noticed. Diagnosis requires biopsy of a gland.

#### ■ Other Lymphomas

There are several other types of lymphoma distinct from Hodgkin's disease *(above)*. These lymphomas typically affect an older age group—those thirty-five and older. Symptoms are similar to those in Hodgkin's disease, with:
• Widespread, painless swollen lymph nodes.
• Weight loss, sweats at night.

Treatment depends on the cell type of lymphoma, which is determined by a blood test, plus bone marrow and lymph node biopsy. The outlook is variable, depending on the cell type involved. Treatments range from simple observation to radiotherapy and chemotherapy.

## ■ Cancer

By the time it causes generalized swelling of nodes, the cancer will be so advanced that it is likely to be obvious from other features. More important from the point of view of early diagnosis is enlargement of a single group of lymph nodes, which may signal the presence of an early cancer in such sites as the breast or the thyroid gland before there are other obvious features. The sites most noticeable are:

• Neck—cancers of lung, thyroid, nose, stomach.
• Groin—cancer of bowel, womb, prostate.
• Armpit—breast cancer.

## ■ Toxoplasmosis

An infection acquired through eating infected meat or sometimes via cat droppings. If caught during pregnancy, it sometimes causes brain and eye damage in the baby.

• In mild cases, generalized, painless, swollen lymph nodes.
• Possibly fever, weakness as well.

## ■ Tuberculosis

The usual glands involved are those around the neck. The swelling is painless and accompanied by general features of TB, such as:

• Prolonged malaise.
• Weight loss.
• Cough, possibly with blood in sputum.

## ■ Leukemia

Leukemia can present with widespread swollen nodes, both in childhood and adulthood. In children, presentation tends to be more dramatic, with:

• Abnormal bleeding, sore throat, malaise.
• Fever, anemia.
• Enlarged liver, spleen.

In adults, the disease tends to have a much slower onset, with:

• Enlarged lymph nodes as a main feature.
• Possibly effects of anemia, and recurrent infection.

Leukemia in childhood often carries a good outlook, with treatment providing excellent prospects of remission or cure. Prognosis in adults depends on the type of leukemia: chronic lymphatic leukemia, which is the most common type, carries a good outlook and often requires no treatment; other types are more insidious with a much worse outlook.

## RARE

### ■ Sarcoidosis

A condition of unknown origin, often discovered by chance from seeing enlarged lymph glands on a chest x-ray. Usually benign, but may cause:

- Rashes, joint pains.
- Malaise.
- Large, painful red lumps on the shin.
- Painful, red eye.
- Breathlessness.

### ■ Secondary Syphilis

A sexually transmitted infection, numerically very uncommon. Risk is increased with multiple casual partners or sex with a sex-industry worker, especially abroad.

- The initial sign is a painless sore on the genitalia.
- General lymph node swelling after several months.
- Wart-like growths around genitalia.
- Vague malaise.

Diagnosis is by blood test. Antibiotic treatment is effective and essential in order to prevent progression to serious nerve disorders, possibly years later.

### ■ Yaws

A syphilis look-alike found in the tropics. Unlike syphilis, it is spread by poor hygiene rather than sexually transmitted.

- Ulcerating skin rash, mainly on the palms and soles of the feet.
- Widespread enlargement of the lymph nodes.

Treatment prevents disfiguring destruction of bone.

### ■ Cat Scratch Fever

An interesting, and probably underrecognized, reason for enlarged glands. Said to be one of the most common causes of persistently swollen glands in the United States. Contact with kittens may pose an increased risk.

- At first, just broken skin from the scratch.
- After a week or two, a small red lump appears.
- Swollen local glands, for example, in the armpit.
- Glands enlarge and may discharge pus.

Illness resolves over a few weeks. Can also be cleared up with antibiotics.

# List of Common Terms

Certain medical or neo-medical terms are used so often in this book that explaining their meaning every time would consume too much space. Thus, we provide the definitions here.

**Acute.** Occurring now; a sudden appearance or exacerbation.

**Anxiety.** "Fear spread thin"; feelings of dread and worry.

**Benign tumor.** A lump that is not cancerous.

**Chronic.** A disease or illness either lasting a long time or present for years.

**Circulatory disease.** Disease of the arteries or veins, which carry blood around the body.

**Cyanosis.** Bluish skin coloration caused by lack of oxygen in the tissues.

**Cyst.** A sac within the body, usually fluid-filled; may also appear as a swelling in or on the body.

**Diagnostic.** Unique to; aiding the diagnosis.

**Follicle.** Glandular structure under skin from which a hair grows.

**Immunosuppression.** The immune system is the body's defense system against infection and other insults; if it is suppressed, either by illness or drugs, its normal function is limited or rendered less effective.

**Indigestion, acidity.** Discomfort after eating.

**Lesion.** A mark, a cut, a wound.

**Malaise.** Feeling generally unwell.

**Malignant.** Cancerous.

**Nodule.** A lump or swelling generally felt on the body's surface.

**Nonspecific.** Usually describes a symptom that does not signify any disease in particular.

**Palpable.** Can be felt by hand.

**Phlegm.** Sticky mucus, produced typically in the lungs as a response to infection.

**Rigor.** A sudden shaking episode, typically accompanied by a fit of shivering.

**Sepsis.** Infection.

**Systemic.** Affecting all of the body's systems; widespread rather than local.

**Tumor.** A growth, often a lump, either benign or malignant.

# Index

Colles' fracture, 299
Color blindness. *See* Blindness, color.
Coma, 12, 386–388
  diabetic, 481
  infections and, 388
Concentration, lack of, 388–389
Confusion, 389–392
Congenital adrenal hyperplasia, 274
Congenital atresia of the esophagus, 117
Congenital contracture, 307
Congenital dislocation of the hip (CDH), 309
Conjunctivitis, 5–6, 7–8, 9, 15, 23, 24, 25, 27
Conn's syndrome. *See* Aldosteronism.
Constipation, 144, 145, 146, 150, 161, 173
Constitutional growth delay, 428
Contact lenses, 8, 27
Contraceptives. *See* Birth control pills.
Convulsions, 108, 392–394
COPD. *See* Chronic obstructive pulmonary disease (COPD).
Copper ring, 5
Cornea, 5, 8, 16, 33, 36
  abrasions, 26, 27
  damaged, 28
  ulcers, 27
Cornea arcus, 5
Corns, 261
Coronary artery bypass grafting, 235
Coronary artery disease, 212, 218, 234–235

Corticosteroids, 278
Cosmetics, 97
Costochondritis, 235–236
Coughs, 221, 223
  drugs and, 223
  dry without phlegm, 222–223
  with bloody phlegm, 225–227
  with bloody phlegm and chest pain, 227
  with phlegm, 223–225
  *See also* Whooping cough.
Cramps, 277
Creutzfeldt-Jakob Disease (CJD) or Variant CJD, 399
Crohn's disease, 125, 150, 151, 155, 158, 166
Croup, 209–210
Crush syndrome, 192
Cushing's syndrome, 273, 278, 352, 488
Cyanosis. *See* Skin, blue.
Cystic fibrosis, 86, 144, 225
Cystitis, 179, 183–184, 187
Cystocele, 178
Cysts, 378
  dermoid, 257
  epididymal, 359
  sebaceous, 130, 136, 257, 295
  thyroglossal, 132
  *See also* Labial cysts; Meibomian cysts; Ovarian cysts.

Da Costa's syndrome, 236
Dacrocystitis, 21, 23
Dandruff, 20, 245, 272
Dapsone, 250
Deafness
  adults, 63–65
  children, 65–67

congenital, 66
Deep vein thrombosis (DVT), 210, 233, 317, 445
Deformities, congenital, 207, 358, 367
Dehydration, 89, 107, 142, 262, 421, 490–493
Delirium, 394
Delusions, 395–396
Dementia, 390, 396–399, 397
  early, 396
  vascular (multi-infarct), 397
  with Lewy bodies, 397–398
Dengue fever, 462
Dental caries, 83
Dentures, 83
Depression, 100, 373, 375, 396, 399–401, 408, 395, 446, 473, 482, 493
Dermatitis. *See* Eczema.
Dermatitis artefacta, 246
Dermatitis herpetiformis, 244, 250
Dermatomyositis, 278
Diabetes, 390, 446, 473, 490, 492, 494
  insipidus, 180, 493
  mellitus, 17, 29, 35, 39, 85, 142, 160, 180, 218, 261, 375
Diarrhea, 150–150, 154–156, 166–168, 173, 489, 491
  AIDS-related, 155
  drugs and, 156
  factitious, 150–151, 155
  traveler's, 155
Diet, 161
Digestive system. *See* Abdomen (digestive system).
Digoxin, 42, 196, 203
Diphtheria, 229–230
Discitis, 294
Discoid lateral meniscus, 315